Methods in Molecular Biology

Series Editor
John M. Walker
School of Life and Medical Sciences
University of Hertfordshire, Hatfield
Hertfordshire, UK

For further volumes:
http://www.springer.com/series/7651

For over 35 years, biological scientists have come to rely on the research protocols and methodologies in the critically acclaimed *Methods in Molecular Biology* series. The series was the first to introduce the step-by-step protocols approach that has become the standard in all biomedical protocol publishing. Each protocol is provided in readily-reproducible step-by-step fashion, opening with an introductory overview, a list of the materials and reagents needed to complete the experiment, and followed by a detailed procedure that is supported with a helpful notes section offering tips and tricks of the trade as well as troubleshooting advice. These hallmark features were introduced by series editor Dr. John Walker and constitute the key ingredient in each and every volume of the *Methods in Molecular Biology* series. Tested and trusted, comprehensive and reliable, all protocols from the series are indexed in PubMed.

Glaucoma

Methods and Protocols

Second Edition

Edited by

Tatjana Jakobs

Mass Eye and Ear, Schepens Eye Research Inst, Boston, MA, USA

Paloma B. Liton

Department of Ophthalmology, Duke University, Durham, NC, USA

Humana Press

Editors
Tatjana Jakobs
Mass Eye and Ear
Schepens Eye Research Inst
Boston, MA, USA

Paloma B. Liton
Department of Ophthalmology
Duke University
Durham, NC, USA

ISSN 1064-3745 ISSN 1940-6029 (electronic)
Methods in Molecular Biology
ISBN 978-1-0716-4139-2 ISBN 978-1-0716-4140-8 (eBook)
https://doi.org/10.1007/978-1-0716-4140-8

This Humana imprint is published by the registered company Springer Science+Business Media, LLC, part of Springer Nature.
The registered company address is: 1 New York Plaza, New York, NY 10004, U.S.A.

Preface

In this second edition of *Glaucoma: Methods and Protocols*, we present an updated and expanded exploration into the methodologies essential for the study of neurodegeneration in glaucoma. Building upon the foundation established in the first edition, this volume integrates updated techniques with a diverse array of new methodologies, offering a comprehensive toolkit for researchers and clinicians alike.

A notable feature of this edition is the expanded focus on ocular hypertension as a critical factor in the pathogenesis of glaucoma. Recognizing the significance of intraocular pressure in disease progression, we have incorporated advanced technologies, methodologies, and in vitro and ex vivo experimental models to investigate its role more comprehensively. Through meticulous experimentation and analysis, this edition aims to elucidate the intricate relationship between elevated intraocular pressure and neurodegeneration, paving the way for targeted therapeutic interventions.

Written for the highly successful *Methods in Molecular Biology* series, chapters provide detailed protocols and implementation guidance. *Glaucoma: Methods and Protocols, Second Edition* serves as an indispensable resource for those engaged in glaucoma research. By integrating updated techniques and embracing new methodologies, this edition aims to propel the field forward, fostering innovation and facilitating progress toward improved understanding and treatment of glaucoma.

Boston, MA, USA — ***Tatjana Jacobs***
Durham, NC, USA — ***Paloma B. Liton***

Contents

Contributors

TED S. ACOTT • *Department of Ophthalmology, Casey Eye Institute, Oregon Health & Science University, Portland, OR, USA*

BRIANNA C. AFIAT • *Department of Optometry and Vision Sciences, University of Melbourne, Parkville, VIC, Australia*

MINI AGA • *Department of Ophthalmology, Casey Eye Institute, Oregon Health & Science University, Portland, OR, USA*

SRIDHAR BAMMIDI • *Department of Ophthalmology, University of Pittsburgh, Pittsburgh, PA, USA*

PETR BARANOV • *Schepens Eye Research Institute of Massachusetts Eye and Ear, Boston, MA, USA*

LARRY I. BENOWITZ • *Department of Neurosurgery and F.M. Kirby Neurobiology Center, Boston Children's Hospital, Boston, MA, USA; Department of Neurosurgery, Harvard Medical School, Boston, MA, USA; Department of Ophthalmology, Harvard Medical School, Boston, MA, USA*

RYAN J. BEVAN • *UK Dementia Research Institute, Hadyn Ellis Building, Cardiff University, Cardiff, UK*

BANG V. BUI • *Department of Optometry and Vision Sciences, University of Melbourne, Parkville, VIC, Australia*

JINGWEN CAI • *Department of Cellular Biology and Anatomy, Medical College of Georgia, Augusta University, Augusta, GA, USA*

WILLIAM O. CEPURNA • *Casey Eye Institute, Oregon Health and Science University, Portland, OR, USA*

JESSICA CHAN • *Department of Biological Sciences, Georgia Institute of Technology, Atlanta, GA, USA*

KAREN CHANG • *Department of Ophthalmology, Harvard Medical School, Schepens Eye Research Institute of Massachusetts Eye and Ear, Boston, MA, USA*

DONG FENG CHEN • *Department of Ophthalmology, Harvard Medical School, Schepens Eye Research Institute of Massachusetts Eye and Ear, Boston, MA, USA*

JULIE CHEN • *Department of Ophthalmology, Harvard Medical School, Schepens Eye Research Institute of Massachusetts Eye and Ear, Boston, MA, USA*

KIN-SANG CHO • *Department of Ophthalmology, Harvard Medical School, Schepens Eye Research Institute of Massachusetts Eye and Ear, Boston, MA, USA*

GLORIA CIMAGLIA • *School of Optometry and Vision Sciences, Cardiff University, Cardiff, UK; UK Dementia Research Institute, Hadyn Ellis Building, Cardiff University, Cardiff, UK*

ABBOT F. CLARK • *Department of Pharmacology & Neuroscience, North Texas Eye Research Institute, University of North Texas Health Science Center, Fort Worth, TX, USA*

J. CRAWFORD DOWNS • *Department of Ophthalmology and Visual Sciences, School of Medicine, University of Alabama at Birmingham, Birmingham, AL, USA*

YIQIN DU • *Department of Ophthalmology, Morsani College of Medicine, University of South Florida, Tampa, FL, USA*

CALEIGH DUNN • *Department of Pathology & Laboratory Medicine, University of Wisconsin School of Medicine and Public Health, Madison, WI, USA*

C. ROSS ETHIER • *Wallace H. Coulter Department of Biomedical Engineering, Georgia Institute of Technology/Emory University, Atlanta, GA, USA*

JENNIFER A. FARALLI • *Department of Pathology & Laboratory Medicine, University of Wisconsin School of Medicine and Public Health, Madison, WI, USA*

M. REZA BAHRANI FARD • *George W. Woodruff School of Mechanical Engineering, Georgia Institute of Technology, Atlanta, GA, USA*

MICHAEL P. FAUTSCH • *Department of Ophthalmology, Mayo Clinic, Rochester, MN, USA*

ANDREW FEOLA • *Wallace H. Coulter Department of Biomedical Engineering, Georgia Institute of Technology/Emory University, Atlanta, GA, USA; Center for Visual and Neurocognitive Rehabilitation, VA Medical Center Atlanta, Decatur, GA, USA; Emory Eye Center, Emory University, Atlanta, GA, USA*

MARK S. FILLA • *Department of Pathology & Laboratory Medicine, University of Wisconsin School of Medicine and Public Health, Madison, WI, USA*

NINA SARA FRATICELLI-GUZMÁN • *George W. Woodruff School of Mechanical Engineering, Georgia Institute of Technology, Atlanta, GA, USA*

PREETHI S. GANAPATHY • *Department of Ophthalmology and Visual Sciences, SUNY Upstate Medical University, Syracuse, NY, USA; Department of Neuroscience and Physiology, SUNY Upstate Medical University, Syracuse, NY, USA; BioInspired Institute, Syracuse University, Syracuse, NY, USA*

MICHAEL P. GEISS • *Department of Ophthalmology and Visual Sciences, SUNY Upstate Medical University, Syracuse, NY, USA; Department of Physics, Syracuse University, Syracuse, NY, USA*

RAJANYA GHOSH • *Department of Ophthalmology and Visual Sciences, SUNY Upstate Medical University, Syracuse, NY, USA; Department of Biochemistry and Molecular Biology, SUNY Upstate Medical University, Syracuse, NY, USA*

SAMUEL HERBERG • *Department of Ophthalmology and Visual Sciences, SUNY Upstate Medical University, Syracuse, NY, USA; Department of Cell and Developmental Biology, SUNY Upstate Medical University, Syracuse, NY, USA; Department of Biochemistry and Molecular Biology, SUNY Upstate Medical University, Syracuse, NY, USA; BioInspired Institute, Syracuse University, Syracuse, NY, USA; Department of Biomedical and Chemical Engineering, Syracuse University, Syracuse, NY, USA*

ANH HOANG • *Department of Optometry and Vision Sciences, University of Melbourne, Parkville, VIC, Australia*

ALEX S. HUANG • *The Viterby Family Department of Ophthalmology, Shiley Eye Institute, University of California, La Jolla, CA, USA*

SIMON W. M. JOHN • *Department of Ophthalmology, Columbia University Irving Medical Center, New York, NY, USA; HHMI, Columbia University Irving Medical Center, New York, NY, USA*

ELAINE C. JOHNSON • *Casey Eye Institute, Oregon Health and Science University, Portland, OR, USA*

STEFANIE KAECH PETRIE • *Department of Neurology, Oregon Health & Science University, Portland, OR, USA*

KATE E. KELLER • *Department of Ophthalmology, Oregon Health & Science University, Portland, OR, USA*

MARY J. KELLEY • *Department of Ophthalmology, Casey Eye Institute, Oregon Health & Science University, Portland, OR, USA*

PEI YING LEE • *Department of Optometry and Vision Sciences, University of Melbourne, Parkville, VIC, Australia*
HAIYAN LI • *Department of Ophthalmology and Visual Sciences, SUNY Upstate Medical University, Syracuse, NY, USA; Department of Cell and Developmental Biology, SUNY Upstate Medical University, Syracuse, NY, USA; Wallace H. Coulter Department of Biomedical Engineering, Georgia Institute of Technology & Emory University, Atlanta, GA, USA*
PALOMA B. LITON • *Department of Ophthalmology, Duke University, Durham, NC, USA*
YUTAO LIU • *Department of Cellular Biology and Anatomy, Medical College of Georgia, Augusta University, Augusta, GA, USA*
DIANA C. LOZANO • *Casey Eye Institute, Oregon Health and Science University, Portland, OR, USA*
RUPALATHA MADDALA • *Department of Ophthalmology, Duke University School of Medicine, Durham, NC, USA*
PRABHAVATHI MADDINENI • *Gavin Herbert Eye Institute-Center for Translational Vision Research, Department of Ophthalmology, Department of Physiology and Biophysics, University of California Irvine School of Medicine, Irvine, California, USA; Department of Ophthalmology, School of Medicine, University of Missouri, Columbia, USA*
VOLHA V. MALECHKA • *Schepens Eye Research Institute of Massachusetts Eye and Ear, Boston, MA, USA*
WEIMING MAO • *Departments of Ophthalmology, Biochemistry & Molecular Biology, and Pharmacology & Toxicology, Eugene and Marilyn Glick Eye Institute, Stark Neurosciences Research Institute, Indiana University School of Medicine, Indianapolis, IN, USA*
FIONA MCDONNELL • *Moran Eye Center, Department of Ophthalmology, University of Utah, Salt Lake City, UT, USA*
COLLEEN M. MCDOWELL • *Department of Ophthalmology, University of Wisconsin-Madison, Madison, WI, USA*
JAMES E. MORGAN • *School of Optometry and Vision Sciences, Cardiff University, Cardiff, UK*
JOHN C. MORRISON • *Casey Eye Institute, Oregon Health and Science University, Portland, OR, USA*
CHRISTINE T. O. NGUYEN • *Department of Optometry and Vision Sciences, University of Melbourne, Parkville, VIC, Australia*
PINKAL D. PATEL • *Department of Pharmacology & Neuroscience, North Texas Eye Research Institute, University of North Texas Health Science Center, Fort Worth, TX, USA*
DONNA M. PETERS • *Department of Pathology & Laboratory Medicine, University of Wisconsin School of Medicine and Public Health, Madison, WI, USA; Department of Ophthalmology & Visual Sciences, University of Wisconsin School of Medicine and Public Health, Madison, WI, USA*
AISHWARYA RAJAGOPALAN • *Department of Ophthalmology, Harvard Medical School, Schepens Eye Research Institute of Massachusetts Eye and Ear, Boston, MA, USA*
P. VASANTHA RAO • *Department of Ophthalmology, Duke University School of Medicine, Durham, NC, USA*
A. THOMAS READ • *Wallace H. Coulter Department of Biomedical Engineering, Georgia Institute of Technology/Emory University, Atlanta, GA, USA*
UTTIO ROY CHOWDHURY • *Department of Ophthalmology, Mayo Clinic, Rochester, MN, USA*

REBECCA M. SAPPINGTON • *Department of Biochemistry, Wake Forest University School of Medicine, Winston-Salem, NC, USA; Department of Ophthalmology, Wake Forest University School of Medicine, Winston-Salem, NC, USA*

MYOUNG SUP SHIM • *Department of Ophthalmology, Duke University, Durham, NC, USA*

AYUSHI SINGH • *Department of Ophthalmology and Visual Sciences, SUNY Upstate Medical University, Syracuse, NY, USA; Department of Cell and Developmental Biology, SUNY Upstate Medical University, Syracuse, NY, USA*

JONATHAN R. SOUCY • *Schepens Eye Research Institute of Massachusetts Eye and Ear, Boston, MA, USA*

W. DANIEL STAMER • *Department of Ophthalmology, Duke University, Durham, NC, USA*

ANA N. STRAT • *Department of Ophthalmology and Visual Sciences, SUNY Upstate Medical University, Syracuse, NY, USA; Department of Neuroscience and Physiology, SUNY Upstate Medical University, Syracuse, NY, USA*

CLEMENS A. STROHMAIER • *Department of Ophthalmology/Optometry, Kepler University Hospital, Johannes Kepler University, Linz, Austria; The Viterby Family Department of Ophthalmology, Shiley Eye Institute, University of California, La Jolla, CA, USA*

YOGAPRIYA SUNDARESAN • *Gavin Herbert Eye Institute-Center for Translational Vision Research, Department of Ophthalmology, Department of Physiology and Biophysics, University of California Irvine School of Medicine, Irvine, California, USA*

KATIE K. N. TRAN • *Department of Optometry and Vision Sciences, University of Melbourne, Parkville, VIC, Australia*

ANNA K. VAN KOEVERDEN • *Department of Optometry and Vision Sciences, University of Melbourne, Parkville, VIC, Australia*

VICKIE H. Y. WONG • *Department of Optometry and Vision Sciences, University of Melbourne, Parkville, VIC, Australia*

ENZHI YANG • *Department of Ophthalmology, Morsani College of Medicine, University of South Florida, Tampa, FL, USA*

YUQIN YIN • *Department of Neurosurgery and F.M. Kirby Neurobiology Center, Boston Children's Hospital, Boston, MA, USA; Department of Neurosurgery, Harvard Medical School, Boston, MA, USA*

HANNAH YOO • *Department of Ophthalmology and Visual Sciences, SUNY Upstate Medical University, Syracuse, NY, USA*

DA ZHAO • *Department of Optometry and Vision Sciences, University of Melbourne, Parkville, VIC, Australia*

GULAB ZODE • *Gavin Herbert Eye Institute-Center for Translational Vision Research, Department of Ophthalmology, Department of Physiology and Biophysics, University of California Irvine School of Medicine, Irvine, California, USA*

Chapter 1

Evaluation of Cross-Linked Actin Networks (CLANs) in Human Trabecular Meshwork Cells and Tissues

Pinkal D. Patel and Abbot F. Clark

Abstract

Elevated intraocular pressure (IOP) is a major risk factor for the development and progression of glaucoma, the leading cause of irreversible vision loss and blindness. An overall increase in resistance to aqueous humor outflow causes sustained elevation in IOP. Glaucomatous insults in the aqueous humor outflow pathway, including the trabecular meshwork (TM), precede such chronic physiological changes in IOP. These insults include ultrastructural changes with excessive extracellular matrix deposition and actin cytoskeletal reorganization that leads to pathological stiffening of the ocular tissues. One of the most common cytoskeletal changes associated with TM tissue stiffness in glaucoma is the increased prevalence of cross-linked actin networks (CLANs) in cells of the trabecular meshwork (TM) and lamina cribrosa (LC). In glaucomatous cells, rearrangement of linear actin stress fibers leads to formation of polygonal arrays within the cytoplasm, resembling a geodesic dome-like structure, that we identified as CLANs. In addition to increased amounts of CLANs in POAG TM cells and tissues, we also discovered that glucocorticoid (GC) and TGFβ2 signaling pathways associated with the development of ocular hypertension (OHT) and glaucoma also induced CLANs in the TM. Despite a clear association, we are yet to completely understand the mechanisms involved in CLAN formation and their direct relevance to disease pathology. In this chapter, we will describe methods to identify and characterize CLANs using fluorescent microscopy in primary TM cell cultures, ex vivo perfusion cultured human anterior segments, and in situ in human donor eyes.

Key words Trabecular meshwork, Cross-linked actin, CLANs, Glaucoma, Dexamethasone, TGFβ2, Cytoskeleton

1 Introduction

Tissues of the aqueous humor outflow pathway, trabecular meshwork (TM) and Schlemm's canal (SC), play an important role in homeostatic regulation of intraocular pressure (IOP). Moreover, there is a definitive correlation between sustained IOP elevation and increased resistance to aqueous humor outflow in these tissues [1, 2]. These chronic physiological changes are preceded by glaucomatous insults leading to disease pathology. Studies have shown that stiffening of the TM and SC tissues as a result of glaucomatous

Tatjana Jakobs and Paloma B. Liton (eds.), *Glaucoma: Methods and Protocols*, Methods in Molecular Biology, vol. 2858,
https://doi.org/10.1007/978-1-0716-4140-8_1,

insults appears to be the cause of increased IOP and aqueous outflow resistance [3–5]. Furthermore, such stiffening has also been observed in the lamina cribrosa (LC) and optic nerve head (ONH) region in the glaucomatous eye causing retinal ganglion cell axonal damage and apoptosis [6].

Increased extracellular matrix (ECM) deposition and reorganization of actin cytoskeleton contribute to stiffening observed in glaucomatous tissues, which leads to biomechanical changes disrupting important cellular processes including cell-ECM interaction, cell-cell interaction, mechanotransduction, and phagocytosis, among other effects [4, 5, 7, 8]. The aqueous humor outflow facility is highly influenced by the structure of the TM and SC cell cytoskeleton, which is further regulated by a myriad of signaling mechanisms and events [9]. For example, the TM and SC cell cytoskeletons are instrumental in transducing external mechanical signals into biochemical signals that regulate cell function. The cytoskeleton is highly dynamic and can maintain continuous tension while rearranging itself geometrically in response to the dynamic microenvironment of the anterior chamber. Aqueous humor outflow resistance heavily depends on the dynamic nature of this cytoskeleton [10]. Depending on the type of anisotropic cues experienced by these cells, the cytoskeleton rearranges to better adapt to the biomechanical stress. These anisotropic cues can be a variety of different entities including change in local ECM composition, cell membrane composition, cell-cell interaction, cell-ECM interaction, cell-substrate interaction, and phagocytosis. In case of TM cells, the ability to dynamically respond to anisotropic cues with cytoskeletal rearrangement is necessary to maintain proper tissue resistance and IOP [11]. One of the most common cytoskeleton changes contributing to stiffness in POAG is the increased prevalence of cross-linked actin networks (CLANs) [12–14]. In glaucomatous cells, rearrangement of linear actin stress fibers leads to formation of polygonal arrays in the cytoplasmic space, initially adjacent to and surrounding the nucleus, resembling a geodesic dome-like structure, that we identify as CLANs [12–14].

Lazerides and his associates were the first to identify and characterize these unique three-dimensional actin structures in freshly plated adherent cells using immunofluorescent microscopy, with the struts staining for actin and tropomyosin and the vertices staining for actin and alpha-actinin [15, 16]. Since then, these CLAN structures have been observed in multiple different cell types [17]. These structures are only transiently formed when cells are first plated to organize their microfilament structures during the adhering and spreading phases of culture and that these structures eventually evolve into linear stress fiber-type arrangement as the cells migrate and become confluent. In contrast to other adherent cells, TM cells differ in that they can reorganize their cytoskeleton to form CLANs in confluent cells, especially in

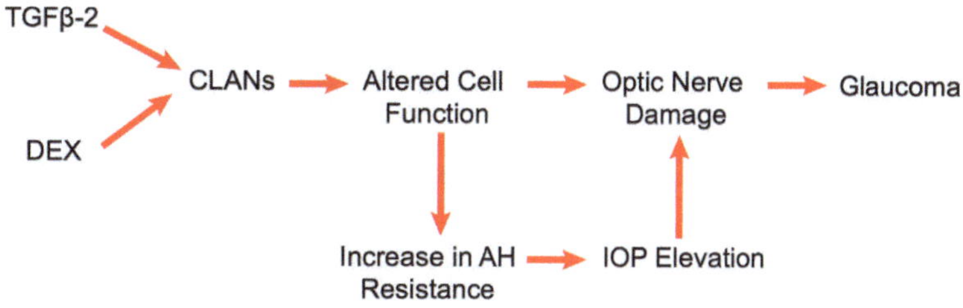

Fig. 1 Schematic of CLAN involvement in glaucoma pathology. (Adapted from Ref. [12])

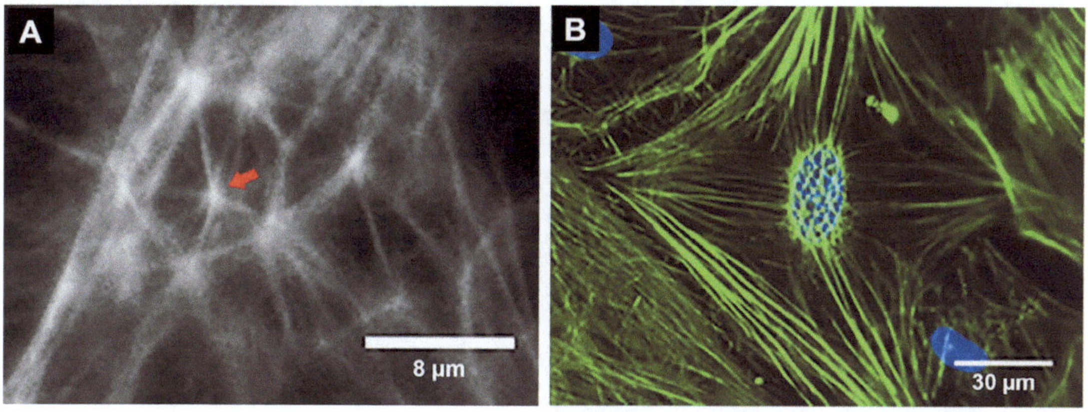

Fig. 2 Examples of phalloidin stained CLANs in HTM cells cultured with TGFβ2 for 7 days [23]. (**a**) Basic CLAN structure with central "hub" (red arrow) and 6 "struts/spokes," each connected to additional hubs. (**b**) Example of CLAN surrounding nucleus in single HTM cell along with linear f-actin stress fibers

TM cells isolated from glaucomatous eyes or when exposed to glaucoma-related insults (Fig. 1). Therefore, studying these structures in confluent TM cells as occurred in TM tissues may be more relevant to the disease pathology. It should be noted that these CLAN structures in cultured TM cells are not artifacts of two-dimensional cell culture because CLANs are also found in TM tissues ex vivo [18] and in situ [14].

Although TM cells have high propensity to form CLANs compared to other cell types in the anterior segment, the level of background CLANs accounts is only 4% in normal human TM cells at confluency [19, 20]. The structure of CLANs can vary greatly from a single CLAN with a central "hub" connected to 5–6 "spokes" (Fig. 2a) to very extensive cross-linked actin networks (Fig. 3a). This low prevalence of CLANs makes it difficult to study CLAN-associated pathology in normal TM cells. The prevalence of CLANs increases to 25–40% in glaucomatous human TM cells [13] (Fig. 3a, d). However, cells and tissues derived from glaucoma donors are less commonly available. We have shown that glaucoma-inducing agents like the glucocorticoid (GC) dexamethasone (DEX) [18–21] (Fig. 3c, d) and transforming growth factor

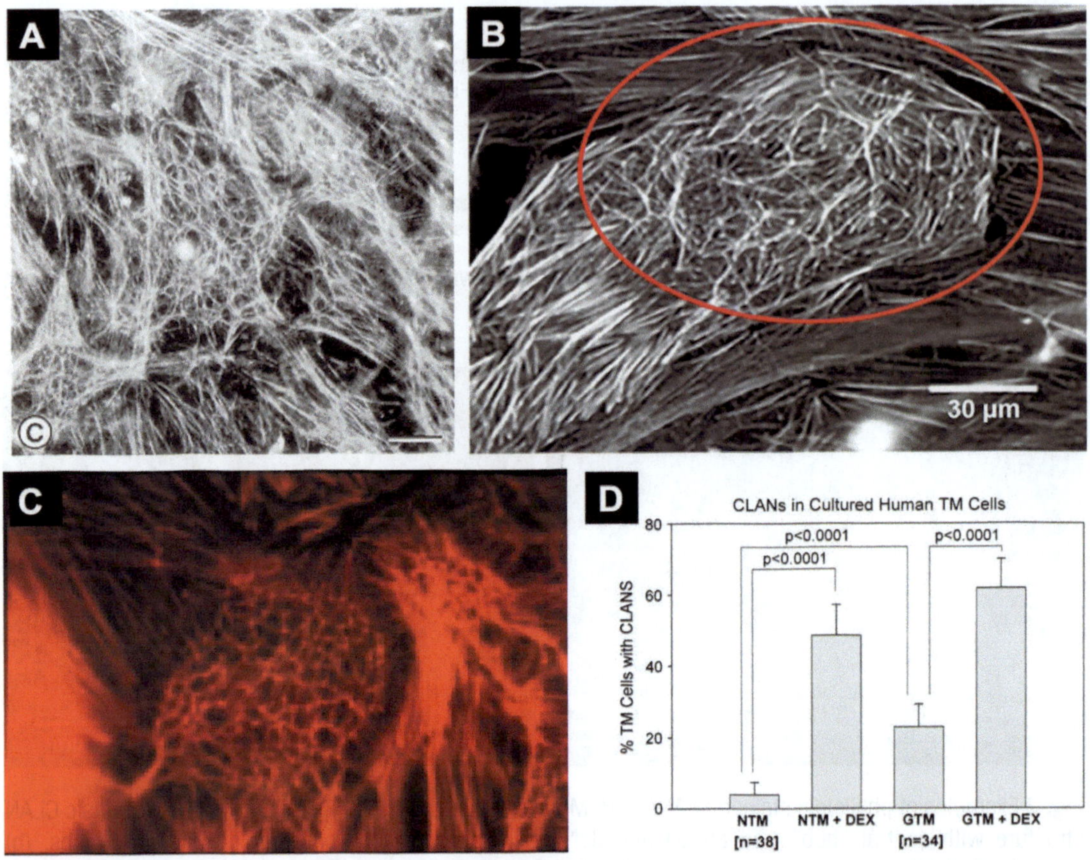

Fig. 3 Examples of CLANs in cultured HTM cells. CLANs in (**a**, **b**) TM cells [13, 23] from human donors. (**c**) Example of CLANs in HTM cells exposed to DEX (100 nM) for 14 days [19]. (**d**) Percent of TM cells with CLANs in normal TM cells (NTM, n = 38 independent cell strains), POAG TM cells (GTM, n = 34 independent cell strains), and both HTM and GTM cells treated with DEX (100 nM) for 14 days [20]. The % TM cells with CLANs was highly statistically different among all four groups of TM cells

β-2 (TGFβ-2) [22, 23] (Fig. 2) can induce CLAN formation in normal TM cells [23]. Experimental induction of CLANs using DEX or TGFβ2 is now commonly used to study the role of CLANs in glaucoma pathology and to test new glaucoma targets.

Glucocorticoids (GCs) are a widely prescribed class of synthetic steroids known for their potent antiinflammatory and immunomodulatory effects. GCs remain the gold standard in treating ocular inflammation associated with disease or surgery. Unfortunately, prolonged GC treatment has been associated with numerous side effects including GC-induced ocular hypertension (GC-OHT) that can lead to iatrogenic secondary open-angle glaucoma [24]. Since the clinical and molecular manifestations of GC-OHT resemble POAG, potent GCs such as DEX have been increasingly used to experimentally probe POAG pathology [20, 25]. DEX treatment increases ECM deposition and induces cytoskeletal reorganization in TM cells causing cell stiffening, which is also observed in cells from POAG patients [1, 13, 14]. We have previously shown that DEX treatment of cultured normal human TM cells can induce CLAN formation [18, 19] (Fig. 2c, d). This experimental induction of CLANs (using 100 nM DEX treatment for 7 days) in now widely used to study CLAN biology and determine its pathological relevance to glaucoma.

The profibrotic cytokine TGFβ2 is elevated in aqueous humor [26–28] and TM cells [29] derived from POAG patients and has been associated with glaucomatous damage to the TM [27, 28, 30]. In addition, TGFβ2 causes ocular hypertension in ex vivo perfusion cultured human anterior segments [30, 31] and in vivo in mice [32, 33]. Furthermore, aqueous humor by itself is also known to induce CLANs formation [22] presumably due to the TGFβ2 in aqueous humor. We previously have shown that both SMAD-dependent and SMAD-independent TGFβ2 signaling contribute to actin cytoskeleton reorganization and induction of CLANs [23].

In this chapter, we will describe methods to induce, identify, and characterize CLANs in TM cells and tissues.

2 Materials

2.1 Cell Culture Medium

1. Normal cell culture medium: Low glucose Dulbecco's modified Eagle's medium (DMEM) supplemented with 10% fetal bovine serum (FBS), 100 units/mL penicillin, 0.1 mg/mL streptomycin, and 0.292 mg/mL L-glutamine.
2. Low-serum cell culture medium: High glucose DMEM supplemented with 0.25–1% FBS, 100 units/mL penicillin, 0.1 mg/mL streptomycin, and 0.292 mg/mL L-glutamine.
3. Perfusion medium: Low glucose DMEM supplemented with penicillin 100 units/mL penicillin, 0.1 mg/mL streptomycin, and 0.292 mg/mL L-glutamine.

2.2 Solutions and Buffers

1. Dexamethasone (DEX) cell treatment solution (10 μM stock): Dissolve 39.247 mg of DEX in 10 mL of 100% ethanol to make a 10 mM DEX solution. Add 10 μL of 10 mM DEX solution to 10 mL 100% ethanol to make the 10 μM DEX stock solution. Sterile filter the 10 μM DEX stock solution using a 0.22 μm syringe filter, and store at 4 °C away from direct light until needed. For final concentration of 100 nM DEX, add 10 μL of 10 μM DEX stock solution to each mL of medium used.
2. Vehicle cell treatment solution (0.01%): Sterile filter 100% ethanol solution using a 0.22 μm syringe filter. For final concentration of 0.01%, add 10 μL of filtered 100% ethanol to each mL of cell culture medium used.

3. Permeabilization buffer: 0.2% Triton-X. Add 20 μL Triton-X to 10 mL of PBS.
4. Blocking buffer: Add 1 mL FBS and 10 μL Triton-X to 9 mL of PBS.

2.3 Reagents and Supplies

1. Human eyes for TM cell isolation and tissue culture can be procured from local tissue/eye bank. We have used Lions Eye (Tampa, Florida) and the UNTHSC Willed Body Program (Fort Worth, Texas) for procuring these gifts (*see* **Note 1**).
2. Autoclaved straight surgical scissors (105–130 mm) and curved surgical scissors (105 mm).
3. Autoclaved Dumont #5 Fine-pointed forceps.
4. Disposable Premier Edge 45° angled Microsurgical Stab knife/blade.
5. Round glass cover slips (12 mm).
6. Nunc Lab-Tek II 4-Chamber glass-bottomed slides with cover.
7. Nunc 24-well plastic cell culture treated plates.
8. Nunc 6-well plastic cell culture treated plates.
9. Micronized dexamethasone.
10. Recombinant human TGFβ2: 20 μg/mL in sterile 4 mM HCl containing 0.1% bovine serum albumin.
11. 4% Paraformaldehyde.
12. 4% Neutral buffer formalin.
13. Dulbecco's phosphate-buffered saline (PBS/DPBS).
14. SuperBlock blocking buffer.
15. Alexa Fluor™ 488 Phalloidin.
16. ProLong Gold Anti-Fade with 4′,6-diamidino-2-phenylindole (DAPI).
17. Tween 20.
18. Propidium iodide.
19. Rhodamine phalloidin.
20. Sytox Green stain: 5 mM solution in DMSO.

3 Methods

3.1 Experimental Induction of CLANs in Confluent TM Cells

3.1.1 Glucocorticoid (GC) Induction of CLANS

1. Plate human TM cells onto 24-well plates at 40–50% confluency and culture them in normal cell culture media until 90–100% confluent (*see* **Notes 1** and **2**). For experiments requiring microscopy, cells are plated on autoclaved round glass coverslips placed in 24-well plates or on chambered slides.

2. Prepare and filter the stock DEX solution and vehicle solution (ethanol) using a 0.22 μm syringe filter as mentioned above in Subheading 2.2. Store sterile stock solution at 4 °C away from direct light.
3. Treat confluent cultures with either vehicle control (0.01% ethanol) or 10 μL of DEX cell treatment solution stock per each mL of medium, added to culture medium.
4. Continue treatment for 7–14 days, replacing with fresh treatment medium 2–3 times per week.

3.1.2 Transforming Growth Factor β2 (TGFβ2)-Mediated Induction of CLANs

For TGFβ2-mediated induction of CLANs, confluent cultured TM cells should be cultured in low serum conditions (0.25–1.0% FBS) to reduce confounding effects from growth factors present in the serum. To enhance cell survival in low serum conditions, use growth medium containing high glucose.

1. Culture the confluent TM cells in low serum medium containing high glucose as described above in Subheading 3.1.
2. For experiments requiring microscopy, plate cells on autoclaved round glass coverslips placed in 24-well plates or on glass-chambered slides.
3. Post acclimation period of 2–3 days, treat with TGFβ2 (5 ng/mL) or vehicle (PBS) for 7–10 days, replacing with fresh medium twice per week.

3.2 Visualization and Quantification of CLANs in Confluent Primary TM Cell Cultures

1. Human primary TM cells are cultured as described previously (*see* **Notes 1** and **2**).
2. When confluent or after DEX or TGFβ2 treatment, fix cells with 2–4% paraformaldehyde in PBS and wash three times with PBS (*see* **Note 3**).
3. Treat cells with permeabilization buffer for 10 min and then wash three times with PBS.
4. Perform blocking for 2 h at room temperature by using Superblock blocking buffer, or alternatively use blocking buffer prepared as shown in Subheading 2.2.
5. Stain cytoplasmic F-actin using phalloidin conjugated with Alexa Fluor-488 (1:100) diluted in Superblock blocking buffer for 1 h at room temperature. If concurrent immunolabeling of other markers is required, stain overnight with primary antibody at 4 °C followed by washing and addition of the relevant fluorescently labelled secondary antibody (*see* **Note 4**).
6. Wash three times with PBS and mount the glass coverslips using ProLong Gold Anti-Fade with DAPI for nuclear counterstaining.

7. Visualize CLANs using an epifluorescence or confocal microscope capable of achieving 600X total magnification. Refer to the representative images (Fig. 2) to aid in identification of CLANs. CLANs are defined as F-actin-containing cytoskeletal structures with at least one triangulated actin arrangement consisting of actin spokes (struts) and at least three identifiable hubs (vertices) (Fig. 2a). Linear fibers of F-actin bundles (i.e., stress fibers) may be more prominent and prevalent in the images, masking the lighter stained CLANs which generally are above the stress fibers. As a result, higher magnification and manual focusing may be required to properly visualize CLANs from the highly fluorescent F-actin linear stress fibers. Capture and evaluate multiple images from each cover slip (take images at ~10 locations with equal cell populations) and 6–10 coverslips per treatment group (generally 100–200 TM cells/slide).
8. Using the images taken, count CLANs in the images in a masked manner. In each image (field of view), count the number of DAPI-positive cells and CLAN-positive cells (CPCs). CLAN-positive cells (CPCs) are defined as any cell in the field of view containing at least one CLAN or multiple CLANs. The formation of CLANs can be compared using the percentage of CPCs, which is calculated by dividing the number of CPCs by the number of DAPI-positive cells.

3.3 Visualizing CLANs In Situ and Ex Vivo in Human Ocular TM Tissues

Visualizing CLANs in TM tissues is more challenging due to the complex three-dimensional structure of the TM, where cells surround the ECM beams and cells within the JCT are somewhat randomly arranged. We have used donor eyes from control and POAG patients [14] as well as our ex vivo perfusion cultured human anterior segment model [18] to visualize CLANs in TM tissues (Fig. 4).

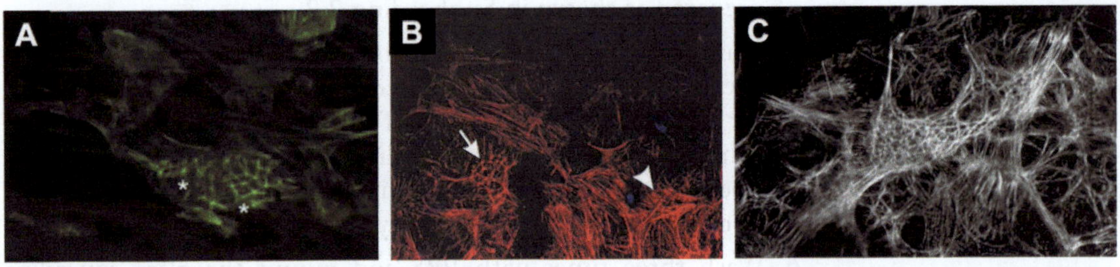

Fig. 4 Examples of TM tissue CLANs: (**a**) in situ visualization of CLANs (*) in TM tissues from POAG donor eyes [14]. (**b, c**) TM tissues from perfusion cultured human anterior segments treated with DEX (100 nM) for 14 days [18]. DEX-induced CLAN containing TM cells within the JCT (arrows) (**b**) and corneoscleral meshwork (**c**)

3.3.1 Visualizing CLANs in Human Donor Eyes In Situ

1. Hemisect the human eye along the equator about 5 mm posterior to the limbus, separating the anterior from the posterior segment using curved scissors (*see* **Note 5**).
2. Remove and discard the lens, iris, and the posterior portion of the ciliary body from the anterior segment using a pair of fine-pointed forceps.
3. In a 6-well plate, immersion fix the remaining anterior segment for 24 h using 4% neutral-buffered formaldehyde, ensuring the entire tissue is submerged in the fixative.
4. After fixation, use a surgical stab blade to make slicing cuts posterior and anterior to the TM toward the Schlemm's canal. These slices are to be made across the entire length of the TM.
5. Using a fine-pointed forceps, lift and peel the sliced tissue strips containing the TM, and place each segment into a well of a 24-well plate.
6. Wash the strips three times with 500 μL of PBS for 10 min each. In the same 24-well plate, incubate the strips overnight at 4 °C in the dark with phalloidin-Alexa 488 diluted 1/20 with PBS/0.1% Tween 20. After overnight incubation, again wash the strips three times with 500 μL of PBS for 10 min each [14]. Incubate samples for 4 h in propidium iodide (diluted 1/10 with 0.1% PBS), and wash an additional three times with 0.1% PBS.
7. Carefully transfer the TM strip to a glass microscope slide to be mounted beneath a coverslip in fluorescence mounting medium. Ensure the orientation of the strip is similar along the entire length of the TM strip.
8. Use a confocal microscope with a 60X oil immersion objective (NA = 1.4) for visualizing CLANs in ex vivo tissues. Optically section the strips at 0.5–1 μm intervals into a z-series of confocal images. Note that the phalloidin-Alexa 488 will fluoresce comparatively more when bound to larger linear actin stress fibers compared to the subcortical CLANs. Manual focus adjustment may be necessary to augment the visibility of CLANs from the linear cortical actin stress fibers during imaging.
9. Use confocal microscope software for processing and evaluating the individual images of the z-stack to identify and determine the size, complexity, and prevalence of CLANs in each field of view. For all the CLANs that occupy more than one z-series (1 μm) image, align the stack images in register; and create composites for analysis. This provides a more robust inclusion/exclusion strategy for CLAN identification and a more precise measurement of the dimensions of these

structures (Fig. 4a). Also be mindful of intraobserver and interobserver variability that can occur in counting CLANs.

10. For quantification, calculate the number of CLANs and number of PI-stained nuclei in a known volume of TM tissue. TM volumes were determined from the area of confocal z-stacks times the number and depth of each optical slice. Be aware that there is an age-related decline in TM cell number [34, 35] that is further acerbated in POAG eyes [36], so that it is important to age-match eyes.

3.3.2 Visualizing CLANs in the TM of Ex Vivo Perfusion Cultured Anterior Segments [18]

1. The technique of ex vivo perfusion culture of human anterior segments varies among labs, but we have been using slight modifications from the original technique [30, 37–41] initially described by Doug Johnson [42] (*see* Chap. 8 in this volume). Dissect the anterior segments from human donor eyes (<24 h post death), with careful removal of the lens, iris, and most of the ciliary body.
2. Place each anterior segment of paired eyes on an island and clamp with an O-ring in a specially engineered Plexiglass dish.
3. Attach one dish cannula to a syringe pump and the other canula to pressure transducer in order to continuously monitor IOP.
4. The covered perfusion dishes are then placed in an incubator at 37 °C with 5% CO_2/air.
5. Then perfuse with the perfusion medium at the constant rate of 2.5 μL/min (approximately the rate of aqueous formation). The IOPs generally stabilize after 24–48 h of perfusion culture.
6. To induce CLANs, treat one eye of each pair with either 100 nM DEX or TGFβ2 (5 ng/mL), while the contralateral eye receives vehicle (0.01% ethanol). Perfusion continues for 7–14 days. Approximately 30–40% of the DEX perfused eyes develop significantly elevated IOP (at least 5 mmHg elevation above baseline) [37], while almost all eyes receiving TGFβ2 develop OHT [30].
7. Alternatively, TM tissues can be transduced with either Ad5 or lentiviral vectors encoding human $TGF\beta2^{C226/228C}$ to generate TGFβ2-induced ocular hypertension.
8. Visualization of CLANs [18] (Fig. 4b, c) within the TM, JCT, and inner wall of Schlemm's canal (SC) can be assessed using two methods. To visualize the uveal and corneoscleral TM, human anterior segments are perfusion fixed at 12 mmHg for 1 h and then immersion fixed for 23 h in neural buffered 4% formalin. The TM tissue is then processed as described above (3.3.1, 4–10).
9. The second method examines the JCT and SC inner wall (IW) endothelium. Anterior segments are perfusion fixed for

2 h and then immersion fixed for 22 h in 3% paraformaldehyde (in PBS).

10. Radial segments for each quadrant are microdissected, making an incision along the posterior margin of SC and opening SC to allow en face visualization of the inner wall endothelium and adjacent JCT.
11. Permeabilize the tissues using the permeabilization buffer (Subheading 2.2) for 5 min and subsequently wash with PBS.
12. Tissues then are stained with rhodamine-phalloidin (diluted 1: 20 in DPBS) for 30 at 37 °C, and nuclei are stained with Sytox Green (1:2400 in TBS) for 5 min at room temperature.
13. After washing tissues in PBS, a thin piece of tissue containing SC, IW, JCT, and remaining meshwork is dissected from remnants of ciliary body and iris root.
14. The thin tissue samples are then mounted on a slide containing a shallow chamber constructed from Parafilm to prevent tissue compression when adding the cover slip.
15. Mounted tissues are then examined by confocal microscopy using the 60X oil immersion lens and optically sectioned at 0.5–1.0 μm intervals to generate Z-stacked images from SC IW through the JCT and into the corneoscleral TM.

4 Notes

1. A general rule of thumb is to retrieve cells and tissues from freshly enucleated eyes, within 24 h postmortem. Uniform precautions and best practices should be used when handling human donor eyes and in the isolation, culture, and characterization of primary human normal TM cells (NTM) and glaucomatous TM cells (GTM) as previously described [43, 44].
2. Great care should be taken in obtaining and characterizing human TM cells (please *see* [43, 45] for details). Human TM cell culture generally occurs through the careful dissection of TM tissue from human donor eyes. The human donor eyes should be obtained from a reputable source that follows the tenets of the Declaration of Helsinki with donor or family consent. TM cells are grown from TM tissue explants [13, 19] or from cells proteolytically isolated from the TM tissue prior to culture [46]. Although culture conditions vary between laboratories, TM cells are usually cultured in DMEM or a DMEM/hybrid medium that contains L-glutamine, antibiotics, and fetal bovine serum (10–20%), with medium changes 2–3 times per week. We have found that the TM cells grow better when some of the conditioned medium is left in

culture (~10–20%) rather than totally replacing the conditioned medium with fresh medium. Although there is no universal marker that differentiates TM cells from other cell types, the consensus recommendation [43, 45] is that the TM cells should be authenticated by a combination of (1) morphology (cells should grow as confluent monolayers with overlapping boundaries), (2) dexamethasone (DEX)-induction of the glaucoma gene *Myocilin* (*MYOC*), and (3) a combination of other markers such as α-smooth muscle actin; collagens I, II, and IV; and laminin. Examination of CLANs should be conducted in confluent TM cells.

3. There are differences in experimental methods used to study CLANs in the TM. Some studies have used adhering and spreading TM cells [47, 48]. CLANs can form in both adherent and spreading TM cells as well as in many other adherent cell types; therefore, these types of CLANs are not unique to TM cells. In contrast, CLAN formation in confluent TM cells is relatively unique to TM cells. The signaling mechanisms involved in CLAN formation can vary depending on the method used. Here we use confluent TM cells as we consider this more representative to the native state of TM cells in TM tissues.
4. Visualization of CLANs in vitro, in ex vivo, and in situ is done by fluorochemical staining with fluorophore-conjugated phalloidin, which binds and labels all F-actin fibers. Antibodies to different types of actin (e.g., smooth muscle actin [19]) or actin-binding proteins [18] can be used to visualize CLANs.
5. Clean the eye ball of adipose tissue and muscles using a curved scissors. Use the insertion points of the extraocular muscles as visual markers for hemisection of the eye globe. Cut along the insertion points to ensure angle tissue is preserved.

Acknowledgments

This work is supported by grants from the NEI/NIH (R01EY016242 and R01EY030967). We would like to thank our numerous colleagues who worked on CLAN research in the Clark lab over a number of years. In addition, we have been very fortunate to collaborate with Prof. Ian Grierson (U. Liverpool) and Prof. Ross Ethier (GIT) in our CLAN studies.

References

1. Rohen JW (1983) Why is intraocular pressure elevated in chronic simple glaucoma? Anatomical considerations. Ophthalmology 90(7): 758–765. https://doi.org/10.1016/s0161-6420(83)34492-4

2. Tamm ER, Braunger BM, Fuchshofer R (2015) Intraocular pressure and the mechanisms involved in resistance of the aqueous humor flow in the trabecular meshwork outflow pathways. Prog Mol Biol Transl Sci 134: 301–314. https://doi.org/10.1016/bs.pmbts.2015.06.007
3. Last JA, Pan T, Ding Y, Reilly CM, Keller K, Acott TS, Fautsch MP, Murphy CJ, Russell P (2011) Elastic modulus determination of normal and glaucomatous human trabecular meshwork. Invest Ophthalmol Vis Sci 52(5): 2147–2152. https://doi.org/10.1167/iovs.10-6342
4. Raghunathan VK, Morgan JT, Chang YR, Weber D, Phinney B, Murphy CJ, Russell P (2015) Transforming growth factor beta 3 modifies mechanics and composition of extracellular matrix deposited by human trabecular meshwork cells. ACS Biomater Sci Eng 1(2):110–118. https://doi.org/10.1021/ab500060r
5. Raghunathan VK, Morgan JT, Park SA, Weber D, Phinney BS, Murphy CJ, Russell P (2015) Dexamethasone stiffens trabecular meshwork, trabecular meshwork cells, and matrix. Invest Ophthalmol Vis Sci 56(8): 4447–4459. https://doi.org/10.1167/iovs.15-16739
6. Hernandez MR, Andrzejewska WM, Neufeld AH (1990) Changes in the extracellular matrix of the human optic nerve head in primary open-angle glaucoma. Am J Ophthalmol 109(2):180–188. https://doi.org/10.1016/s0002-9394(14)75984-7
7. Keller KE, Aga M, Bradley JM, Kelley MJ, Acott TS (2009) Extracellular matrix turnover and outflow resistance. Exp Eye Res 88(4): 676–682. https://doi.org/10.1016/j.exer.2008.11.023
8. Bradley JM, Kelley MJ, Zhu X, Anderssohn AM, Alexander JP, Acott TS (2001) Effects of mechanical stretching on trabecular matrix metalloproteinases. Invest Ophthalmol Vis Sci 42(7):1505–1513
9. Braunger BM, Fuchshofer R, Tamm ER (2015) The aqueous humor outflow pathways in glaucoma: a unifying concept of disease mechanisms and causative treatment. Eur J Pharm Biopharm 95(Pt B):173–181. https://doi.org/10.1016/j.ejpb.2015.04.029
10. Tan JC, Peters DM, Kaufman PL (2006) Recent developments in understanding the pathophysiology of elevated intraocular pressure. Curr Opin Ophthalmol 17(2):168–174. https://doi.org/10.1097/01.icu.0000193079.55240.18
11. Acott TS, Kelley MJ, Keller KE, Vranka JA, Abu-Hassan DW, Li X, Aga M, Bradley JM (2014) Intraocular pressure homeostasis: maintaining balance in a high-pressure environment. J Ocul Pharmacol Ther 30(2–3): 94–101. https://doi.org/10.1089/jop.2013.0185
12. Bermudez JY, Montecchi-Palmer M, Mao W, Clark AF (2017) Cross-linked actin networks (CLANs) in glaucoma. Exp Eye Res 159:16. https://doi.org/10.1016/j.exer.2017.02.010
13. Clark AF, Miggans ST, Wilson K, Browder S, McCartney MD (1995) Cytoskeletal changes in cultured human glaucoma trabecular meshwork cells. J Glaucoma 4:183–188
14. Hoare MJ, Grierson I, Brotchie D, Pollock N, Cracknell K, Clark AF (2009) Cross-linked actin networks (CLANs) in the trabecular meshwork of the normal and glaucomatous human eye in situ. Invest Ophthalmol Vis Sci 50(3):1255–1263. https://doi.org/10.1167/iovs.08-2706
15. Lazarides E (1976) Actin, alpha-actinin, and tropomyosin interaction in the structural organization of actin filaments in nonmuscle cells. J Cell Biol 68(2):202–219. https://doi.org/10.1083/jcb.68.2.202
16. Lazarides E (1976) Two general classes of cytoplasmic actin filaments in tissue culture cells: the role of tropomyosin. J Supramol Struct 5(4):531(383)–563(415). https://doi.org/10.1002/jss.400050410
17. Wade NC, Grierson I, O'Reilly S, Hoare MJ, Cracknell KP, Paraoan LI, Brotchie D, Clark AF (2009) Cross-linked actin networks (CLANs) in bovine trabecular meshwork cells. Exp Eye Res 89(5):648–659. https://doi.org/10.1016/j.exer.2009.06.006
18. Clark AF, Brotchie D, Read AT, Hellberg P, English-Wright S, Pang IH, Ethier CR, Grierson I (2005) Dexamethasone alters F-actin architecture and promotes cross-linked actin network formation in human trabecular meshwork tissue. Cell Motil Cytoskeleton 60(2): 83–95. https://doi.org/10.1002/cm.20049
19. Clark AF, Wilson K, McCartney MD, Miggans ST, Kunkle M, Howe W (1994) Glucocorticoid-induced formation of cross-linked actin networks in cultured human trabecular meshwork cells. Invest Ophthalmol Vis Sci 35(1):281–294
20. Clark AF, Wordinger RJ (2009) The role of steroids in outflow resistance. Exp Eye Res 88(4):752–759. https://doi.org/10.1016/j.exer.2008.10.004
21. Peng M, Rayana NP, Dai J, Sugali CK, Baidouri H, Suresh A, Raghunathan VK, Mao

W (2022) Cross-linked actin networks (CLANs) affect stiffness and/or actin dynamics in transgenic transformed and primary human trabecular meshwork cells. Exp Eye Res 220: 109097. https://doi.org/10.1016/j.exer.2022.109097

22. O'Reilly S, Pollock N, Currie L, Paraoan L, Clark AF, Grierson I (2011) Inducers of cross-linked actin networks in trabecular meshwork cells. Invest Ophthalmol Vis Sci 52(10): 7316–7324. https://doi.org/10.1167/iovs.10-6692
23. Montecchi-Palmer M, Bermudez JY, Webber HC, Patel GC, Clark AF, Mao W (2017) TGFbeta2 induces the formation of cross-linked actin networks (CLANs) in human trabecular meshwork cells through the Smad and non-Smad dependent pathways. Invest Ophthalmol Vis Sci 58(2):1288–1295. https://doi.org/10.1167/iovs.16-19672
24. Clark AF (1995) Basic sciences in clinical glaucoma: steroids, ocular hypertension, and glaucoma. J Glaucoma 4(5):354–369
25. Wordinger RJ, Clark AF (1999) Effects of glucocorticoids on the trabecular meshwork: towards a better understanding of glaucoma. Prog Retin Eye Res 18(5):629–667
26. Tripathi RC, Li J, Chan WF, Tripathi BJ (1994) Aqueous humor in glaucomatous eyes contains an increased level of TGF-beta 2. Exp Eye Res 59(6):723–727. https://doi.org/10.1006/exer.1994.1158
27. Fuchshofer R, Tamm ER (2012) The role of TGF-beta in the pathogenesis of primary open-angle glaucoma. Cell Tissue Res 347(1): 279–290. https://doi.org/10.1007/s00441-011-1274-7
28. Lutjen-Drecoll E (2005) Morphological changes in glaucomatous eyes and the role of TGFbeta2 for the pathogenesis of the disease. Exp Eye Res 81(1):1–4. https://doi.org/10.1016/j.exer.2005.02.008
29. Tovar-Vidales T, Clark AF, Wordinger RJ (2011) Transforming growth factor-beta2 utilizes the canonical Smad-signaling pathway to regulate tissue transglutaminase expression in human trabecular meshwork cells. Exp Eye Res 93(4):442–451. https://doi.org/10.1016/j.exer.2011.06.011
30. Fleenor DL, Shepard AR, Hellberg PE, Jacobson N, Pang IH, Clark AF (2006) TGFbeta2-induced changes in human trabecular meshwork: implications for intraocular pressure. Invest Ophthalmol Vis Sci 47(1): 226–234. https://doi.org/10.1167/iovs.05-1060
31. Gottanka J, Chan D, Eichhorn M, Lutjen-Drecoll E, Ethier CR (2004) Effects of TGF-beta2 in perfused human eyes. Invest Ophthalmol Vis Sci 45(1):153–158. https://doi.org/10.1167/iovs.03-0796
32. Shepard AR, Millar JC, Pang IH, Jacobson N, Wang WH, Clark AF (2010) Adenoviral gene transfer of active human transforming growth factor-{beta}2 elevates intraocular pressure and reduces outflow facility in rodent eyes. Invest Ophthalmol Vis Sci 51(4):2067–2076. https://doi.org/10.1167/iovs.09-4567
33. McDowell CM, Tebow HE, Wordinger RJ, Clark AF (2013) Smad3 is necessary for transforming growth factor-beta2 induced ocular hypertension in mice. Exp Eye Res 116:419–423. https://doi.org/10.1016/j.exer.2013.10.017
34. Grierson I, Howes RC (1987) Age-related depletion of the cell population in the human trabecular meshwork. Eye (Lond) 1(Pt 2): 204–210. https://doi.org/10.1038/eye.1987.38
35. Alvarado J, Murphy C, Polansky J, Juster R (1981) Age-related changes in trabecular meshwork cellularity. Invest Ophthalmol Vis Sci 21(5):714–727
36. Alvarado J, Murphy C, Juster R (1984) Trabecular meshwork cellularity in primary open-angle glaucoma and nonglaucomatous normals. Ophthalmology 91(6):564–579. https://doi.org/10.1016/s0161-6420(84)34248-8
37. Clark AF, Wilson K, de Kater AW, Allingham RR, McCartney MD (1995) Dexamethasone-induced ocular hypertension in perfusion-cultured human eyes. Invest Ophthalmol Vis Sci 36(2):478–489
38. Wordinger RJ, Fleenor DL, Hellberg PE, Pang IH, Tovar TO, Zode GS, Fuller JA, Clark AF (2007) Effects of TGF-beta2, BMP-4, and gremlin in the trabecular meshwork: implications for glaucoma. Invest Ophthalmol Vis Sci 48(3):1191–1200. https://doi.org/10.1167/iovs.06-0296
39. Pang IH, McCartney MD, Steely HT, Clark AF (2000) Human ocular perfusion organ culture: a versatile ex vivo model for glaucoma research. J Glaucoma 9(6):468–479
40. Wang WH, McNatt LG, Pang IH, Hellberg PE, Fingert JH, McCartney MD, Clark AF (2008) Increased expression of serum amyloid A in glaucoma and its effect on intraocular pressure. Invest Ophthalmol Vis Sci 49(5): 1916–1923. https://doi.org/10.1167/iovs.07-1104

41. Wang WH, McNatt LG, Pang IH, Millar JC, Hellberg PE, Hellberg MH, Steely HT, Rubin JS, Fingert JH, Sheffield VC, Stone EM, Clark AF (2008) Increased expression of the WNT antagonist sFRP-1 in glaucoma elevates intraocular pressure. J Clin Invest 118(3): 1056–1064. https://doi.org/10.1172/JCI33871
42. Johnson DH, Tschumper RC (1987) Human trabecular meshwork organ culture. A new method. Invest Ophthalmol Vis Sci 28(6): 945–953
43. Keller KE, Bhattacharya SK, Borras T, Brunner TM, Chansangpetch S, Clark AF, Dismuke WM, Du Y, Elliott MH, Ethier CR, Faralli JA, Freddo TF, Fuchshofer R, Giovingo M, Gong H, Gonzalez P, Huang A, Johnstone MA, Kaufman PL, Kelley MJ, Knepper PA, Kopczynski CC, Kuchtey JG, Kuchtey RW, Kuehn MH, Lieberman RL, Lin SC, Liton P, Liu Y, Lutjen-Drecoll E, Mao W, Masis-Solano M, McDonnell F, McDowell CM, Overby DR, Pattabiraman PP, Raghunathan VK, Rao PV, Rhee DJ, Chowdhury UR, Russell P, Samples JR, Schwartz D, Stubbs EB, Tamm ER, Tan JC, Toris CB, Torrejon KY, Vranka JA, Wirtz MK, Yorio T, Zhang J, Zode GS, Fautsch MP, Peters DM, Acott TS, Stamer WD (2018) Consensus recommendations for trabecular meshwork cell isolation, characterization and culture. Exp Eye Res 171:164–173. https://doi.org/10.1016/j.exer.2018.03.001
44. Stamer DW, Roberts BC, Epstein DL, Allingham RR (2000) Isolation of primary open-angle glaucomatous trabecular meshwork cells from whole eye tissue. Curr Eye Res 20(5): 347–350
45. Stamer WD, Clark AF (2017) The many faces of the trabecular meshwork cell. Exp Eye Res 158:112–123. https://doi.org/10.1016/j.exer.2016.07.009
46. Stamer WD, Seftor RE, Williams SK, Samaha HA, Snyder RW (1995) Isolation and culture of human trabecular meshwork cells by extracellular matrix digestion. Curr Eye Res 14(7): 611–617. https://doi.org/10.3109/02713689508998409
47. Filla MS, Clark R, Peters DM (2014) A syndecan-4 binding peptide derived from laminin 5 uses a novel PKCepsilon pathway to induce cross-linked actin network (CLAN) formation in human trabecular meshwork (HTM) cells. Exp Cell Res 327(2):171–182. https://doi.org/10.1016/j.yexcr.2014.07.035
48. Filla MS, Schwinn MK, Nosie AK, Clark RW, Peters DM (2011) Dexamethasone-associated cross-linked actin network formation in human trabecular meshwork cells involves beta3 integrin signaling. Invest Ophthalmol Vis Sci 52(6): 2952–2959. https://doi.org/10.1167/iovs.10-6618

Chapter 2

Three-Dimensional Extracellular Matrix Protein Hydrogels for Human Trabecular Meshwork Cell Studies

Ayushi Singh, Rajanya Ghosh, Haiyan Li, Michael P. Geiss, Hannah Yoo, Ana N. Strat, Preethi S. Ganapathy, and Samuel Herberg

Abstract

The extracellular microenvironment plays a crucial role in regulating a wide range of cell behaviors. Biopolymer hydrogels are ideally suited to present a realistic three-dimensional extracellular milieu to cells in vitro. Here, we describe the fabrication and use of soft tissue-mimetic extracellular matrix protein hydrogels for investigations of human trabecular meshwork cell biology.

Key words Bioengineering, Biopolymers, Photo-crosslinking, Outflow tract, Glaucoma

1 Introduction

Our collective understanding of many trabecular meshwork (TM) cell processes is derived from studies performed using nonphysiological culture conditions. Conventional polystyrene or glass substrates lack dimensionality and are orders of magnitude stiffer [1] than the native TM tissue [2]. While most researchers acknowledge that standard two-dimensional cell culture materials are not ideal to recapitulate the TM cellular microenvironment, there is currently a knowledge barrier toward the application of three-dimensional cell culture systems. Here, we describe extracellular matrix (ECM) protein hydrogels to those who may be unfamiliar with procedures to culture and study TM cells in a soft tissue-like three-dimensional microenvironment.

ECM hydrogels, that is, water-swollen biopolymer networks, provide a simplistic version of the native three-dimensional tissue environment and allow for accurate in vitro modeling of cellular, biochemical, and biomechanical behaviors [3]. Polymer precursors

---

Authors Ayushi Singh, Rajanya Ghosh, Haiyan Li have equally contributed to this chapter.

Tatjana Jakobs and Paloma B. Liton (eds.), *Glaucoma: Methods and Protocols*, Methods in Molecular Biology, vol. 2858,
https://doi.org/10.1007/978-1-0716-4140-8_2,

containing photoactive functional groups can be chemically crosslinked by short exposure to ultraviolet (UV) or blue light in the presence of a photoinitiator in a cytocompatible manner [4]. The resulting hydrogel network provides a supportive three-dimensional environment enabling normal cell behaviors. Using a reductionist approach, we focused on key ECM components present in the native TM [5]. Our aim was to partially recapitulate the juxtacanalicular tissue (JCT) region that is most critical for aqueous humor outflow resistance regulation. JCT-TM cells reside embedded in a fibrillar ECM containing collagen type I and elastin, with the narrow spaces between TM cells and ECM fibers filled with a ground substance rich in the glycosaminoglycan hyaluronic acid [6].

Collagen type I and hyaluronic acid are widely used in biomedical applications and photo-crosslinkable polymers are commercially available. Native elastin is insoluble, preventing its direct use in biomaterials [7]. Therefore, different types of soluble elastin-like polypeptides have been engineered [8]. Of particular interest is a version that contains an elastic core sequence flanked by a short peptide to render it photo-crosslinkable [9]. To fabricate ECM hydrogels simulating the JCT-TM region, human TM cells are mixed with the functionalized precursors and photoinitiator, followed by photo-crosslinking using conditions optimized to maintain high cell viability. Our well-defined soft tissue-mimetic ECM hydrogel [10–16] overcomes critical limitations of previous TM models made from either undefined or overly simplistic biopolymers [17–19] that do not properly address the natural ECM composition and three-dimensional tissue architecture.

2 Materials

1. Methacrylate-conjugated bovine collagen type I (PhotoCol®, Fig. 1a): Add 16.7 mL of sterile 20 mM acetic acid to the lyophilized methacrylated collagen to achieve a concentration of 6 mg/mL (*see* **Note 1**). Transfer the vial to a shaker table or rotator plate and mix at 4 °C overnight to fully solubilize. After solubilization, the collagen solution is stable for 2 months when stored at 4 °C (*see* **Note 2**). The sterile neutralization buffer (i.e., alkaline 10X phosphate buffered saline) will be required immediately prior to use (*see* Subheading 3.1).
2. Thiol-conjugated hyaluronic acid (Glycosil®, Fig. 1b): Using a syringe and needle, add 1.0 mL of sterile reconstitution buffer (i.e., 1X phosphate-buffered saline) to the lyophilized thiolated hyaluronic acid to achieve a concentration of 10 mg/mL at a pH of ~7.4. Briefly vortex and transfer the vial to a cell culture incubator at 37 °C for ~45 min to fully solubilize. The

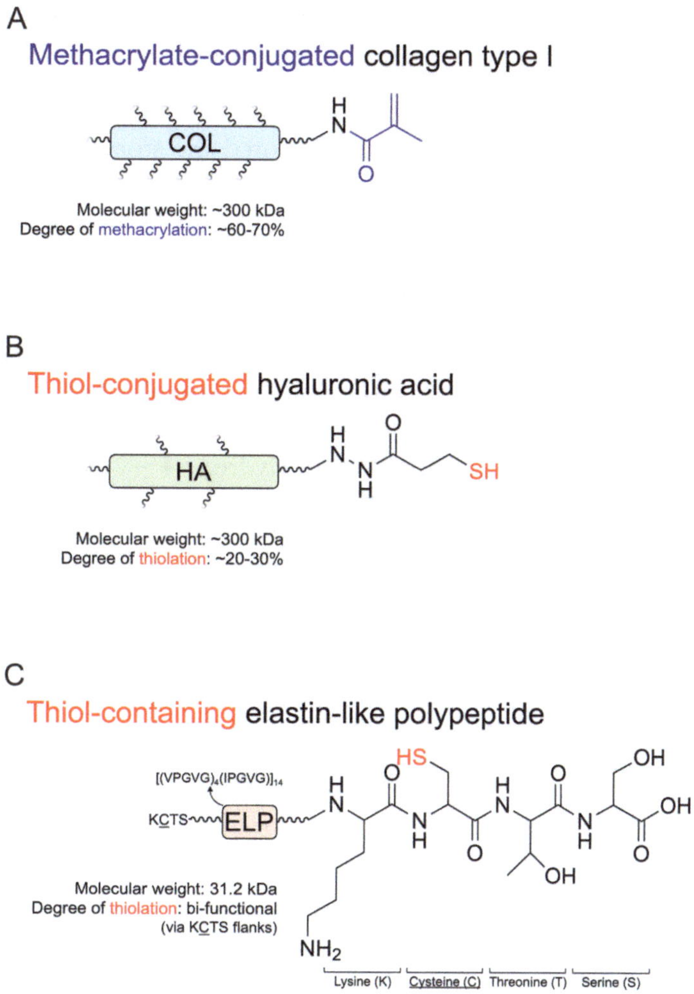

Fig. 1 ECM hydrogel precursors. Schematic of (**a**) methacrylate-conjugated collagen type I, (**b**) thiol-conjugated hyaluronic acid, and (**c**) thiol-containing elastin-like polypeptide (thiol via KCTS flanks). The photoactive polymers can form chemical crosslinks via methacrylate, thiol-ester, or disulfide linkages

hyaluronic acid solution should be used fresh/same day and not be frozen (*see* **Note 3**).

3. Thiol-containing elastin-like polypeptide (Fig. 1c): It consists of 70 repeats of the pentapeptide VPGVG, in which the first valine is replaced with isoleucine in every fifth pentapeptide (i.e., ([VPGVG]4[IPGVG])14), flanked by KCTS residues to render the elastin-like polypeptide photo-crosslinkable (original design and expression/purification details described in Ref. [9]; modified expression and purification details described in Ref. [10]; *see* **Note 4**). Add appropriate volume of chilled sterile 1X phosphate-buffered saline to the lyophilized elastin-like polypeptide to achieve a concentration of 10 mg/mL at a

pH of ~7.4 (*see* **Note 5**). Transfer the 50 mL tube to a shaker table or rotator plate and mix at 4 °C overnight to fully solubilize. Sterilize using a 0.2 μm syringe filter in the cold (*see* **Note 6**). The elastin-like polypeptide solution is stable for 2 months when aliquoted and stored at 4 °C (*see* **Note 7**).

4. LAP (lithium phenyl-2,4,6-trimethylbenzoylphosphinate) photoinitiator: Add 5 mL of sterile TM cell growth media (Dulbecco's Modified Eagle's Medium) containing 10% fetal bovine serum and 1% penicillin/streptomycin/glutamine to the lyophilized photoinitiator to achieve a concentration of 2.0% (w/v) or 20 mg/mL. Vortex to fully solubilize. The LAP photoinitiator solution (wrapped in aluminum foil) is stable for 2 weeks when stored protected from light at 4 °C.
5. IRG (2-Hydroxy-4′-(2-hydroxyethoxy)-2-methylpropiophenone) photoinitiator: Add 20 mL of sterile TM cell growth media to the lyophilized photoinitiator to achieve a concentration of 0.5% (w/v) or 5 mg/mL (*see* **Note 8**). Vortex and transfer the vial (wrapped in aluminum foil) to a cell culture incubator at 37 °C for ~45–60 min to fully solubilize (periodically remove and vortex). The IRG photoinitiator solution is stable for 2 weeks when stored protected from light at 4 °C.
6. Thoroughly characterized [20] primary human TM cells.
7. Trypsinization solution: 0.25% trypsin/EDTA.
8. Aluminum foil.
9. UV/Vis spot curing lamp with calibrated radiometer.
10. Polydimethylsiloxane (Sylgard 184)-coated 24-well culture plates.
11. SurfaSil-coated 18 × 18-mm square glass coverslips.

3 Methods

The following protocol describes the fabrication of soft tissue-mimetic ECM hydrogels (elastic modulus: ~0.3 kPa) in two principal configurations (droplets on 24 well-plates and thin films on glass coverslips) [10–15] according to a specific formulation using two different types of photoinitiators with tailored photo-cross-linking protocols (Table 1). This formulation is used to calculate the volumes required for each polymer precursor for any given experiment. It is recommended to always calculate for ~20% extra volume to account for unavoidable losses in pipette tips due to the viscosity of the polymer solutions.

Table 1
ECM hydrogel formulation and photo-crosslinking conditions

Collagen neutralization				
	Stock concentration (mg/mL)	**Volume (μL)**		
Methacrylate-conjugated collagen type I (stock from vial; 6 mg/mL)	6.0	1000		
Neutralization buffer		85		
*Methacrylate-conjugated collagen type I (adjusted stock; 5 5 mg/mL)	5.5	*1085*	*SUM*	
Hydrogel preparation (LAP)				
	Stock concentration (mg/mL)	**Volume part**	**Ratio**	**Final concentration (mg/mL)**
*Methacrylate-conjugated collagen type I (adjusted stock)	5.5	13	0.65	3.6
Thiol-containing elastin-like polypeptide	10	5	0.25	2.5
Thiol-conjugated hyaluronic acid	10	1	0.05	0.5
Photoinitiator media +/– TM cells	*(2.0% LAP)*	1	0.05	*(0.1% LAP)*
Photo-cross linking conditions (LAP) 320 mW/cm^2; 10 s @405 nm (blue light)				
Hydrogel preparation (IRG)				
	Stock concentration (mg/mL)	**Volume part**	**Ratio**	**Final concentration (mg/mL)**
*Methacrylate-conjugated collagen type I (adjusted stock)	5.5	13	0.65	3.6
Thiol-containing elastin-like polypeptide	10	5	0.25	2.5
Thiol-conjugated hyaluronic acid	10	1	0.05	0.5
Photoinitiator media +/– TM cells	*(0.5% IRG)*	1	0.05	*(0.025% IRG)*
Photo-crosslinking conditions (IRG) 2.2 W/cm^2; 5 s @320–500 nm (UV light)				

3.1 Hydrogel Mixing

1. Remove the desired volume of the thiol-conjugated hyaluronic acid solution from the vial (1/20th volume part, Table 1), and transfer to a sterile sample tube on ice (wrapped in aluminum foil).
2. Remove the desired volume of the thiol-containing elastin-like polypeptide solution from the 50 mL tube (5/20th volume part, Table 1) and transfer to the sample tube on ice containing the hyaluronic acid.

3. Trypsinize (0.25% trypsin/EDTA) a suitable flask of human TM cells (passage 2–6, at ~80% confluence) and count the cells (*see* **Note 9**). Transfer the calculated volume of cell suspension for a final concentration of TM cells in the hydrogel mixture of 1.0×10^6 cells/mL to a 15 mL (or 50 mL) tube, and pellet the cells by centrifugation (1000× *g*, 5–10 min). Reconstitute the TM cell pellet in the calculated volume of photoinitiator (LAP or IRG)-containing TM cell growth media (20×10^6 cells/mL; 1/20th volume part, Table 1), and transfer to the sample tube on ice containing the hyaluronic acid and elastin-like polypeptide.
4. To prepare the working stock of methacrylate-conjugated bovine collagen type I, remove the desired volume of the collagen solution from the vial and transfer to a sterile tube on ice (wrapped in aluminum foil). To achieve a pH of ~7.4, add 85 μLof chilled neutralization buffer (i.e., alkaline 10X phosphate-buffered saline) per 1.0 mL of collagen, mix thoroughly by pipetting, and keep on ice (*see* **Note 10**). Remove the desired volume of neutralized methacrylate-conjugated bovine collagen type I solution (13/20th volume part, Table 1), and transfer to the sample tube on ice containing the hyaluronic acid, elastin-like polypeptide, photoinitiator, and TM cells.
5. Thoroughly yet carefully (avoid air bubbles) mix the final hydrogel-cell suspension in the sample tube by pipetting and keep on ice.

3.2 UV Spot Curing System Calibration

1. To ensure a repeatable photo-crosslinking process, measure and calibrate the light output from the UV/Vis spot curing lamp before each use with a calibrated radiometer.
2. The light intensity (in mW/cm^2 or W/cm^2) is a function of the absolute power output at the tip of the light guide (in mW or W) and its distance from the hydrogel sample that determines the surface area (in cm^2) of the light circle.
3. It is important to optimize the photo-crosslinking conditions (i.e., wavelength, light intensity, and exposure time) for each hydrogel and cell type (*see* **Note 11**). In addition, it is recommended that the light guide be mounted in such a way that the emitted light circle covers no more than the surface area of the respective well the hydrogel sample is in to avoid accidental reexposure of samples in adjacent wells of the culture plate.

3.3 Hydrogel Crosslinking: Droplets

1. Pipette 10 μL of the hydrogel-cell suspension into one well of a polydimethylsiloxane (Sylgard 184)-coated 24-well culture plate. Immediately return the sample tube on ice. The hydrophobized well surface facilitates stable droplet formation for a defined dome-shaped hydrogel construct.

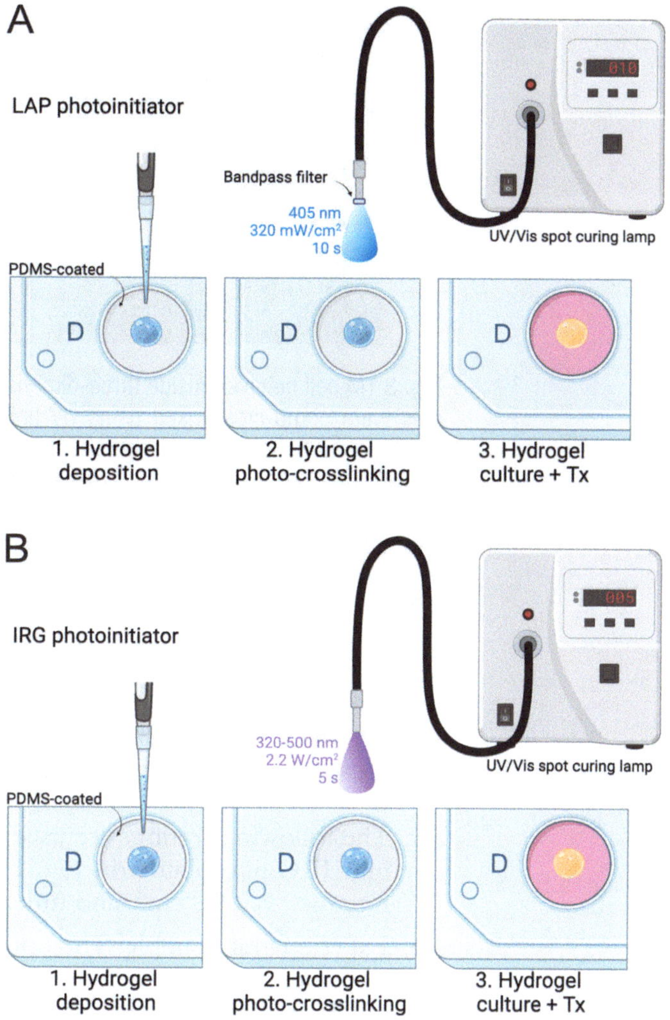

Fig. 2 Schematic of ECM hydrogel droplet formation. Ten μL of the TM cell-containing hydrogel precursor solution are plated on PDMS-coated 24-well plates. Hydrogels are photo-crosslinked using (**a**) blue light (LAP photoinitiator, 405 nm bandpass filter, 320 mW/cm^2, 10 s) or (**b**) UV light (IRG photoinitiator, 320–500 nm, 2.2 W/cm^2, 5 s) and cultured in TM cell growth media in absence/presence of any treatments. (Created with BioRender.com)

2. Position the 24-well plate under the UV/Vis spot curing lamp with the hydrogel-containing well directly underneath the mounted light guide.
3. Wearing UV safety goggles, activate the UV/Vis spot curing lamp to photo-crosslink the TM cell-encapsulated ECM hydrogel (*see* **Note 12**).
4. The following settings are used for blue light photo-crosslinking (LAP photoinitiator, Fig. 2a): wavelength, 405 nm using a bandpass filter attached to the light guide; intensity, 320 mW/cm^2; and time, 10 s.

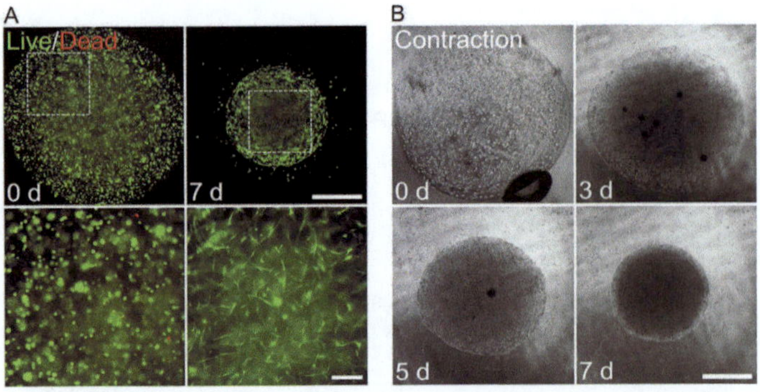

Fig. 3 TM cell behavior inside three-dimensional ECM hydrogel droplets. Hydrogels were photo-crosslinked using UV light (IRG photoinitiator, 320–500 nm, 2.2 W/cm^2, 5 s). (**a**) Representative fluorescence micrographs of TM cell-encapsulated ECM hydrogels at 0 day (i.e., immediately after photo-crosslinking) showing negligeable cytotoxicity (~90% live cells) from UV light exposure, and after 7 days cultured in TM cell growth media showing prominent cell spreading in the three-dimensional hydrogel network. Hydrogels were stained using a LIVE/DEAD™ Viability/Cytotoxicity Kit (Invitrogen; Thermo Fisher Scientific; live cells = green; dead cells = red). Scale bars, 1 mm (top) and 250 μm (bottom). (**b**) Representative brightfield images of TM cell-encapsulated ECM hydrogels at 0 days, 3 days, 5 days, and 7 days. Hydrogels significantly contracted over time, reaching ~40% of their original size by 7 days. Scale bar, 1 mm. (Images reproduced from Ref. [10] with permission from Elsevier)

5. The following settings are used for UV light photo-crosslinking (IRG photoinitiator, Fig. 2b): wavelength, 320–500 nm; intensity, 2.2 W/cm^2; and time, 5 s.
6. Experimental example: The optimized UV crosslinking conditions were shown to be cytocompatible [10]. High cell viability of ~90% was observed immediately after photo-crosslinking (i.e., 0 day) (Fig. 3a). The ECM hydrogel was found to provide a supportive three-dimensional environment with prominent cell spreading observed after a 7-day culture in TM cell growth media (Fig. 3a). Longitudinal contractility analyses showed significant hydrogel contraction over time, reaching ~40% of their original size by 7 days (Fig. 3b).

3.4 Hydrogel Crosslinking: Thin Films

1. Pipette 30 μL of the hydrogel-cell suspension onto SurfaSil-coated 18 × 18 mm square glass coverslips followed by placing 12 mm round glass coverslips onto the hydrogels to facilitate even spreading of the polymer solution. Immediately return the sample tube on ice. The hydrophobized square coverslip surface facilitates easy removal of the hydrogel-adhered round glass coverslip.
2. Position the coverslip-hydrogel-coverslip "sandwich" directly underneath the mounted UV/Vis spot curing lamp light guide.

3. Wearing UV safety goggles, activate the UV/Vis spot curing lamp to photo-crosslink the TM cell-encapsulated ECM hydrogel (*see* **Note 12**) using the same conditions for blue light (LAP photoinitiator, Fig. 4a) or UV light (IRG photoinitiator, Fig. 4b) photo-crosslinking as described in Subheading. 3.3.
4. Experimental example: To assess TM cell pathobiology in a soft tissue-mimetic three-dimensional microenvironment in absence of any biochemical stimuli, glaucomatous TM cells derived from a patient with a documented history of primary open-angle glaucoma (kindly provided by Dr. Kate Keller at the Oregon Health and Sciences University; characterized in Ref. [21]) were encapsulated and directly compared to healthy normal TM cells (best possible age match, characterized in Ref. [13]). Confocal microscopy analyses showed that glaucomatous TM cells retain an inherent pathological cellular phenotype that mirrors key features of the diseased tissue. Glaucomatous TM cells displayed qualitatively more abundant and more disorganized or "tangled" filamentous-actin stress fibers in the three-dimensional hydrogel compared to normal TM cells (Fig. 5).

4 Notes

1. Consult the manufacturer's instructions for the appropriate volume of 20 mM acetic acid to be added to the lyophilized methacrylate-conjugated bovine collagen type I if a stock concentration other than 6.0 mg/mL is desired.
2. We find that the methacrylate-conjugated bovine collagen type I solution is stable for up to 4 months when stored at 4 °C.
3. We find that the thiol-conjugated hyaluronic acid solution can be aliquoted in 1.5 mL tubes, parafilm-wrapped to limit oxygen exposure, and stored frozen at −20 °C for up to 3 months.
4. The glycerol stock of transformed (thiol-containing elastin-like polypeptide plasmid construct) Tuner (DE3) competent cells can be obtained from the corresponding author upon request.
5. The thiol-containing elastin-like polypeptide precipitates at high temperatures and solubilizes at low temperatures, with a thermal transition temperature of 29 °C for a 1% (w/v) solution [9]. Therefore, the thiol-containing elastin-like polypeptide solution must be always kept on ice to avoid undesired coagulation.
6. In lieu of sterile filtration, the lyophilized thiol-containing elastin-like polypeptide can be UV sterilized in the biosafety cabinet for 20 min before solubilization.

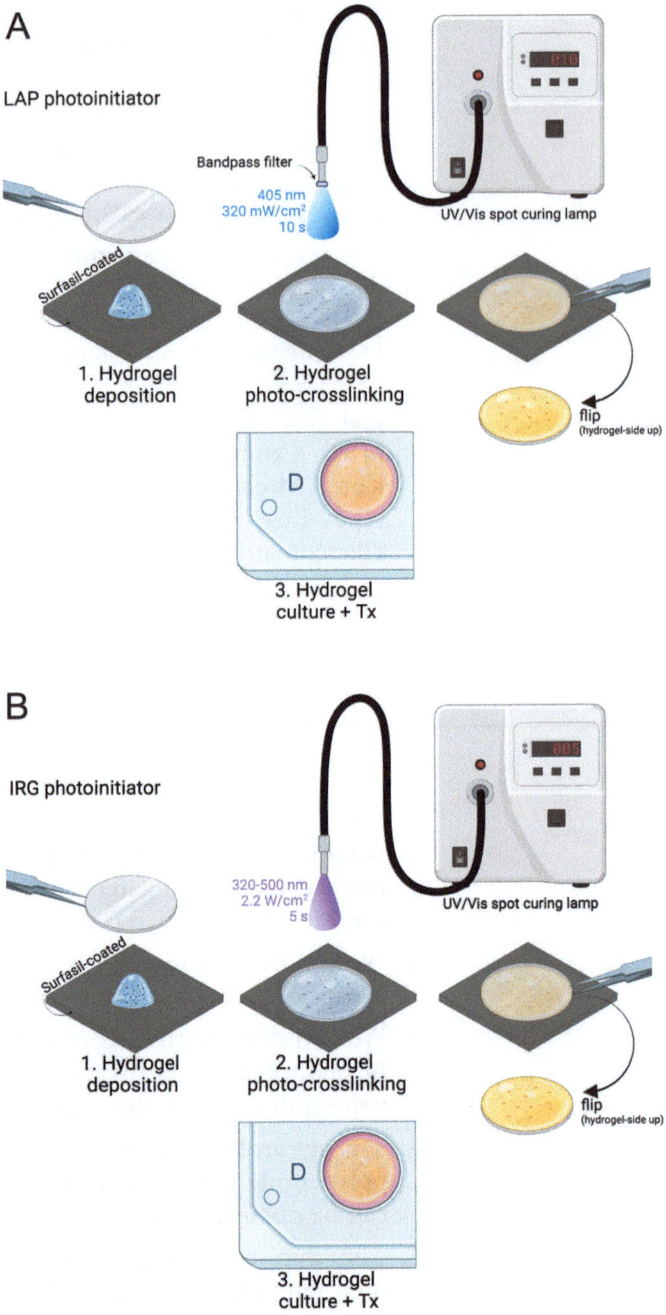

Fig. 4 Schematic of ECM hydrogel thin film formation. Thirty μL of the TM cell-containing hydrogel precursor solution are plated on Surfasil-coated 18 × 18 mm square coverslips followed by placing regular 12 mm round coverslips atop. Hydrogels are photo-crosslinked using (**a**) blue light (LAP photoinitiator, 405 nm bandpass filter, 320 mW/cm^2, 10 s) or (**b**) UV light (IRG photoinitiator, 320–500 nm, 2.2 W/cm^2, 5 s) and cultured (hydrogel-side facing up) in TM cell growth media in absence/presence of any treatments. (Created with BioRender.com)

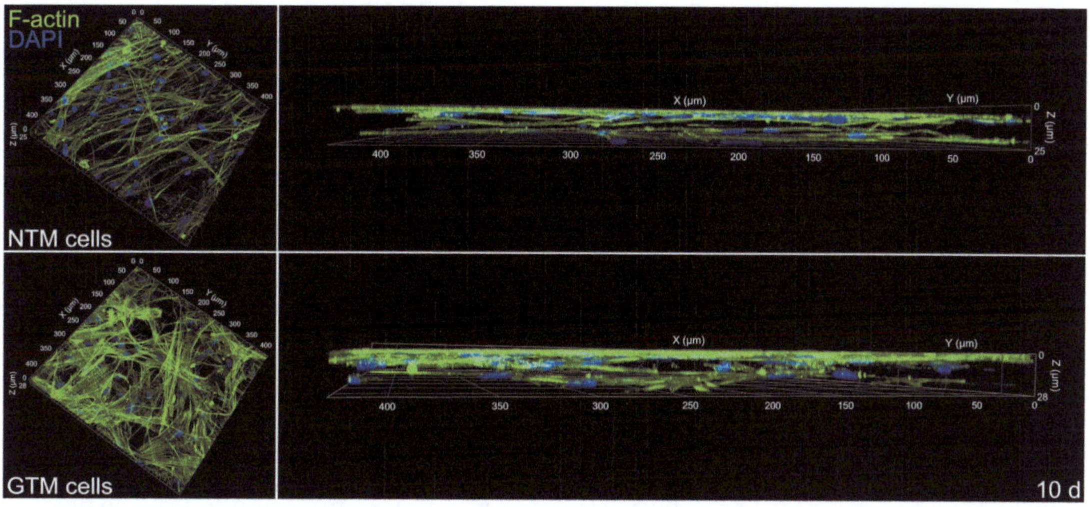

Fig. 5 TM cell behavior inside three-dimensional ECM thin film hydrogels. Hydrogels were photo-crosslinked using blue light (LAP photoinitiator, 405 nm, 320 mW/cm^2, 10 s). (**a**) Representative confocal fluorescence micrographs (Zeiss LSM 780 (Zeiss, Germany); resolution: 2.4089 pixels per μm; voxel size: 0.4151 × 0.4151 × 0.8159 μm^3) of normal TM (NTM; ID: HTM36; female, 56 years of age; characterized in Ref. [13]) or glaucomatous TM (GTM; ID: GTM 2018–1672; male, 57 years of age; characterized in Ref. [20]) cell-encapsulated ECM hydrogels at 10 days showing qualitatively more intense/thicker Phalloidin 488-stained (Abcam, Waltham, MA, USA) filamentous (F)-actin stress fibers (DAPI = nuclear stain) in glaucomatous TM cells with a greater degree of disorganization inside the three-dimensional hydrogel compared to normal TM cells

7. We find that the thiol-containing elastin-like polypeptide solution is stable for up to 6 months when stored at 4 °C.
8. In lieu of reconstituting at a low concentration of 0.5% (w/v) or 5 mg/mL in growth media, the IRG photoinitiator can be solubilized at a high concentration in neat methanol at 10% (w/v) or 100 mg/mL according to the manufacturer's instructions.
9. Ensure that the laboratory is compliant with all institutional biosafety requirements when working with primary human tissues and cells.
10. Consult the manufacturer's instructions for the appropriate volume of neutralization buffer to be added to the reconstituted methacrylate-conjugated bovine collagen type I solution if a stock concentration other than 6.0 mg/mL is used.
11. The photo-crosslinking conditions directly affect TM cell viability and ECM hydrogel stiffness. Higher light intensity and/or longer exposure time can cause increased cell death (undesired) and increased ECM stiffness (potentially undesired). Therefore, careful optimization of the photo-crosslinking conditions is required if changes are desired.

12. We find that activating the UV/Vis spot curing system with the foot pedal switch is more efficient, especially when running larger experiments, than using the start/stop button on the lamp body to open the shutter.

Acknowledgments

This work was supported by National Institutes of Health grants K08EY031755 (to P.S.G.), R01EY034096 and R21EY036189 (to S.H.), American Glaucoma Society Young Clinician Scientist Award (to P.S.G.), BrightFocus Foundation National Glaucoma Research Award G2024006S (to S.H.), a Syracuse University BioInspired Pilot Grant (to S.H.), unrestricted grants to the SUNY Upstate Medical University Department of Ophthalmology and Visual Sciences from Research to Prevent Blindness (RPB) and from Lions Region 20-Y1, and RPB Career Development Awards (to P.S.G. and S.H.).

References

1. Baker BM, Chen CS (2012) Deconstructing the third dimension: how 3D culture microenvironments alter cellular cues. J Cell Sci 125 (Pt 13):3015–3024. https://doi.org/10.1242/jcs.079509
2. Wang K, Read AT, Sulchek T, Ethier CR (2017) Trabecular meshwork stiffness in glaucoma. Exp Eye Res 158:3–12. https://doi.org/10.1016/j.exer.2016.07.011
3. Caliari SR, Burdick JA (2016) A practical guide to hydrogels for cell culture. Nat Methods 13(5):405–414. https://doi.org/10.1038/nmeth.3839
4. Zhang YS, Khademhosseini A (2017) Advances in engineering hydrogels. Science 356(6337): eaaf3627. https://doi.org/10.1126/science.aaf3627
5. Abu-Hassan DW, Acott TS, Kelley MJ (2014) The trabecular meshwork: a basic review of form and function. J Ocul Biol 2(1):9
6. Keller KE, Acott TS (2013) The juxtacanalicular region of ocular trabecular meshwork: a tissue with a unique extracellular matrix and specialized function. J Ocul Biol 1(1):3
7. Mithieux SM, Weiss AS (2005) Elastin. Adv Protein Chem 70:437–461. https://doi.org/10.1016/S0065-3233(05)70013-9
8. Nettles DL, Chilkoti A, Setton LA (2010) Applications of elastin-like polypeptides in tissue engineering. Adv Drug Deliv Rev 62(15): 1479–1485. https://doi.org/10.1016/j.addr.2010.04.002
9. Zhang YN, Avery RK, Vallmajo-Martin Q, Assmann A, Vegh A, Memic A, Olsen BD, Annabi N, Khademhosseini A (2015) A highly elastic and rapidly crosslinkable elastin-like polypeptide-based hydrogel for biomedical applications. Adv Funct Mater 25(30): 4814–4826. https://doi.org/10.1002/adfm.201501489
10. Li H, Bague T, Kirschner A, Strat AN, Roberts H, Weisenthal RW, Patteson AE, Annabi N, Stamer WD, Ganapathy PS, Herberg S (2021) A tissue-engineered human trabecular meshwork hydrogel for advanced glaucoma disease modeling. Exp Eye Res 205: 108472. https://doi.org/10.1016/j.exer.2021.108472
11. Li H, Raghunathan V, Stamer WD, Ganapathy PS, Herberg S (2022) Extracellular matrix stiffness and TGFbeta2 regulate YAP/TAZ activity in human trabecular meshwork cells. Front Cell Dev Biol 10:844342. https://doi.org/10.3389/fcell.2022.844342
12. Li H, Henty-Ridilla JL, Bernstein AM, Ganapathy PS, Herberg S (2022) TGFbeta2 regulates human trabecular meshwork cell contractility via ERK and ROCK pathways with distinct signaling crosstalk dependent on the culture substrate. Curr Eye Res 47:1–41. https://doi.org/10.1080/02713683.2022.2071943
13. Bagué T, Singh A, Ghosh R, Yoo H, Kelly C, deLong MA, Kopczynski CC, Herberg S

(2022) Effects of netarsudil-family rho kinase inhibitors on human trabecular meshwork cell contractility and actin remodeling using a bioengineered ECM hydrogel. Front Ophthalmol 2:948397. https://doi.org/10.3389/fopht.2022.948397

14. Yoo H, Singh A, Li H, Strat AN, Bague T, Ganapathy PS, Herberg S (2023) Simvastatin attenuates glucocorticoid-induced human trabecular meshwork cell dysfunction via YAP/-TAZ inactivation. Curr Eye Res 48(8): 736–749. https://doi.org/10.1080/02713683.2023.2206067

15. Li H, Singh A, Perkumas KM, Stamer WD, Ganapathy PS, Herberg S (2022) YAP/TAZ mediate TGFβ2-induced Schlemm's canal cell dysfunction. Invest Ophthalmol Vis Sci 63(12):15. https://doi.org/10.1167/iovs.63.12.15

16. Li H, Kuhn M, Kelly RA, Singh A, Palanivel KK, Salama I, De Ieso ML, Stamer WD, Ganapathy PS, Herberg S (2024) Targeting YAP/TAZ mechanosignaling to ameliorate stiffness-induced Schlemm's canal cell pathobiology, Am J Physiol Cell Physiol 326(2): C513–C528

17. Bouchemi M, Roubeix C, Kessal K, Riancho L, Raveu AL, Soualmia H, Baudouin C, Brignole-Baudouin F (2017) Effect of benzalkonium chloride on trabecular meshwork cells in a new in vitro 3D trabecular meshwork model for glaucoma. Toxicol In Vitro 41:21–29. https://doi.org/10.1016/j.tiv.2017.02.006

18. Waduthanthri KD, He Y, Montemagno C, Cetinel S (2019) An injectable peptide hydrogel for reconstruction of the human trabecular meshwork. Acta Biomater 100:244–254. https://doi.org/10.1016/j.actbio.2019.09.032

19. Saccà SC, Tirendi S, Scarfì S, Passalacqua M, Oddone F, Traverso CE, Vernazza S, Bassi AM (2020) An advanced in vitro model to assess glaucoma onset. ALTEX – Alternatives to Animal Experimentation 37(2):265–274. https://doi.org/10.14573/altex.1909262

20. Keller KE, Bhattacharya SK, Borras T, Brunner TM, Chansangpetch S, Clark AF, Dismuke WM, Du Y, Elliott MH, Ethier CR, Faralli JA, Freddo TF, Fuchshofer R, Giovingo M, Gong H, Gonzalez P, Huang A, Johnstone MA, Kaufman PL, Kelley MJ, Knepper PA, Kopczynski CC, Kuchtey JG, Kuchtey RW, Kuehn MH, Lieberman RL, Lin SC, Liton P, Liu Y, Lutjen-Drecoll E, Mao W, Masis-Solano M, McDonnell F, McDowell CM, Overby DR, Pattabiraman PP, Raghunathan VK, Rao PV, Rhee DJ, Chowdhury UR, Russell P, Samples JR, Schwartz D, Stubbs EB, Tamm ER, Tan JC, Toris CB, Torrejon KY, Vranka JA, Wirtz MK, Yorio T, Zhang J, Zode GS, Fautsch MP, Peters DM, Acott TS, Stamer WD (2018) Consensus recommendations for trabecular meshwork cell isolation, characterization and culture. Exp Eye Res 171:164–173. https://doi.org/10.1016/j.exer.2018.03.001

21. Sun YY, Bradley JM, Keller KE (2019) Phenotypic and functional alterations in tunneling nanotubes formed by glaucomatous trabecular meshwork cells. Invest Ophthalmol Vis Sci 60(14):4583–4595. https://doi.org/10.1167/iovs.19-28084

Chapter 3

Protocol for the Extraction and Characterization of Trabecular Meshwork Cell Cytoskeleton Fraction

Rupalatha Maddala and P. Vasantha Rao

Abstract

Among various cellular attributes modulating aqueous humor (AH) outflow through the trabecular pathway and eventually intraocular pressure, the involvement of actomyosin regulated cellular contraction and relaxation, cell-extracellular matrix adhesion and cell-cell junctions, and mechanotransduction are well recognized. Although various biological and pharmacological agent-modulated AH outflows were associated with altered actin cytoskeletal organization and cell adhesive interactions of trabecular meshwork (TM) cells, these changes were analyzed largely with a biased approach to examine the specific proteins, but there were very few efforts in examining them with hypothesis-free unbiased approach in their native state. Therefore, in this chapter, we describe a protocol tailored to characterize the cytoskeleton of TM cells. This simple protocol can be applied to identifying the differentially regulated TM cell cytoskeleton proteins under any given treatment condition in conjunction with quantitative proteomic analysis.

Key words Trabecular meshwork, Cytoskeleton, Aqueous humor, Glaucoma, Intraocular pressure

1 Introduction

Elevated intraocular pressure (IOP) due to impaired aqueous humor (AH) drainage through the trabecular pathway is a major and modifiable risk factor for glaucoma (optic nerve atrophy), a leading cause of irreversible blindness worldwide [1]. In humans, AH drainage through the trabecular pathway consisting of trabecular meshwork (TM), juxtacanalicular tissue, and Schlemm's canal accounts for more than 80% of total AH outflow, and blockage in this pathway is the primary cause for elevated IOP in glaucoma patients [2]. Although elevated IOP is multifactorial, and dysregulation of various cellular processes account for the increased resistance to AH outflow through the trabecular pathway, changes in TM tissue contractile characteristics, cell adhesive interactions, barrier activity, phagocytic activity, and material properties are well recognized to influence AH outflow and eventually IOP [3].

Tatjana Jakobs and Paloma B. Liton (eds.), *Glaucoma: Methods and Protocols*, Methods in Molecular Biology, vol. 2858,
https://doi.org/10.1007/978-1-0716-4140-8_3,

Importantly, lowering of elevated IOP is the mainstay of treatment for glaucoma, and various biological and pharmacological agents modulating cell morphology, actomyosin cytoskeletal organization, cell adhesive interactions, and permeability of trabecular meshwork cells are demonstrated to influence AH outflow and IOP [3]. However, our understanding of the regulation of actomyosin organization, actin cytoskeletal dynamics, cell-ECM adhesion, and cell-cell interactions of TM cells is limited, and we have a scanty knowledge on the cellular and molecular basis for the changes in these cellular attributes in TM cells of glaucoma [3]. Especially the cytoskeleton is insoluble and its extraction in its native state is a challenging task, thus currently the cytoskeleton characteristics of TM are poorly understood. Therefore, it is imperative to use improved methods and determine the cytoskeletal and cell adhesive changes in both normal, glaucoma, and drug-treated TM cells to better understand their role in AH outflow and IOP and to develop efficacious IOP-lowering agents to treat glaucoma.

For example, there were several studies reporting the cytoskeletal changes induced by glucocorticoids (e.g., dexamethasone), TGF-β2, and extracellular matrix in TM cells and their association with increased resistance to AH outflow through the TM; however, in most of these studies, there was a lack of effort on a comprehensive and unbiased approach to identify various dysregulated cytoskeletal and cytoskeletal-associated proteins [3]. Recently, we extracted the cytoskeleton fraction of human TM cells in its native state using a protocol originally described for the extraction and characterization of mouse embryonic fibroblasts by Choi et al. [4] and characterized this fraction further by LC/MS/MS proteomic analysis. Moreover, we have performed a label-free quantification to identify various proteins whose levels were altered under dexamethasone treatment in TM cells [5]. This hypothesis-free and unbiased approach helped us to identify the specific proteins involved in actin network crosslinking, formation of actin stress fibers, and actin bundling in TM cells under Dex treatment [5].

Therefore, in this chapter, we describe the reproducible protocol that we used to isolate and characterize the changes in the TM cell cytoskeleton profile which can be used readily.

2 Materials

2.1 Cell Culture

1. Human trabecular meshwork cells (HTM) isolated from the corneal rims or human cadaver eyes.
2. Culture medium: DMEM (Dulbecco's Modified Eagle Medium) low glucose media supplemented with 10% heat-inactivated fetal bovine serum (FBS), penicillin-streptomycin

(100 U and 100 μg/500 mL media, respectively), and glutamine (4 mM).

3. Trypsin-EDTA (0.25%) and phenol red.
4. Cell culture plates (100 mm, tissue culture-treated surface).
5. Cell lifter.
6. Inverted cell culture microscope.
7. Cell culture incubator, humidified with 5% CO_2.

2.2 Cell Treatments

1. Dexamethasone (Dex): 500 mM in ethyl alcohol.
2. Ethyl alcohol, pure.

2.3 Cytoskeleton Extraction

1. Phosphate-buffered saline (1X PBS).
2. Cell lysis buffer: 50 mM Pipes (piperazine-N, N′-bis), 50 mM NaCl, 5% glycerol, 0.1% NP-40, 0.1% Triton X-100, 0.1% Tween20, 5 mM sodium fluoride, 2 mM sodium orthovanadate, protease inhibitors, phosphatase inhibitors, 50 mM Tris–HCl, and pH 7.5.
3. Nuclease buffer: 50 mM Tris–HCl buffer, pH 7.5, 10 mM $MgCl_2$, 2 mM $CaCl_2$, and 10 U/mL Benzonase nuclease.
4. 1% SDS (sodium dodecyl sulfate)
5. Pierce™ BCA Protein Assay Kit or other protein quantification kits.

2.4 Antibodies

1. Antihuman GAPDH.
2. Antihuman α-actinin.

2.5 Reagents for Proteomic Analysis

1. 50 mM ammonium bicarbonate
2. Bovine casein.
3. 20% SDS (sodium dodecyl sulfate)
4. Dithiothreitol (DTT).
5. 20 mM iodoacetamide
6. Phosphoric acid.
7. S-Trap (Protifi) binding buffer: 90% methanol, 100 mM triethyl ammonium bicarbonate buffer (TEAB).
8. S-Trap microcartridge.
9. Sequencing grade trypsin.
10. 50 mM triethyl ammonium bicarbonate buffer (TEAB)
11. Formic acid.
12. Suspension buffer: 1% TriFluoroAcetic acid (TFA), 2% acetonitrile, and 25 fmol/μL of yeast aldehyde dehydrogenase.

2.6 Equipment and Lab Supplies

1. 96-Well Non-Treated Plates Flat Bottom Wells, Polystyrene
2. Microcentrifuge tubes (Protein Low Bind tubes, 0.6 mL).
3. Fisher Vortex genie2.
4. Bench-top centrifuge.
5. Savant Speedvac with refrigerated vapoTrap.
6. Multi-Mode Microplate Reader.
7. Mass tandem mass spectrometer: We used nanoAcquity UPLC system (Waters Corp) coupled with a Thermo Orbitrap Fusion Lumos high-resolution accurate mass tandem mass spectrometer equipped with a FAIMSPro device via a nanoelectrospray ionization source but any other high end mass spectrometry from the institutional core resources would be ideal.

3 Methods

All the reagents are prepared fresh with laboratory grade deionized water.

3.1 Cell Culture Treatment

1. Grow early passage HTM cells to confluence in 10 cm Eppendorf tissue culture-treated plastic dishes. Monitor cell growth and confluence on a daily basis under a cell culture scope (*see* **Note 1**).
2. Treat with 0.5 μM Dex on daily basis for 7 days in the presence of 2% FBS (*see* **Note 2**). Control cells are treated with ethanol (1 μL/mL) also on a daily frequency (*see* **Note 3**).
3. Change culture media on alternate days for both control and Dex-treated cells.

3.2 Cytoskeleton Extraction

1. Rinse cells twice with ice cold 1XPBS.
2. Add 5 mL of freshly prepared ice-cold cell lysis buffer to each plate and incubate for 1.5 min on ice, swirling around.
3. Collect cell lysates into Eppendorf tubes and label them as cytosolic fractions. Keep these fractions on ice until **step 6**.
4. Gently rinse the residual gel in the plates twice with ice-cold 50 mM Tris–HCl buffer (pH 7.5).
5. Add 5 mL of nuclease buffer and incubate the gel at room temperature for 10 min. Make sure the entire gel is covered with the nuclease buffer (*see* **Note 4**).
6. Remove the buffer and add the cytosolic cell lysate collected in **step 3** back to the respective plates.
7. Incubate for an additional 30 sec on ice to release and solubilize both DNA/RNA binding protein. Collect the cell lysates back into the same tube as cytosolic fractions.

8. Gently rinse plates again with ice-cold Tris–HCl buffer three more times.
9. Add 500 μL of 1% SDS and scrape the cytoskeletal fraction remaining on the plates with a cell lifter. Collect fraction into low binding tubes and label as cytoskeletal fractions.
10. Quantify protein concentrations using a Pierce™ BCA kit.
11. Check crosscontamination of cytoskeletal fractions with cytosolic proteins by Western blot/immunoblotting against known cytosolic markers, that is, GAPDH.
12. Confirm cytoskeleton enrichment by immunoprobing for α-actinin antibody. Cytoskeletal fractions devoid of crosscontamination are further processed for proteomic analysis.

3.3 Sample Preparation for Proteomics

1. Dissolve cytoskeletal protein fraction (15 μg) in 50 mM ammonium bicarbonate (100 μL) and spike with undigested bovine casein at a total of either 1 or 2 pmol to serve as an internal quality control standard.
2. Supplement protein fractions with 29.4 μL of 20% SDS. Add 10 mM DTT (final concentration) and reduce for 30 min at 80 °C.
3. Add 20 mM iodoacetamide and let the proteins alkylate for 30 min at room temperature.
4. Supplement samples with a final concentration of 1.2% phosphoric acid and 1004 μL of S-Trap (Protifi) binding buffer.
5. Trap proteins on a S-Trap microcartridge and digest with sequencing grade trypsin (20 ng/μL) for 1 h at 47 °C.
6. Elute protein samples with 20 μL each of 50 mM TEAB, followed by 0.2% formic acid, and finally with 50% acetonitrile (ACN)/0.2% formic acid.
7. Lyophilize eluted protein samples to dryness using Savant Speedvac and resuspend in 30 μL of suspension buffer.
8. For additional quality control purposes, prepare a study pool QC (SPQC) samples by pooling equal amounts of each individual sample into a single sample (three replicate SPQC samples) and run it periodically throughout the total acquisition window.

3.4 LC-MS/MS Analysis

Here, we describe quantitative LC/MS/MS performed on 2 μL of sample, using a nanoAcquity UPLC system coupled with a Thermo Orbitrap Fusion Lumos high-resolution accurate mass tandem mass spectrometer equipped with a FAIMSPro device via a nanoelectrospray ionization source. Similar equipment can be used.

1. Trap 2 µL of each sample on a Symmetry C18 20 mm × 180 µm trapping column (5 µL/min at 99.9/0.1 v/v water/acetonitrile).
2. Perform analytical separation using a 1.8 µm Acquity HSS T3 C18 75 µm × 250 mm column with a 90-min linear gradient of 5–30% acetonitrile with 0.1% formic acid at a flow rate of 400 nanoliters/minute (nL/min) with a column temperature of 55 °C.
3. Collect data for three difference compensation voltages (CV): −40 v, −60 v, and −80 v.
4. Within each CV, perform a data-dependent acquisition (DDA) mode of acquisition with an $r = 120{,}000$ (@ m/z 200) full MS scan from m/z 375–1500 with a target AGC value of 4e5 ions. Acquire MS/MS scans in the linear ion trap in "rapid" mode with a target AGC value of 1e4 and max fill time of 35 milliseconds.

3.5 Quantitative Data Analysis

1. Import data from the UPLC-MS/MS into Proteome Discoverer 2.4.
2. Align each individual LCMS data files based on the accurate mass and retention time of detected precursor ions ("features") using Minora Feature Detector algorithm in Proteome Discoverer.
3. Measure relative peptide abundance based on peak intensities of selected ion chromatograms of the aligned features across all runs.
4. Search the MS/MS data against the SwissProt Homo sapiens database.
5. Use Mascot Distiller and Mascot Server to produce fragment ion spectra and to perform the database searches. Include fixed modification on Cys (carbamidomethyl) and variable modification on Met (oxidation) in the database search parameters.
6. Annotate the data at a maximum 1% protein false discovery rate based on q-value calculations using Peptide Validator and Protein FDR Validator nodes in Proteome Discoverer. Address peptide homology using razor rules in which a peptide matched to multiple different proteins is exclusively assigned to the protein has more identified peptides. Address protein homology by grouping proteins that have the same set of peptides to account for their identification. Assign a master protein within a group based on % coverage.

4 Notes

1. Early cell passages work best for cytoskeletal fraction isolation, as the higher passage cells lose their cell type-specific selective protein expression.
2. Here we have described the experiments with Dex treatments, but any other treatment regimen could be performed either for shorter or longer durations, as long as the cells are healthy and not lifting from the culture dishes.
3. Preferably, treatments were added daily at a fixed time.
4. Nuclease buffer was always prepared fresh with Benzonase, which had optimal enzyme activity and shelf life, and precautions should be taken to make sure the entire gel was covered with the nuclease buffer, to get efficient degradation of all types of DNA and RNA and effectively removing all the nucleic acids from protein samples.

Acknowledgments

We thank Erik J. Soderblom, PhD, from the Proteomics and Metabolomics Shared Resource, Duke University School of Medicine, Duke Center for Genomic and Computational Biology, for his help in mass spectrometry analysis. This work was supported by the National Institutes of Health grants—R01EY018590, R01EY028823, and P30EY005722.

References

1. Weinreb RN, Aung T, Medeiros FA (2014) The pathophysiology and treatment of glaucoma: a review. JAMA 311(18):1901–1911
2. Tamm ER, Braunger BM, Fuchshofer R (2015) Intraocular pressure and the mechanisms involved in resistance of the aqueous humor flow in the trabecular meshwork outflow pathways. Prog Mol Biol Transl Sci 134:301–314
3. Rao PV, Pattabiraman PP, Kopczynski C (2017) Role of the rho GTPase/rho kinase signaling pathway in pathogenesis and treatment of glaucoma: bench to bedside research. Exp Eye Res 158:23–32
4. Choi S, Kelber J, Jiang X, Strnadel J, Fujimura K, Pasillas M et al (2014) Procedures for the biochemical enrichment and proteomic analysis of the cytoskeletome. Anal Biochem 446:102–107
5. Maddala R, Eldawy C, Bachman W, Soderblom EJ, Rao PV (2023) Glypican-4 regulated actin cytoskeletal reorganization in glucocorticoid treated trabecular meshwork cells and involvement of Wnt/PCP signaling. J Cell Physiol 238(3):631–646

Chapter 4

Measurements of Phagocytosis in Trabecular Meshwork Cells

Jennifer A. Faralli, Mark S. Filla, Caleigh Dunn, and Donna M. Peters

Abstract

The restriction in the movement of aqueous humor through the trabecular meshwork is known to play an important role in the pathogenesis of glaucomas. Among the functions of the trabecular meshwork that help to prevent this restriction and maintain the movement of aqueous humor is phagocytosis. Cells in the trabecular meshwork actively phagocytose pigment, cellular debris, and other materials in order to help keep the drainage pathway clear. A decrease in phagocytosis has thus been implicated in the development of glaucomas. In this chapter, we outline two methods using fluorescent markers that can be used to measure the phagocytic properties of trabecular meshwork cells in culture.

Key words Phagocytosis, Trabecular meshwork, Glaucoma, Cell cultures, Immunofluorescence microscopy

1 Introduction

Phagocytosis is the process by which a cell ingests or engulfs apoptotic cells and foreign matter in its microenvironment. Almost all cell types are capable of performing phagocytosis, but only professional phagocytes (macrophages, neutrophils, monocytes, dendritic cells, and osteoclasts) are capable of phagocytosis at a high efficiency. Interestingly, despite the presence of macrophages and monocytes in the trabecular meshwork (TM) of the anterior segment of the human eye [1, 2], phagocytosis in the TM appears to be performed by the TM cells themselves. This phagocytic property of TM cells is thought to play an important role in maintaining intraocular pressure by keeping the outflow pathway free of cellular debris and degraded extracellular matrix proteins that can restrict outflow and cause an elevation in intraocular pressure [3–7]. Hence, phagocytosis plays an essential role in maintaining tissue homeostasis.

Tatjana Jakobs and Paloma B. Liton (eds.), *Glaucoma: Methods and Protocols*, Methods in Molecular Biology, vol. 2858, https://doi.org/10.1007/978-1-0716-4140-8_4,

Among the substances reported to be engulfed by TM cells is autogenous blood present in aqueous humor [1, 8], photocoagulation debris from the iris [9, 10], melanin granules [11], and degradation products of extracellular matrix proteins such as collagens, proteoglycans, etc. [12]. Abnormalities in the phagocytic properties of TM cells are believed to contribute to several different glaucomas, including exfoliation, pigmentary, and glucocorticoid-induced glaucoma.

The phagocytotic properties of TM cells have been measured using a number of different markers including India ink [13], latex beads coated with FITC and antibodies [14–16], zymosan particles [17], pigment [18], and red blood cells [6, 19]. In this chapter, we will describe two methods using fluorescent probes to measure phagocytosis in TM cells in culture [20–24].

2 Materials

1. pHrodo™ fluorescent-conjugated red, *S. aureus* BioParticles™ (2 mg/vial),
2. 10X Hank's balanced salt solution (HBSS) with calcium and magnesium and without phenol red
3. 100 mM HEPES buffer, pH 7.4
4. Phosphate-buffered saline (PBS).
5. Human TM cells (provided by you).
6. Cell culture media: Low-glucose Dulbecco's modified Eagle's medium (DMEM), 15% FBS, 2 mM-glutamine, 1% amphotericin B, 0.05% gentamicin, and 1 ng/mL FGF-2 [25–27].
7. CellMask™ Green plasma membrane stain.
8. Non-CO_2 incubator set at 37 °C.
9. Alexa 488-conjugated *S. aureus* BioParticles™ (Ex/Em 495/519).
10. Opsonizing reagent: Purified rabbit polyclonal antibodies that are specific for *S. aureus*.
11. Secondary anti-rabbit IgG labeled with an Alexa 546 fluorophore.
12. DAPI.
13. Tissue culture CO_2 incubator set at 37 °C and 8 % CO_2.
14. Inverted fluorescent microscope capable of detecting the Alexa 488 fluorophore and Alexa 546 fluorophore or flow cytometer capable of detecting fluorophore (red or green).

3 Methods

3.1 Detection of Phagocytosis Using pHrodo™ Red-Conjugated Staphylococcus aureus BioParticles™ (See Fig. 1)

The pHrodo™ Red dye is nonfluorescent at neutral pH, but it turns bright red upon acidification into the phagosome, thus selectively detecting internalized material. Quantification can be done using a variety of approaches. In this review, we provide instructions on how to use fluorescence-activated cell sorter (FACS) analysis or standard fluorescent microscopy to determine the level of fluorescence in cells challenged with the pHrodo™ red-conjugated *S. aureus* bioparticles. The assay can be easily adapted to a 96-well format and analyzed using a fluorescent microplate reader (*see* **Note 1**).

All procedures with human trabecular meshwork cells should be carried out under sterile conditions in a biological safety cabinet.

3.1.1 Incubation of Trabecular Meshwork Cells with pHrodo™ Bioparticles

1. Plate the TM cells at desired cell density. The final cell density depends on how the level of phagocytosis will be determined. For example, if analysis will be done by FACS, cells can be plated at a nearly confluent density of 5.0×10^5 cells/9.6 cm^2 (6-well plate) to insure enough cells for analysis. For analysis using an upright fluorescent microscope, cells should be plated subconfluently, so individual cells can be identified and counted. For this type of experiment, usually 2.5×10^4 cells/2.0 cm^2 (4-well plate) is enough.
2. Allow cells to attach for at least 4–24 h before starting assay. Cells can be serum starved at this time if desired by placing cells in DMEM containing 0–1% FBS.
3. Add the treatment (siRNA, pharmacological reagents, etc.) to affect phagocytosis taking care to set up appropriate control-treated wells of cells (scrambled siRNA, vehicle buffers, etc.).
4. Make a solution of 1X HBSS, 25 mM HEPES, pH 7.4 containing 1% FBS (*see* **Note 2**).
5. Resuspend a single vial of lyophilized pHrodo™ red-conjugated *S. aureus* BioParticles™ in a sterile solution of 2 mL of HBSS. This will generate a 10X stock solution at 1 mg/mL. The recommended working solution is 100 μg/mL.
6. Vortex or sonicate the solution well in order to get a homogenous dispersion of the pHrodo™ BioParticles™. The manufacturer's recommendation is 10 min in a bath sonicator.
7. Prepare a working solution of the BioParticles™ in 1X HBSS/25 mM HEPES, pH 7.4 buffer containing 1% FBS for the assay (*see* **Note 3**). The manufacturer recommends a 1:10 dilution or 10 μL of BioParticles™ per 100 μL of cell culture medium. However, the optimal dilution may have to be empirically

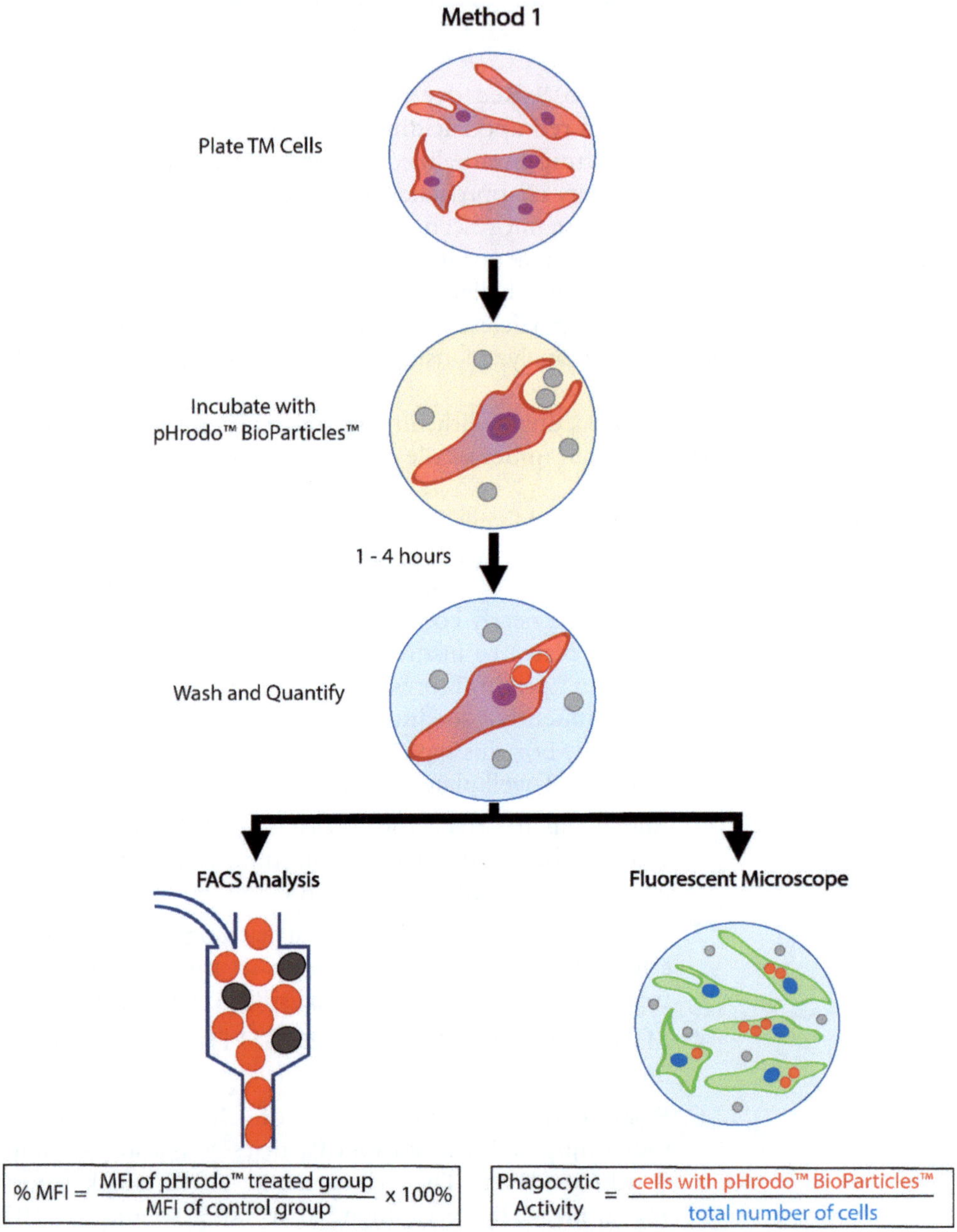

Fig. 1 Schematic showing method 1 to measure phagocytosis. TM cells are plated and incubated with pHrodo™ beads. Cells are washed and phagocytosis is measured using either FACS or an inverted fluorescent microscope. Geometric mean fluorescence intensity (MFI)

determined and, depending on your analysis, it may be necessary to use a 1:5 dilution. Keep the buffer and the BioParticles™ at 37 °C until ready to use.

8. Remove the existing culture medium from the wells and wash the cells well (~2 times) with sterile HBSS prewarmed to 37 °C.

9. Remove the wash buffer and add the pHrodo™ BioParticles™ in the HBSS/HEPES/FBS solution prepared in **step 7** to each well. Add enough buffer to cover the cell monolayer.
10. Incubate the cells with the BioParticles™ for 1–4 h in a bench-top, non-CO_2 incubator at 37 °C in order to maintain the pH of the HBSS/HEPES buffer and then process the cells for analysis (*see* **Note 4**).
11. At the end of the desired incubation period, remove the assay buffer, and wash the cells at least two times with sterile HBSS prewarmed to 37 °C.

3.1.2 Detection and Quantification of Phagocytosis in Cultures Using Fluorescence-Activated Cell Sorter (FACS) Analysis [20]

1. Lift cells from tissue culture dishes using either a nonenzymatic commercial product (Cell Dissociation Solution, Sigma) or 2 mM EDTA in HBSS (*see* **Note 5**).
2. Analyze unfixed cell suspensions with a flow cytometer. The pHrodo™ red dye can be detected using a filter set of 560/585 nm (Ex/Em).
3. Quantification of phagocytosis is then done by comparing the geometric mean fluorescence intensity (MFI) of cells containing pHrodo™-labeled *S. aureus*™ relative to their respective control. Percent MFI is calculated by dividing the MFI of phagocytized pHrodo™-labeled BioParticles™ of the treated group by that of the control group × 100%.

3.1.3 Quantification Using a Standard Upright Fluorescent Microscope [23]

1. To view the live, unfixed cells, cells can be stained with CellMask™ Green diluted 1/1000 in the phagocytosis buffer for 10 min in a non-CO_2 incubator.
2. Wash the cells at least two times with sterile HBSS/25 mM HEPES, pH 7.4 buffer.
3. Place fresh 1X HBSS/25 mM HEPES, pH 7.4 buffer on the cells, and immediately view the unfixed cells under an inverted fluorescence microscope.
4. The CellMask™ green stain can be detected using a standard FITC filter set (522/535 nm) and will last for 60–90 min.
5. The pHrodo™ red dye can be detected using a filter set of 560/585 nm.
6. The phagocytic activity is calculated by determining the ratio of cells containing pHrodo™ labeled BioParticles™ versus total number of cells from three to five separate randomly chosen areas per slide.

The Alexa-488 fluorophore is fluorescent over a pH range from 3 to 10. The fluorescence of BioParticles™ conjugates that are bound to the surface of the cell (but not internalized) therefore need to be quenched in this assay. The probes can be quenched using ethidium bromide or trypan blue [28]. Alternatively, a secondary antibody that binds to the extracellular bioparticles opsonized with rabbit IgG can be used to identify and exclude the unphagocytosed BioParticles™ from the quantification [24]. As in the other method, this fluorescent BioParticles™ product can be used to study phagocytosis using fluorescence microscopy, quantitative spectrofluorometry, or flow cytometry.

3.2 Detection of Phagocytosis Using Alexa 488-Conjugated S. aureus BioParticles™ [24] (See Fig. 2)

1. If using a fluorescent microscope to quantify the assay, it is important that the cells be subconfluent so that individual cells can be visualized and counted.
2. Place sterile 12 mm round glass coverslips into the wells of 24-well dish. Then plate TM cells at a cell density of approximately 25,000 cells/coverslip into each well. We typically cultured our TM cells in low-glucose DMEM containing 15% FBS, 2 mM-glutamine,1% amphotericin B, 0.05% gentamicin, and 1 ng/mL FGF-2 [25–27].
3. Allow the cells to grow for 3–24 h, before adding the BioParticles™.
4. Prior to the start of the assay, reconstitute the Alexa 488-conjugated *S. aureus* BioParticles™ in sterile PBS at a concentration of 20 mg/mL. Gently swirl the BioParticles™ into suspension. Then vortex the solution for ~15 s as recommended by the manufacturer to obtain a homogenous solution. If BioParticles™ are not to be immediately used, sodium azide should be added to the solution at a final concentration of 2 mM.
5. After a homogenous solution of the BioParticles™ is obtained, determine the number of BioParticles™ per mL using a hemocytometer to count the number of particles.
6. Next, reconstitute the vial of opsonizing reagent (rabbit IgG to *S. aureus*) with 0.5 mL of tissue culture grade water as recommended by the manufacturer.
7. Preincubate the Alexa 488-conjugated *S. aureus* BioParticles™ (from heat- or chemically killed *S. aureus*) with an equal volume of the opsonizing reagent at 37 °C for 1 h to conjugate the opsonizing reagent to the BioParticles™. In this case, the opsonizing reagent is purified rabbit IgG antibody that is specific for *S. aureus*.
8. Wash unbound IgG from the bioparticle-IgG complex by centrifuging the solution at low speed (800–1500× *g*) for 15–20 min. Resuspend the BioParticles™-IgG in PBS and repeat the centrifugation 2–3 times with fresh PBS to remove excess unbound antibody.
9. To set up the phagocytosis assay, remove the medium from the plated TM cells, and replace it with serum-free medium

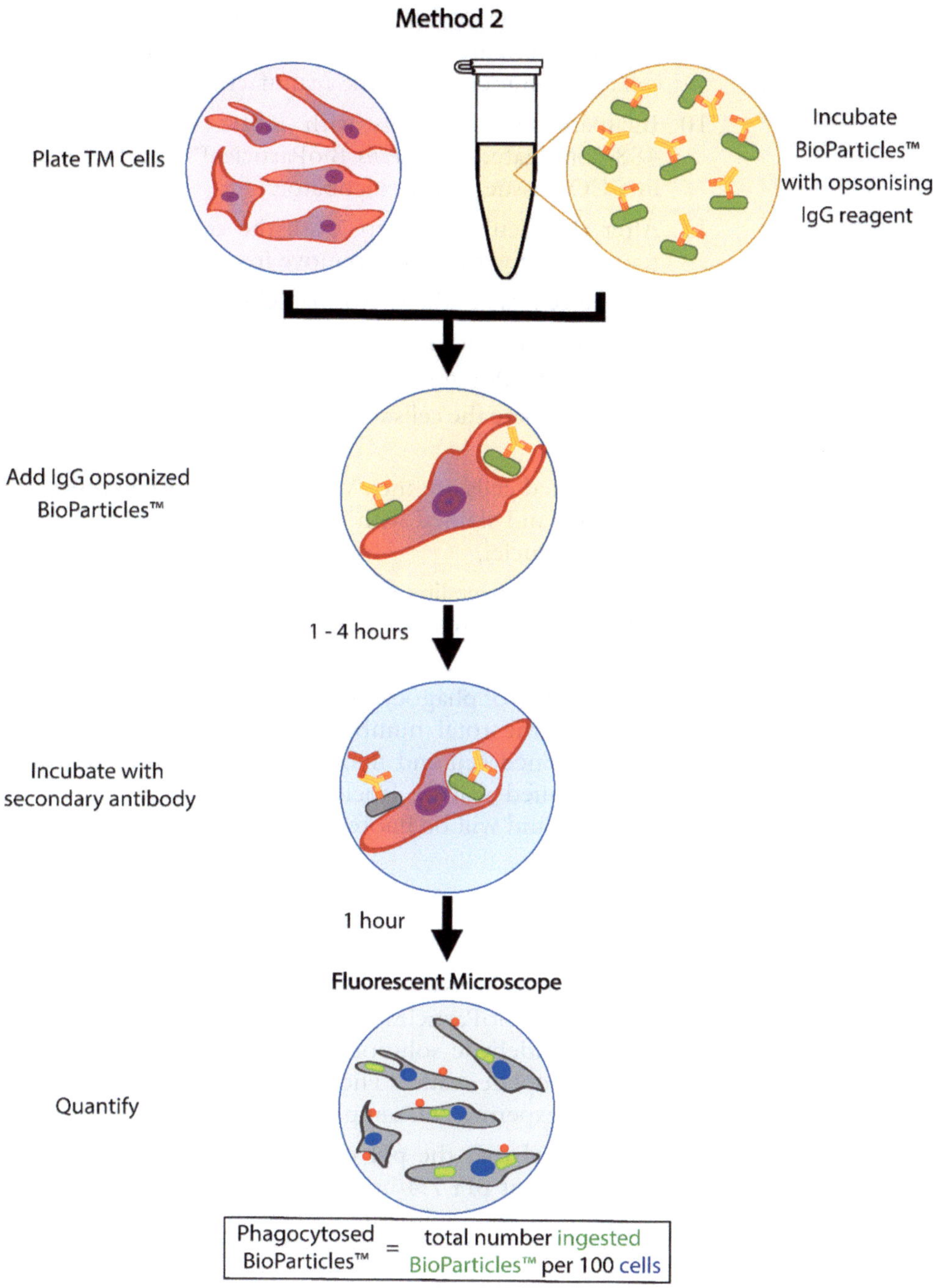

Fig. 2 Schematic showing method 2 to measure phagocytosis. TM cells are plated and incubated with opsonized *S. aureus* BioParticles™. Cells are washed and BioParticles™ not engulfed but bound to cell surface are labeled with a secondary antibody and will fluoresce red. BioParticles™ engulfed by cells will fluoresce green. Phagocytosis is measured using an inverted fluorescent microscope

containing the rabbit IgG-opsonized Alexa 488-conjugated *S. aureus* BioParticles™. Use a ratio of 50 BioParticles™ per cell as recommended by the manufacturer.

10. Incubate the TM cells with rabbit IgG-opsonized Alexa 488-conjugated *S. aureus* BioParticles™ for 1–4 h at 37 °C in a CO_2 tissue culture incubator.
11. After the incubation step, wash the cells 2–3 times at room temperature with PBS to remove free BioParticles™.
12. Fix the cells with 4% paraformaldehyde in PBS for 30 min.
13. Wash the cells with PBS 2–3 times and then block with 5% BSA and 5% goat preimmune serum in PBS for 30 min.
14. Next, incubate the cells with Alexa 546 goat anti-rabbit IgG for 1 h.
15. The labeled cells are then washed to remove excess secondary antibody and stained with DAPI (1 μg/mL) for 5–10 min to stain the nuclei.
16. Mount the coverslips onto a glass slide. Visualize and image cellular phagocytosis of the BioParticles™ with a fluorescent microscope.
17. The number of phagocytosed bioparticles can be quantified by counting the total number of BioParticles™ ingested by a DAPI-stained cell and fluorescent at 488 nm. Bioparticles™ not engulfed will be labeled with the secondary anti-rabbit antibody and will be fluorescent at 546 nm.

4 Notes

1. When doing the assay in a 96-well format, cells incubated with pHrodo™ BioParticles™ can be fixed with standard 2–4% paraformaldehyde solutions for later analysis using a fluorescent microplate reader. The differences in signal between control and experimental samples should remain for up to 48 h.
2. It is critical that the pH of the buffer used for the assay be maintained at pH 7.4 in order to minimize background fluorescence from noningested pHrodo BioParticles™. Noningested bioparticles can become fluorescent if pH drops below pH 7.4.
3. The 1% FBS is added to support the metabolic activity of the cells during the assay. Alternatively, the manufacturer's Live Imaging solution can be used in lieu of the HBSS/HEPES/FBS buffer.
4. If you are using the manufacturer's Live Imaging Solution, a CO_2 incubator at 37 °C with 5% CO_2 should be used.
5. At this time, cells can be labeled with an antibody, if desired, as performed in [20].

Acknowledgments

This work was supported by NEI grants EY017006, EY026009, and EY032905 (DMP) and a Core grant to the Department of Ophthalmology and Visual Sciences (P30 EY016665).

References

1. Grierson I, Lee WR (1973) Erythrocyte phagocytosis in the human trabecular meshwork. Br J Ophthalmol 57:400–415
2. Alvarado JA, Katz J, Trivedi MS (2010) Monocyte modulation of aqueous outflow and recruitment to the trabecular meshwork following selective laser trabeculoplasty. JAMA Ophthalmol 128:731–737
3. Bill A (1975) Editorial: the drainage of aqueous humor. Invest Ophthalmol Vis Sci 14:1–3
4. Murphy CG, Johnson M, Alvarado JA (1992) Juxtacanalicular tissue in pigmentary and primary open angle glaucoma. The hydrodynamic role of pigment and other constituents. Arch Ophthalmol 110:1779–1785. https://doi.org/10.1001/archopht.1992.01080240119043
5. Johnson DH, Richardson TM, Epstein DL (1989) Trabecular meshwork recovery after phagocytic challenge. Curr Eye Res 8:1121–1130
6. Buller C, Johnson DH, Tschumper RC (1990) Human trabecular meshwork phagocytosis. Observations in an organ culture system. Invest Ophthalmol Vis Sci 31:2156–2163
7. Schlotzer-Schrehardt U, Naumann GO (1995) Trabecular meshwork in pseudoexfoliation syndrome with and without open-angle glaucoma. A morphometric, ultrastructural study. Invest Ophthalmol Vis Sci 36:1750–1764
8. Shabo AL, Maxwell DS (1972) The structure of the trabecular meshwork of the primate eye: a light and electron microscopic study with peroxidase. Microvasc Res 4:384–398
9. MacRae D, Sears ML (1970) Peroxidase passage through the outflow channels of human and rhesus eyes. Exp Eye Res 10:15–16
10. Grierson I, Chisholm IA (1978) Clearance of debris from the iris through the drainage angle of the rabbit's eye. Br J Ophthalmol 62:694–704
11. Richardson TM, Hutchinson BT, Grant WM (1977) The outflow tract in pigmentary glaucoma: a light and electron microscopic study. Arch Ophthalmol 95:1015–1025
12. Acott TS, Wirtz MK (1996) Biochemistry of aqueous outflow. In: Ritch R, Shields MB, Krupin T (eds) The Glaucomas. Mosby-Year Book, St. Louis, pp 281–305
13. Rohen JW, van der Zypen E (1968) The phagocytic activity of the trabecular meshwork endothelium. An electron-microscopic study of the vervet (Cercopithecus aethiops). Albrecht Von Graefes Arch Klin Exp Ophthalmol 175: 143–160
14. Grierson I, Day J, Unger WG, Ahmed A (1986) Phagocytosis of latex microspheres by bovine meshwork cells in culture. Graefes Arch Clin Exp Ophthalmol 224:536–544
15. Matsumoto Y, Johnson DH (1997) Dexamethasone decreases phagocytosis by human trabecular meshwork cells in situ. Invest Ophthamol Vis Sci 38:1902–1907
16. Matsumoto Y, Johnson DH (1997) Trabecular meshwork phagocytosis in glaucomatous eyes. Ophthalmologica 211:147–152
17. Sherwood ME, Richardson TM (1988) Phagocytosis by trabecular meshwork cells: sequence of events in cats and monkeys. Exp Eye Res 46: 881–895
18. Epstein DL, Freddo TF, Anderson PJ, Patterson MM, Bassett-Chu S (1986) Experimental obstruction to aqueous outflow by pigment particles in living monkeys. Invest Ophthamol Vis Sci 27:387–395
19. Goldberg MF, Tso MOM (1978) Rubeosis iridis and glaucoma associated with sickle cell retinopathy: a light and electron microscopic study. Ophthalmol 85:1028–1041
20. Gagen D, Filla MS, Clark R, Liton P, Peters DM (2013) Activated αvβ3 integrin regulates αvβ5 integrin-mediated phagocytosis in trabecular meshwork cells. Invest Ophthamol Vis Sci 54:5000–5011. https://doi.org/10.1167/iovs.13-12084
21. Du Y, Rob DS, Mann MM, Funderburgh ML, Funderburgh JL, Schuman JS (2012) Multipotent stem cells from trabecular meshwork become phagocytic TM cells. Invest Ophthalmol Vis Sci 53:1566–1575. https://doi.org/10.1167/iovs.11-9134

22. Porter K, Lin Y, Liton PB (2013) Cathepsin B is up-regulated and mediates extracellular matrix degradation in trabecular meshwork cells following phagocytic challenge. PLoS ONE 8(7):e68668. https://doi.org/10.1371/journal.pone.0068668
23. Faralli JA, Desikan H, Peotter J, Kanneganti N, Weinhaus B, Filla MS, Peters DM (2019) Proteomic analyses of phagocytosis in dexamethasone (DEX)-treated human trabecular meshwork (TM) cells reveals a role for Gulp1 and ABR. Mol Vis 25:237–254
24. Zhang X, Ognibene CM, Clark AF, Yorio T (2007) Dexamethasone inhibition of trabecular meshwork cell phagocytosis and its modulation by glucocorticoid receptor beta. Exp Eye Res 84:275–284. https://doi.org/10.1016/j.exer.2006.09.022
25. Polansky JR, Weinreb R, Alvarado JA (1981) Studies on human trabecular cells propagated in vitro. Vis Res 21(1):155–160
26. Polansky JR, Weinreb RN, Baxter JD, Alvarado J (1979) Human trabecular cells. I. Establishment in tissue culture and growth characteristics. Invest Ophthamol Vis Sci 18(10):1043–1049
27. Keller KE, Bhattacharya SK, Borrás T, Brunner TM, Chansangpetch S, Clark AF, Dismuke WM, Du Y, Elliott MH, Ethier CR, Faralli JA, Freddo TF, Fuchshofer R, Giovingo M, Gong H, Gonzalez P, Huang A, Johnstone MA, Kaufman PL, Kelley MJ, Knepper PA, Kopczynski CC, Kuchtey JG, Kuchtey RW, Kuehn MH, Lieberman RL, Lin SC, Liton P, Liu Y, Lütjen-Drecoll E, Mao W, Masis-Solano M, McDonnell F, McDowell CM, Overby DR, Pattabiraman PP, Raghunathan VK, Rao PV, Rhee DJ, Chowdhury UR, Russell P, Samples JR, Schwartz D, Stubbs EB, Tamm ER, Tan JC, Toris CB, Torrejon KY, Vranka JA, Wirtz MK, Yorio T, Zhang J, Zode GS, Fautsch MP, Peters DM, Acott TS, Stamer WD (2018) Consensus recommendations for trabecular meshwork cell isolation, characterization and culture. Exp Eye Res 171:164–173. https://doi.org/10.1016/j.exer.2018.03.001
28. Ninkovic J, Roy S (2014) High throughput fluorometric technique for assessment of macrophage phagocytosis and actin polymerization. J Vis Exp 93:e52195. https://doi.org/10.3791/52195

Chapter 5

Nanotubules and Cellular Communication in Trabecular Meshwork Cells

Kate E. Keller and Stefanie Kaech Petrie

Abstract

Glaucoma causes dysfunction to tissues located in the anterior and posterior eye. In the anterior eye, the trabecular meshwork (TM) is the site of pathogenesis, where decreased TM cell numbers and alterations to the amount and composition of extracellular matrix hinder outflow of aqueous humor fluid from the anterior chamber. This causes intraocular pressure (IOP) elevation. Elevated IOP, a main risk factor for primary open-angle glaucoma, damages the axons of retinal ganglion cells in the posterior eye, which ultimately leads to blindness. Thus, clinical treatment paradigms for glaucoma are focused on reducing IOP. Normotensive IOPs are established by balancing the production of aqueous fluid from the ciliary body with drainage through the TM to Schlemm's canal. When IOP becomes elevated, TM cells coordinate a homeostatic response to lower IOP, which requires effective and efficient cellular communication. Tunneling nanotubes (TNTs) are transient specialized structures that allow cells to communicate with one another. Actin-rich tubes allow direct transmission of signals and cargoes between cells. This is important to overcome limitations of diffusion-based signaling in aqueous environments such as the anterior eye. Here, we describe a live-cell imaging method for monitoring TNTs in primary TM cells.

Key words Glaucoma, Trabecular meshwork, Cytoskeleton, Tunneling nanotubes, Live-cell imaging, Cell biology, Cellular communication, Protocol

1 Introduction

1.1 Trabecular Meshwork and Intraocular Pressure

The trabecular meshwork (TM) tissue regulates the outflow of aqueous humor fluid from the anterior chamber of the eye [1, 2]. When outflow is hindered, due to dysfunction of the TM, intraocular pressure (IOP) becomes elevated, which increases the risk for glaucoma [3]. As IOP increases, there is continual feedback between the extracellular matrix, to which TM cells attach, and receptors on the TM cell membrane, which detect and respond to the biomechanical cues exerted on the tissue by elevated IOP. To launch a homeostatic response to return IOP to normal ranges, the cells must communicate with each other. Most signaling mechanisms rely on secretion of signals from one cell, diffusion through the

Tatjana Jakobs and Paloma B. Liton (eds.), *Glaucoma: Methods and Protocols*, Methods in Molecular Biology, vol. 2858, https://doi.org/10.1007/978-1-0716-4140-8_5,

extracellular milieu, and binding to receptors on an adjacent target cell [4]. However, this diffusion-based signaling suffers from an inherent problem: The further away the target cell resides from the signal source, the lower concentration of signal reaching it. This deficiency is exacerbated in the fluid environment of the anterior eye, where secreted signals are diluted in aqueous humor and can be washed into Schlemm's canal without reaching their intended targets. Thus, additional communication mechanisms must exist to efficiently transfer IOP-related signals between TM cells in situ.

1.2 Tunneling Nanotubes

Tunneling nanotubes (TNTs) are physical tubular connections between cells through which cellular cargoes are passed [5, 6]. TNTs have been detected in cell cultures of adherent ocular cells, including TM cells and retinal epithelial cells [7, 8]. In addition, TNTs are detected in eye tissues in situ such as the mouse cornea and in retinal pericytes, where they regulate neurovascular coupling [9–11]. Studies using live-cell imaging show that these unique, transient structures are formed by fusion of filopodia emanating the cell surface of two individual cells [5, 12]. Once a nanotubule has formed, cargoes such as organelles (mitochondria, endosomes, lysosomes) or signals (miRNA, viruses, growth factors, prions) are directly communicated between cells. Actin filaments stabilize the core of the tubule [13]. TNTs are typically thin (50–200 nm in diameter) but can extend >200 μm in length [14, 15]. Thus, TNTs allow cells to signal long distances, overcoming limitations of diffusion-based signaling [10, 16].

1.3 Live-Cell Imaging and Microscope Considerations

Live-cell imaging is a powerful technique to follow the behavior of cells in normal culture conditions, as well as their responses to drug treatments [17]. This technique is especially useful for interrogating dynamics of the actin cytoskeleton and was imperative for describing TNT formation [5]. Live imaging of fluorescently labeled cells requires special considerations for maintaining cell health during time-lapse recording to ensure that phototoxic effects do not interfere with the biology under investigation. Exposure to intense excitation light can induce phototoxicity, resulting in cellular stress and altered biological responses [18]. Modern imaging systems are configured with state-of-the-art features to ensure cell health is maintained and to minimize phototoxicity. The following features should be considered when choosing a microscope setup for live-cell imaging experiments:

1. The environment on inverted microscope stands can be equipped with heated stage incubators, or larger microscope enclosures, to control temperature of the sample. A humidified air and gas mixture is circulated over the stage to replicate the CO_2 atmosphere of a regular tissue culture incubator. However, care must be taken when using high-resolution and high

magnification lenses, which require an immersion liquid between the front of the lens and the coverslip, to avoid creating an effective heatsink through the large microscope body. This can create an area, where the lens connects to the sample, that has a significantly lower temperature than the physiological temperature setpoint of the chamber. To overcome this, objectives are heated directly, or the microscope body is heated through a larger stage enclosure. Alternatively, so-called "dry" lenses leave an insulating air gap between the front of the lens and the vessel support and can be deployed during time-lapse recordings, albeit with lower resolution and generally lower magnification.

2. For cells cultured directly on glass coverslip supports, a standard widefield microscope in combination with computational light reassignment through iterative deconvolution is a cost-effective alternative to more expensive laser-based imaging systems. Fluorescent signals from single cell layers are effectively deblurred and optically sectioned without the involvement of pinholes, implicated in conventional confocal microscopy, that eliminate many of the photons emitted from fluorescent labels from being detected.
3. Excitation using a light-emitting diode (LED) is preferred because the combination of a band-pass excitation barrier filter and a tuned excitation peak of an LED more effectively eliminates unwanted excitation light, particularly harmful UV rays present in high-intensity arc light sources. Furthermore, the fast on/off latency of LEDs allows for triggered coupling of light exposure to active data collection of the digital camera.
4. Well-priced modern sCMOS cameras have good quantum efficiency to detect photons across a wide range of wavelengths. Their chip sizes are larger and more densely packed with detector elements compared to those of expensive EMCCD detectors.
5. Motorized field diaphragms can be deployed to limit the illumination area to only the field of view captured on the detector array.
6. Plating cells into vessels with thin glass coverslip bottoms positions the cells within the working distance of high-numerical aperture lenses, which collect more light and afford more resolution when correctly mapped to the pixel density of the camera chip.
7. High-precision piezo-driven stage automation expands the number of cells that can be followed in a single time-lapse recording through point revisiting and/or montaging of adjacent fields of view into stitched images.

8. Active hardware-based focus devices eliminate the need for software-based autofocusing routines, which require acquisition of multiple images to compensate for focus drift over time.

Together, these features reduce phototoxicity, aid the execution of live-cell imaging experiments, and ensure high-quality time-lapse recordings of challenging samples, such as flat TM cells. Here, we describe live-cell imaging methods to monitor TNT formation in primary TM cell cultures. In these studies, we use the high-affinity, membrane-permeable, SiR – actin stain to label the actin cytoskeleton of TM cells and a Zeiss Celldiscoverer 7 microscope to perform live-imaging studies [8, 19, 20]. The methods described herein can be applied to any adherent cell type, while additional approaches to characterize TNTs may also be of value [21].

2 Materials

2.1 Cells, Culture Media, and Supplements

1. Early-passage primary TM cells: Primary TM cells are cultured from dissected TM tissue from human normal or glaucoma cadaver eyes (Lions Vision Gift, Portland, OR) under the rules of the Declaration of Helsinki of 1975 (*see* **Note 1**).
2. Low-glucose culture media: Dulbecco's Modified Eagle Medium (DMEM) with 1 g/L D-glucose, 4 mM L-glutamine, and 110 mg/L sodium pyruvate.
3. High-glucose culture media: DMEM with 4 g/L D-glucose, 4 mM L-glutamine, and 110 mg/L sodium pyruvate.
4. Antibiotic-antimycotic solution 100×: 10,000 units/mL penicillin, 10,000 μg/mL streptomycin, and 25 μg/mL Amphotericin B.
5. Hyclone-characterized fetal bovine serum (FBS), endotoxin-free.
6. Phosphate-buffered saline (PBS), pH 7.4, sterile: 1 mM potassium phosphate monobasic, 155 mM sodium chloride, and 3 mM sodium phosphate dibasic.
7. 0.25% Trypsin-EDTA (1×).

2.2 Cell Culture Plates and Staining Reagents

1. Six-well plates with 35 mm wells and #1.5 cover glass bottoms with lid (*see* **Note 2**).
2. Spirochrome SiR – Actin labeling kit: SiR – actin is detected similar to standard "far-red" channel dyes, such as Cy5, or Alexa Fluor 647 (*see* **Note 3**).
3. Verapamil: Supplied in the SiR – actin kit. It is a broad-spectrum efflux pump inhibitor that improves staining intensity of SiR – actin in live cells.
4. Cell culture-grade dimethyl sulfoxide (DMSO).

2.3 Instrumentation Overview

For the experiments described here, we use the ZEISS Celldiscoverer 7 (CD7). CD7 is a purposely designed instrument for live-cell imaging that incorporates the design features discussed above (Subheading 1.3). Herein, we describe the protocol for time-lapse imaging of SiR – actin using the CD7, but any inverted research microscope configured with similar features will facilitate success in capturing nanotube dynamics. The CD7 includes a heated sample chamber and heated objectives. A mixture of CO_2 and air is bubbled through a water bottle for humidification and pumped into the sample chamber. The illumination light path includes a square field diaphragm that is adjusted to limit LED illumination to the field of view captured on the camera by the large diameter objectives uniquely designed for the CD7. A 5×/0.35 objective is used for initial focusing, and a Plan APO 20×/0.95 high-resolution objective is deployed for time-lapse recordings. Fluorescent signals are detected on a Hamamatsu Orca Flash 4.0v3 sCMOS camera at a pixel resolution of 0.324 μm per pixel and a field of view of 663 μm by 663 μm. Hardware-based focusing is used to find focus and is engaged during time-lapse imaging to compensate for focus drifts. Additional description of these features as they pertain to imaging nanotubes in TM cells is incorporated into the setup steps in the protocol below.

3 Methods

3.1 Preparation of Culture Media and Cell Staining Reagents

1. Prepare complete media by mixing low- and high-glucose DMEM 1:1 and then adding 1% antibiotic-antimycotic solution and 10% fetal bovine serum.
2. Dissolve 1 vial of SiR – actin in 50 μL DMSO to prepare a 1 mM stock solution. Store the stock solution at −20 °C for up to 3 months (*see* **Note 4**).
3. Prepare a 1000× stock solution of verapamil by resuspending the vial in 100 μL DMSO. The final concentration of this stock solution is 10 mM verapamil. Store the stock solution at −20 °C.
4. To prepare the SiR – actin staining solution, add 0.3 μL SiR – actin and 3 μL verapamil to 3 mL prewarmed DMEM supplemented with 10% FBS. The final SiR – actin concentration is 100 nM, and this volume is sufficient to stain all wells of one 6-well plate. Staining solution should be prepared fresh for each experiment and should not be reused.

3.2 Cell Labeling with SiR – Actin

1. The day prior to imaging, trypsinize a flask of TM cells, wash with PBS + 10% FBS to neutralize any remaining trypsin, and plate at 1×10^5 cells per well of a glass coverslip 6-well plate.

2. Add additional prewarmed media to a volume of 2 mL per well and gently swirl dishes so cells are evenly distributed.
3. Incubate cells overnight at 37 °C, 5% CO_2, in a humidified environment.
4. Remove spent media and wash the cells once with PBS (*see* **Note 5**).
5. Add 100 nM SiR – actin solution to the well (500 μL per well) and incubate for 1 h at 37 °C. If organelle stains are desired, cells can be labeled with those (*see* **Note 6**).
6. Wash cells twice with PBS and add 1 mL prewarmed medium (DMEM +10% FBS) to each well (*see* **Note 7**).

3.3 Microscope Setup and Sample Loading

1. Turn on and warm up the microscope. Check and refill the humidifier water bottle, open the ZEN software, set the temperature in the environmental controls to 37 °C, and equilibrate the system for at least 30 min. Just prior to sample loading, turn on the CO_2 controller and adjust the fan speed of the air pump to continuously circulate CO_2-equilibrated air through the humidifier bottle and into the sample chamber.
2. Load the plate onto the instrument stage. The CD7 system includes automated steps that measure the refractive index and thickness of the sample support and detect the vessel format. The determined values are used to define limits for stage and objective movement, which are based on the lens's working distance and the recess of the vessel bottom from the outer well plate walls. This prevents collision of the lens with the bottom of the plate and surrounding support (*see* **Note 8**). The instrument acquires an overview image of the plate and the holder for navigation, and defaults to the 5×/0.35 objective for initial navigation and focusing.
3. Wait at least 15 min for the cells to equilibrate to the chamber environment before starting a time-lapse recording.

3.4 Define Time-Lapse Acquisition Parameters

1. Configure the light path and channels. The CD7 assists this process with a "Smart Setup" wizard in the ZEN software. Preset optical configurations for Cy5 or Alexa 647, which have similar spectral properties as SiR – actin, are selected in the wizard. Specifically, LED excitation with a peak at 625 nm with a quadband reflective multiband-pass dichroic (RQBS 405 + 493 + 575 + 653) is used to excite the fluorescent label, while a quadband emission filter (EM QBP 425/30 + 514/30 + 592/25 + 709/100) detects fluorescence.
2. If a transmitted light image of the cells is desired, select "TL" in the dye wizard and choose "TL Phase Gradient." Transmitted illumination with an IR-LED, with a peak intensity at 725 nm

and passed through a rotating half-moon pupil, creates a high-contrast phase-gradient contrast image of even the thinnest parts of TM cells.

3. Determine the LED intensity for excitation and the exposure time for detection. This is important to generate image data with a signal-to-noise sufficient to see necessary detail and detect dim signals above background but without bleaching the fluorophore and inducing phototoxicity (*see* **Note 9**). As a starting point, recommended acquisition parameters are 20% LED settings for intensity and 400 ms for camera exposure time for the fluorescence channel and 10% LED and 5 ms camera exposure for the transmitted light image. Lower light intensities and longer exposure times are less phototoxic than higher light intensities and short exposure times [18].
4. To focus on your sample, start by using a low-magnification lens. The CD7 defaults to a 5×/0.35 objective. This poses less risk of inadvertently driving the lens too close to the sample. Also, lower magnification lenses generally have a larger depth of focus and focus at a larger distance from the bottom of the vessel (*see* **Note 10**). Use the automated "Find Surface" function in the ZEN software for initial focusing.
5. Select your lens of choice for data acquisition. For flat TM cells, we chose the 20×/0.95 objective. This 2x tube lens is useful for more brightly labeled cultures as the extra magnification increases the nominal numerical aperture of the lens, yielding an image with a tighter depth of focus and more contrast. The lens also features an automated correction collar, which is fine-tuned during software initialization to the thickness of the sample support. This maximizes contrast and resolution by minimizing lens aberrations.
6. Define z-stack parameters. To determine the number and spacing of focus planes to capture during the time-lapse recording, select a representative field of view and focus to the bottom and top of the range to capture to set the lower and upper limits for the z-stack. Considering the depth of focus of the lens (*see* **Note 10**), select the spacing and the number of z-planes to capture during the recording. For flat TM cells, two or three focal planes, 0.7 μm apart, can capture the depth of the cytoplasm and nanotube extensions. When including a transmitted light channel, choose to acquire only one transmitted image at the center of the z-stack.
7. Find representative fields of view to image in each well, and store their x, y, and z-coordinates for recall during time-lapse recording. The CD7 can store single positions, or tiled arrays, and it offers a number of ways to automate the revisiting and refocusing on the stored positions. In our case, each well in the

6-well plate represented a different condition, so we chose to store four positions per well. Therefore, a total of 24 stored positions were set for recall during recording.

8. In "Live" acquisition mode, use the keyboard controls to fine-tune the focus, and "store" the new focus z-value for the first position. The "Store Focus" function records the offset against the reflecting interface so that when moved to another area of the same well, or a different well, the "Recall Focus" function focuses to the same distance from the vessel support and brings the sample into focus.
9. Take advantage of any autofocusing strategies supported on your microscope setup to compensate for inevitable small focal drifts during the recording. For the CD7, the hardware-based "Definite Focus" stabilizes the focus position across time points. It is important to verify that the z-value of each stored x, y position is based on the offset of the first position. To do this, start at the first position, and then engage the stored offset by selecting the "Recall Focus" function. Verify the z-positions for the other stored positions and update their z-values after fine-focusing where needed. When setting up the time-lapse recording, instruct the software to engage the "Definite Focus" at each position prior to acquiring the image.
10. Set the time interval and length of the recording. The time interval should be matched to the rate of change of the biological event to be captured (*see* **Note 11**). For imaging nanotubes in TM cells, we imaged every 2 min for 2 h total. To estimate the total time needed to acquire one full set of images at all positions, select "Measure Speed" in the ZEN software. For the 24 position points selected in **step 8**, the software predicted that it would take 1 min and 50 s to acquire three z-slices on two channels for all of these points, indicating that a complete loop could be acquired within the desired 2 min. Adjustments to the above parameters (z-slices, number of positions, selected channels) may be needed if it is not possible to acquire one full set within the chosen interval time.
11. Define a storage location for the data. We recommend saving the data directly to the hard drive instead of keeping it in volatile RAM of the computer. Files can be very large if multiple positions, with multiple channels and z-stacks, are chosen. For the example given in Subheading 3.4, **step 8**, the file size was ~56 GB.
12. Start the time-lapse recording. Imaging proceeds according to the parameters you have selected and ends automatically after the final time point is acquired. Time-lapse recordings can also be paused if needed (*see* **Note 12**).

3.5 Time-Lapse Data Visualization

1. To review the multidimensional time-lapse recording, use your system's software control to choose a position, a z-slice, a channel, or a channel overlay, and play the result over time for visual inspection within the software. Use display adjustments to enhance contrast and brightness to identify an event worth exporting for dissemination.
2. Find the positional, slice, and time-point information that captures the event you want to showcase in a multidimensional file. Extract the underlying images into a new subset for further processing. This keeps the original "raw" dataset unmodified for future deposition into a publicly shared data repository. If you acquired a z-stack, consider flattening the volume information into a two-dimensional view by applying a maximum intensity projection along the z-axis. After subset creation, you might need to fine-tune the display adjustments to again highlight the event you want to showcase.
3. Use a built-in video export function in your setup's software to export a time-lapse movie. Alternatively, export the images as an RGB TIFF series and import them into a third-party software capable of creating a video file. Beware that this step burns in any display adjustments made, so it is important to make sure that you replicate the same adjustments to all data files that you want your audience to compare side by side. TIFF images of fluorescence and phase gradient PGC channels can be used in publications to highlight TNT formation over time (*see* Fig. 1).
4. Determine the replay speed of your video by selecting how many of the time points should be used per second of the final video. For time-lapse recordings of TM cells, a replay speed of 3–5 frames per second has been used, which condenses the time-lapse recording 360–600-fold. The resulting videos were 12–20 s long. To reduce the file size, opt to use a common compression/decompression algorithm and file format (*see* **Note 13**).

4 Notes

1. Primary cell strains are established and characterized by monitoring cellular morphology and by dexamethasone induction of myocilin, as outlined in the guidelines for culturing primary TM cells [22]. It is important to evaluate at least three biological replicates because primary cell strains can differ in their growth properties. Also, cellular senescence should be evaluated by β-galactosidase staining [20]. Primary TM cells are used between passages 2 and 6 for cells derived from normal eyes and between 2 and 5 for glaucomatous TM cells.

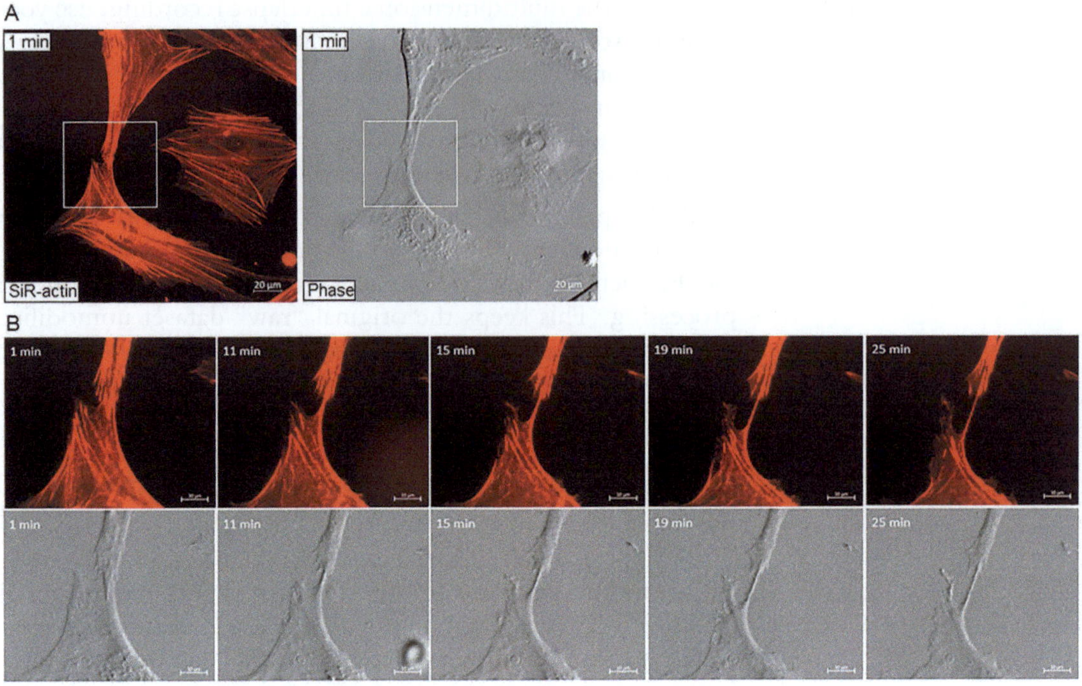

Fig. 1 (**a**) Still images of TM cells stained with SiR – actin (red) or imaged with phase gradient PGC (gray). Scale bar = 20 μm. (**b**) Boxed area in (**a**) is selected as a region of interest. The time points (1, 11, 15, 19, and 25 min) show a thin, actin-rich TNT forming as two TM cells slowly edge away from one another. The phase gradient PGC images show the plasma membrane of the TM cell and the rounded appearance of the nanotubule between the two cells

2. Different size plates and slides can be used, but it is important to use glass with nominal 170 μm thickness, equivalent to so-called #1.5 coverslips. This thickness is used by all major microscope manufacturers in their lens design. Failure to match this standard results in suboptimal correction of chromatic and spherical aberrations and loss of contrast and resolution in the acquired digital data.
3. Actin can be fluorescently labeled by other methods [23]. There are advantages and disadvantages of each stain, and researchers should consider image contrast (e.g., Lifeact-TagGFP binds globular actin as well as F-actin, which can produce high cytoplasmic background that drowns out filamentous actin staining), delivery method (e.g., some require transfection or infection), and membrane permeability (e.g., the classic F-actin stain, phalloidin, has low cell membrane permeability and is not recommended for live-cell imaging) [24].
4. The methods and concentrations of SiR – actin described herein work well for staining primary TM cells. If other adherent cell types are being used, it is advised to perform a series of

exploratory experiments to determine the best concentration and incubation time for the stain. Suggested incubation times and concentrations can be found in the SiR – actin manufacturer's datasheet. Some cell types are sensitive to verapamil treatment, so it is advised to design initial experiments to determine if verapamil is detrimental to cell health.

5. When exchanging media, or washing adherent cells with PBS, tip the plate so that the media accumulates on one side of the well, and gently remove the liquid. When replacing fluid, add the liquid so that it drains down the side of the well and then flows across the surface of the cells. These practices are essential so that the adherent cells are not dislodged from the surface of the coverslip.
6. As mentioned in the introduction, TNTs can transport organelles between cells [5, 6, 15]. Organelles can be stained with fluorescent dyes. We have used Vybrant DiO cell labeling solution [8, 19, 20] with success, but other fluorescent membrane dyes are available. If researchers are interested in monitoring mitochondria transport via TNTs, several fluorescent mitochondrial dyes are available, such as MitoTracker. Organelle stains can be used in conjunction with SiR – actin, but it is important to carefully select reagents to ensure there is no spectral overlap of their fluorophores with SiR – actin. Fluorescent organelle stains should be applied prior to placing the vessel in the microscope.
7. DMEM can be used for experiments with SiR – actin in the far-red range of the visual spectrum. However, if using fluorescent reagents with shorter wavelengths, the culture medium should have reduced riboflavin content to minimize autofluorescence and allow dim signals to be detected [25]. A commonly available medium with low riboflavin content is Ham's F-12. However, specialty media formulations with no riboflavin are also available from several manufacturers.
8. Multiwell plates usually feature a recessed bottom, which makes the edges of the plate inaccessible to objectives that focus close to the vessel bottom. The geometry of the plate recess and the lens determine the exact exclusion range, but it is generally the case that the outermost rows and columns of 96 well plates are inaccessible to lenses with numerical apertures higher than 0.45 and free working distances below 0.5 mm.
9. The CD7 is equipped with LED light sources, which, unlike lasers, do not substantially heat the glass coverslip or the sample. However, it is important to evaluate whether the LED intensity and exposure settings are gentle enough when applied continuously. For each fluorescence channel, find a sacrificial

area with signal in your sample and start "Live" imaging. Scrutinize the image for a noticeable decrease of the maximum intensity level and a shift of the intensity histogram to lower intensities. If you observe this during the "live" image, your settings are bleaching the fluorophores and contributing to phototoxicity. To rectify, lower the light intensity (e.g., from 20% to 15%) until no changes are observed during continuous illumination. Compensate by increasing exposure times (e.g., from 400 to 500 ms) to maintain acceptable signal to noise in the image.

10. The depth of focus of a lens is linked to the numerical aperture of the objective, which describes the angle of diffracted light rays that emanate from the sample captured by the lens. The larger the angle, the higher the lateral resolution, the narrower the depth of focus, and the shorter the free working distance of the lens. Fluorescence microscopy benefits from imaging with high numerical aperture lenses because they collect more light emanating from the sample, but their narrow depth of focus increases the risk that the observer misses the sample when focusing through a thin sample. It is therefore safer to initially focus with a low-magnification lens with lower numerical aperture and a wider depth of focus and then to use the parfocality settings stored in the motorized microscope to bring the sample into the shallow focus depth of a high numerical aperture lens.
11. In all live-cell imaging experiments, there is a balancing act to consider when choosing detection, z-stack parameters, and the number of positions to follow because their combined acquisition time needs to fall within the limits of the data acquisition rate required to accurately digitize the dynamics under investigation. According to the Nyquist-Shannon sampling theorem, to reconstruct a continuous time event with a discontinuous digital recording, the image frequency must be sampled with at least twice the frequency of change. Aim to set the camera exposure time in each channel short. Keep in mind that in live-cell imaging, the aim is not to stretch intensity values in the image across the full dynamic range of the detector but to detect signals with sufficient signal-to-noise ratio to visualize and possibly quantify intensities. Changing the number of channels, their respective exposure times, and the number of z-slices will affect the length of time it takes for the microscope to revisit all the points. If monitoring rapid dynamics, such as actin in nanotubes, limits to these parameters are quickly reached. However, if your experimental question is not related to capturing rapid dynamics, then you can choose more data points to acquire in your experiment. For thin TM cells, a

z-stack may not be needed, and imaging of TNTs can often be acquired on a single plane, which may allow more positions to be monitored.

12. The CD7 is ideal to evaluate the effects of drug treatments on TNTs because there is a port on top of the instrument through which drugs can be pipetted directly into the wells. To do this, click "pause" in the software during recording, add the drug (or vehicle control) through the port, and then "resume" imaging. Acquisition continues as previously set up. When adding drugs/treatments through the CD7 port, it is important that the solutions are prewarmed because adding cold substances can cause temperature fluctuations that can have dramatic effects on cellular responses. We have used the CD7 to study TM cell responses to netarsudil, a Rho kinase inhibitor drug that is FDA-approved under the brand name Rhopressa® for reducing elevated IOP in glaucoma patients [19].
13. Unfortunately, a compression/decompression algorithm (codec) that works across a variety of computing platforms and operating systems has never been widely agreed upon. The most commonly deployed codecs to play videos in web browsers are the H.264 and H.265 codecs in .mp4 format. These are poised to become the quasistandards going forward. However, because of the lack of standards, and the continuing development of new codecs that can compress videos to smaller size without apparent loss in quality, the microscope manufacturers often do not offer video export that deploy these newer codecs. Therefore, we recommend exporting images to a commercial third-party software. Since codecs include executables for decoding, they are very prone to security issues. We discourage downloading open-source software and converters.

Acknowledgments

This work was supported by NIH NEI grants R01 EY019643, R01 EY032590, and P30 EY010572 and an unrestricted grant to the Casey Eye Institute, OHSU, from the Research to Prevent Blindness.

References

1. Stamer WD, Clark AF (2017) The many faces of the trabecular meshwork cell. Exp Eye Res 158:112–123. https://doi.org/10.1016/j.exer.2016.07.009
2. Vranka JA, Kelley MJ, Acott TS, Keller KE (2015) Extracellular matrix in the trabecular meshwork: intraocular pressure regulation and dysregulation in glaucoma. Exp Eye Res 133:112–125. https://doi.org/10.1016/j.exer.2014.07.014
3. Acott TS, Vranka JA, Keller KE, Raghunathan V, Kelley MJ (2021) Normal and glaucomatous outflow regulation. Prog Retin Eye Res 82:100897. https://doi.org/10.1016/j.preteyeres.2020.100897

4. Muller P, Rogers KW, Yu SR, Brand M, Schier AF (2013) Morphogen transport. Development 140(8):1621–1638. https://doi.org/10.1242/dev.083519
5. Rustom A, Saffrich R, Markovic I, Walther P, Gerdes HH (2004) Nanotubular highways for intercellular organelle transport. Science 303(5660):1007–1010. https://doi.org/10.1126/science.1093133
6. Davis DM, Sowinski S (2008) Membrane nanotubes: dynamic long-distance connections between animal cells. Nat Rev Mol Cell Biol 9(6):431–436. https://doi.org/10.1038/nrm2399
7. Wittig D, Wang X, Walter C, Gerdes HH, Funk RH, Roehlecke C (2012) Multi-level communication of human retinal pigment epithelial cells via tunneling nanotubes. PLoS One 7(3): e33195. https://doi.org/10.1371/journal.pone.0033195
8. Keller KE, Bradley JM, Sun YY, Yang YF, Acott TS (2017) Tunneling nanotubes are novel cellular structures that communicate signals between trabecular meshwork cells. Invest Ophthalmol Vis Sci 58(12):5298–5307. https://doi.org/10.1167/iovs.17-22732
9. Chinnery HR, Pearlman E, McMenamin PG (2008) Cutting edge: membrane nanotubes in vivo: a feature of MHC class II+ cells in the mouse cornea. J Immunol 180(9):5779–5783
10. Chinnery HR, Keller KE (2020) Tunneling nanotubes and the eye: intercellular communication and implications for ocular health and disease. Biomed Res Int 2020:7246785. https://doi.org/10.1155/2020/7246785
11. Alarcon-Martinez L, Villafranca-Baughman D, Quintero H, Kacerovsky JB, Dotigny F, Murai KK et al (2020) Interpericyte tunnelling nanotubes regulate neurovascular coupling. Nature 585(7823):91–95. https://doi.org/10.1038/s41586-020-2589-x
12. Gerdes HH, Carvalho RN (2008) Intercellular transfer mediated by tunneling nanotubes. Curr Opin Cell Biol 20(4):470–475. https://doi.org/10.1016/j.ceb.2008.03.005
13. Ljubojevic N, Henderson JM, Zurzolo C (2021) The ways of actin: why tunneling nanotubes are unique cell protrusions. Trends Cell Biol 31(2):130–142. https://doi.org/10.1016/j.tcb.2020.11.008
14. Abounit S, Zurzolo C (2012) Wiring through tunneling nanotubes--from electrical signals to organelle transfer. J Cell Sci 125(Pt 5): 1089–1098. https://doi.org/10.1242/jcs.083279
15. Gurke S, Barroso JF, Gerdes HH (2008) The art of cellular communication: tunneling nanotubes bridge the divide. Histochem Cell Biol 129(5):539–550. https://doi.org/10.1007/s00418-008-0412-0
16. Sherer NM (2013) Long-distance relationships: do membrane nanotubes regulate cell-cell communication and disease progression? Mol Biol Cell 24(8):1095–1098. https://doi.org/10.1091/mbc.E12-08-0622
17. Ettinger A, Wittmann T (2014) Fluorescence live cell imaging. Methods Cell Biol 123:77–94. https://doi.org/10.1016/B978-0-12-420138-5.00005-7
18. Hockberger P (2000) Sources and remedies of phototoxicity in live cell microscopy. Microsc Today 8:30–32. https://doi.org/10.1017/S1551929500063434
19. Keller KE, Kopczynski C (2020) Effects of netarsudil on actin-driven cellular functions in normal and glaucomatous trabecular meshwork cells: a live imaging study. J Clin Med 9(11). https://doi.org/10.3390/jcm9113524
20. Sun YY, Bradley JM, Keller KE (2019) Phenotypic and functional alterations in tunneling nanotubes formed by glaucomatous trabecular meshwork cells. Invest Ophthalmol Vis Sci 60(14):4583–4595. https://doi.org/10.1167/iovs.19-28084
21. Abounit S, Delage E, Zurzolo C (2015) Identification and characterization of tunneling nanotubes for intercellular trafficking. Curr Protoc Cell Biol 67:11–21. https://doi.org/10.1002/0471143030.cb1210s67
22. Keller KE, Bhattacharya SK, Borras T, Brunner TM, Chansangpetch S, Clark AF et al (2018) Consensus recommendations for trabecular meshwork cell isolation, characterization and culture. Exp Eye Res 171:164–173. https://doi.org/10.1016/j.exer.2018.03.001
23. Melak M, Plessner M, Grosse R (2017) Actin visualization at a glance. J Cell Sci 130(3): 525–530. https://doi.org/10.1242/jcs.189068
24. Flores LR, Keeling MC, Zhang X, Sliogeryte K, Gavara N (2019) Lifeact-GFP alters F-actin organization, cellular morphology and biophysical behaviour. Sci Rep 9(1):3241. https://doi.org/10.1038/s41598-019-40092-w
25. Ludin B, Doll T, Meili R, Kaech S, Matus A (1996) Application of novel vectors for GFP-tagging of proteins to study microtubule-associated proteins. Gene 173(1 Spec No):107–111. https://doi.org/10.1016/0378-1119(95)00899-3

Chapter 6

Isolation and Characterization of Exosomes from Ocular Samples

Jingwen Cai and Yutao Liu

Abstract

Exosomes are microsize vesicles secreted by nearly all cells to the extracellular space. The vesicles transport cell signaling and communicate with other cells. Ultracentrifugation is the standard method to isolate exosomes from culture media or body fluid. Without ultracentrifuge, exosomes can be precipitated by polyethylene glycol or separated by size exclusion chromatography. After isolation, nanoparticle tracking analysis can help to estimate the size and concentration of exosome samples. Transmission electron microscopy can directly show the size and morphology of exosomes. Moreover, the sample should be characterized by the expression of several exosome biomarker proteins. Exosomal contents such as proteins and miRNAs could be profiled using appropriate technologies.

Key words Exosomes, Extracellular vesicles, Ultracentrifuge, Polyethylene glycol, Size exclusion chromatography, Transmission electron microscopy, Nanoparticle tracking analysis

1 Introduction

All cells can secrete membrane vesicles that carry proteins, DNA, RNA, lipids, and other cell information to the extracellular space [1]. Currently, there are two main categories, exosomes and microvesicles, characterized by their different biogenesis [1–3]. Exosomes are formed by the inward budding of the endosomal membrane and are secreted when the multivesicular endosomes fuse with the cell surface. Microvesicles are formed by outward budding and direct shedding of the plasma membrane [4–6]. The exosomes exist in all body fluids, including tears, aqueous humor, and vitreous humor in the eye [7, 8]. The contents in these vesicles may reveal the physiological condition of their origin cells and may interact with other target cells. A primary interest in this field is to examine vesicle contents to study their role as signaling vehicles. This chapter will describe the brief procedure for exosome isolation and characterization. There is no single optimal isolation method to isolate

Tatjana Jakobs and Paloma B. Liton (eds.), *Glaucoma: Methods and Protocols*, Methods in Molecular Biology, vol. 2858,
https://doi.org/10.1007/978-1-0716-4140-8_6,

exosomes. Depending on the study's downstream applications and specific aims, the investigators need to select an appropriate method matched to the study. The characterization of exosomes is fundamental for following steps, suggesting that findings result from isolated exosomes, not from cells, proteins, or lipids.

2 Materials

2.1 Preparation of Culture Media for Purification of Exosomes

1. Polyallomer or polycarbonate ultracentrifuge tubes.
2. Ultracentrifuge and fixed-angle or swinging-bucket rotors (*see* Table 1).
3. Fetal bovine serum (FBS).
4. Cell culture media: Dulbecco's Modified Eagle's Medium (DMEM) containing low glucose (1 mg/L), 2 mM L-glutamine, and antibiotics [0.5% gentamicin or penicillin (100 units/ml) and streptomycin (100 μg/ml)].
5. 0.22 μm vacuum filter sterilization apparatus
6. Sterile glass bottle (100 mL to 1 L).

2.2 Ultra-centrifugation of Fluid Samples

1. Biological samples, that is, culture media, aqueous humor, and vitreous humor.
2. 15 mL or 50 mL polypropylene centrifuge tubes
3. Refrigerated centrifuge.
4. Phosphate-buffered saline (PBS).
5. Polyallomer or polycarbonate ultracentrifuge tubes.
6. Ultracentrifuge and fixed-angle or swinging-bucket rotor (Table 1).
7. Two-sided balance.
8. Micropipettors.
9. −80 °C freezer.

Table 1
Ultracentrifuge rotor[a] information for exosome purification

Rotor (Thermo Fisher)	Tubes (Thermo Fisher)	Max vol/tube (mL)	Max RCF (×g)
TFT-80.4	Polyallomer Thin Wall	3.3	468,246
SureSpin 630 (17 mL)	Polyallomer Thin Wall	16	166,880
SureSpin 630 (36 mL)	Polyallomer Thin Wall	35	166,880
Fiberlite F40L-8 × 100	Polycarbonate bottle	76	213,000

[a]The ultracentrifuge is Thermo Fisher Sorvall WX Ultra 80

2.3 Precipitation with ExoQuick

1. ExoQuick-TC.
2. Conditional culture media: Collected from the cell culture, clarified by centrifugation.
3. 15 mL polypropylene centrifuge tubes
4. Countertop centrifuge.
5. Micropipettors.
6. Phosphate-buffered saline (PBS).

2.4 Characterization of Exosomes by Transmission Electron Microscopy (TEM)

1. 4% paraformaldehyde (PFA).
2. Formvar carbon-coated EM grids.
3. Phosphate-buffered saline (PBS).
4. Parafilm.
5. Forceps.
6. 1% glutaraldehyde solution in H_2O.
7. Distilled water.
8. Uranyl-oxalate solution, pH 7.0.
9. Glass dish.
10. Methyl cellulose-uranyl acetate solution, pH 4.0: Mix 2% methyl cellulose with 4% uranyl acetate at 9:1 ratio just before use.
11. Small stainless-steel loop (*see* **Note 1**).
12. Whatman no. 1 filter paper.
13. Transmission electron microscope.

2.5 Characterization of Exosomes by Immunoelectron Microscopy

1. Materials listed in Subheading 2.4.
2. 50 mM glycine solution in PBS
3. Blocking buffer: 5% BSA in PBS or 10% fetal calf serum in PBS.
4. Primary antibody and (optional) secondary antibody.
5. Wash buffer: 0.1% BSA in PBS or 0.1% fetal calf serum in PBS.
6. Protein A-gold conjugate.

2.6 Characterization of Exosomes by Nanoparticle Tracking Analysis

1. Zetaview PMX 120 and corresponding software or other nano-tracker device.
2. UltraPure distilled water.
3. 15 mL and 50 mL polypropylene centrifuge tubes
4. 1 mL and 5 mL syringes
5. Nanosphere size standards.
6. 1xPBS.

2.7 Characterization of Exosomes by Immunoblotting

1. Exosome pellet.
2. RIPA buffer.
3. Protease inhibitor.
4. 1.5 mL Eppendorf tube
5. Phosphate-buffered saline (PBS).
6. 4× Laemmli buffer
7. Primary antibodies against exosomal proteins: CD171, CD63, and CD9.
8. Standard reagents and equipment for total protein quantification and Western blotting.

3 Methods

3.1 Preparation of Exosome-Production Culture Media

It is well-known that the common culture media complement, fetal bovine serum (FBS), carries undefined exosomes that will interrupt the analysis of cell-derived exosomes. Therefore, it is necessary to remove FBS-derived exosomes in the culture media for exosome-related studies. There are four options to avoid FBS-derived exosome contamination:

1. If the cells can tolerate FBS-free media for the defined time, collect the exosomes from serum-free media.
2. Substitute FBS by bovine serum albumin (BSA),
3. Use commercial exosome-depleted media.
4. Prepare exosome-depleted media as follows:
   (a) Add FBS to serum-free culture media to make 20% FBS media (*see* **Note 2**).
   (b) Centrifuge this media overnight at 100,000× *g* at 4 °C.
   (c) Connect a 0.22 μm filter to the vacuum and put it on top of the sterile glass bottle. Filter the supernatant carefully without disturbing the pellet to produce sterile exosome-depleted culture media containing 20% FBS.
   (d) Add the exosome-depleted FBS media to serum-free media to reach the final FBS concentration (*see* **Note 3**). The final media or the exosome-depleted FBS media can be stored for up to 4 weeks at 4 °C.

3.2 Isolation of Exosomes by Ultracentrifugation

Serial ultracentrifugation is the general method to purify exosomes by centrifugation at increasing forces to eliminate potential contaminants at different weights (e.g., cells, dead cells, cell debris, proteins). Then the supernatant is centrifuged at ultrahigh speed (≥100,000× *g*) to pellet exosomes. We will describe the methods for ultracentrifugation of low-viscose fluid (i.e., conditioned culture media) and high-viscose fluid (i.e., aqueous humor, vitreous).

3.2.1 Ultracentrifugation of Low-Viscose Fluid

1. Collect culture media into 15 mL or 50 mL centrifuge tubes.
2. Centrifuge at 2000× *g* for 20 min at 4 °C.
3. Using a pipet, carefully transfer the supernatant to new tubes. Do not pour the supernatant. To ensure that the pellet is not disturbed, leave behind 0.5–1.0 cm of liquid above the pellet to avoid any contamination.
4. Centrifuge supernatant at 10,000× *g* for 30 min at 4 °C.
5. Using a pipet, carefully transfer the supernatant to the ultracentrifuge tubes appropriate for the rotor, without disturbing the pellet. The pellet may not be visible, so do not touch the side or bottom of the tube and stop removing supernatant when 0.5–1 cm of liquid is left behind.
6. Label each tube with the number of locations in the ultracentrifuge rotor.
7. On a two-sided balance, put two sample tubes that will be directly opposite in the ultracentrifuge rotor on each side. Add PBS to fill the tube and balance these paired samples. Repeat until all opposite samples are balanced (*see* **Note 4**).
8. Centrifuge at 100,000× *g* for 70 min at 4 °C.
9. Carefully remove supernatant using a pipette, leaving 2–5 mm of liquid above the bottom.
10. Resuspend the pellet in 1 mL PBS by pipetting up and down many times from the upper side toward bottom of the tube. If multiple tubes are used, pool the resuspended pellets into one tube. Then add PBS to fill the tube and balance opposite samples.
11. Centrifuge at 100,000× *g* for 70 min at 4 °C.
12. Remove most of the supernatants using a pipet. The remaining liquid is aspirated using a micropipettor. Slowly turn the tube downward and aspirate the liquid on the side of the tube.
13. Resuspend the pellet in 25–100 μL PBS or appropriate lysis buffer.
14. Store suspensions up to 1 year at −80 °C. Avoid multiple freezing and thawing cycles.

3.2.2 Ultracentrifugation of High-Viscous Fluid

1. Dilute biofluid with an equal volume of PBS and transfer to a 1.5 mL centrifuge tube (*see* **Note 5**).
2. Centrifuge at 2000× *g* for 30 min at 4 °C.
3. Using a micropipette, carefully transfer the supernatant, without disturbing the pellet, to a new 1.5 mL centrifuge tube.
4. Centrifuge supernatant at 12,000× *g* for 45 min at 4 °C.
5. Again, carefully transfer the supernatant to an ultracentrifuge tube appropriate for the rotor. Add PBS to fill the tube and to balance opposite samples.

6. Centrifuge at 110,000× *g* for 2 h at 4 °C.
7. Carefully remove the supernatant using a micropipettor and resuspend the pellet in 1 mL PBS. Add PBS to fill the tube and balance opposite samples.
8. Centrifuge at 100,000× *g* for 70 min at 4 °C.
9. Using a micropipettor, carefully remove the supernatant and resuspend the pellet in 25–100 μL PBS or appropriate lysis buffer.
10. Exosome suspensions can be stored for up to 1 year at −80 °C. Avoid repeated freezing and thawing.

3.3 Isolation of Exosomes by Sedimentation

Polyethylene glycol (PEG) has been used to purify viruses with similar biophysical properties to exosomes. Compared to ultracentrifugation, precipitation-based methods do not need specific equipment and produce visible pellets to avoid excessive loss. Many commercial kits mixed different molecular weights of PEG at various concentrations to precipitate particles between 30 and 200 nm. The higher PEG concentration will precipitate smaller particles, so 8% PEG is recommended to isolate culture media exosomes for downstream applications [9]. Here, we will describe isolation of exosomes using the commercially available kit, ExoQuick-TC, widely used in the exosome field.

1. Collect 5 mL culture media in a 15 mL tube.
2. Centrifuge 3000× *g* for 15 min to remove cells and cell debris.
3. Using a pipet, carefully transfer the supernatant to a new 15 mL tube. Add 1 mL of ExoQuick-TC and mix by inverting the tube several times.
4. Keep the tube upright and incubate overnight at 4 °C.
5. Centrifuge at 1500× *g* for 30 min.
6. Pour the supernatant and then centrifuge at 1500× *g* for 5 min.
7. Using a micropipettor, carefully remove the remaining fluid without disturbing the pellet.
8. Resuspend the exosome pellet in 100–500 μL PBS or an appropriate lysis buffer.
9. Store suspensions for up to a year at −80 °C. Avoid multiple freezing and thawing cycles.

3.4 Characterization of Exosome by Electron Microscopy

The major biophysical characteristic of exosomes is the nanometer size, which is too small to be detected by a stereo microscope. Therefore, transmission electron microscopy (TEM) is the primary choice to observe the morphology of exosomes. Since other small particles have similar sizes as exosomes, the expression of protein markers that indicate vesicle origin is crucial and can be detected by immunoelectron microscopy, described in Subheading 3.5.

1. Mix the exosome suspension with an equal volume of 4% paraformaldehyde (PFA) (*see* **Note 6**).
2. Pipet 5 μL of exosome/2% PFA solution onto several Formvar-coated EM grids. It is better to have 2–3 replicates for each sample. Cover the grid and let the membrane absorb for 20 min in a dry area (*see* **Note 7**).
3. Pipet 100 μL of PBS on a sheet of parafilm. Using clean forceps, carefully transfer the grid (membrane side down) onto the PBS to wash.
4. Pipet 50 μL of the 1% glutaraldehyde solution onto a sheet of parafilm. Then, carefully transfer the grid onto the solution for 5 min.
5. Pipet 100 μL of distilled water onto a sheet of parafilm. Then carefully transfer the grid onto the water for 2 min to wash. Change the distilled water on the parafilm, and rinse again. Repeat for a total of eight washes.
6. Pipet 50 μL of the uranyl-oxalate solution (pH 7) onto a sheet of parafilm. Then carefully transfer the grid onto the solution for 5 min.
7. Place a glass dish on ice. Place a sheet of parafilm onto the cold glass surface. Add 50 μL of methyl cellulose-uranyl acetate solution (pH 4) onto the parafilm. Carefully transfer the grid onto the solution and incubate on a cold surface for 10 min.
8. Carefully remove the EM grid using the stainless-steel loop. Then blot excess liquid by gently pushing the loop to the Whatman no. 1 filter paper at a 90° angle and slowly drag the loop across the filter paper. Stop and lift the loop before the remaining liquid is completely absorbed by the filter paper, so a thin film is left behind over the exosome side of the grid (*see* **Note 8**).
9. Air-dry the grid in the stainless-steel loop at room temperature for 5–10 min.
10. The grids can be stored for many years in an appropriate grid storage box.
11. Examine the prepared grids under the TEM at 80 kV. Exosomes will appear as round-shaped vesicles with a diameter of 40–150 nm (*see* **Note 9**).

3.5 Characterization of Exosome by Immuno-EM

1. Mix the exosome suspension with an equal volume of 4% PFA.
2. Pipet 5 μl of the exosome/2% PFA solution onto several Formvar-coated EM grids. It is better to have 2–3 replicates for each sample. Cover the grid and let the membrane absorb for 20 min in a dry area.

3. Pipet 100 μL of PBS on a sheet of parafilm. Using clean forceps, carefully transfer the grid (membrane side down) onto the PBS to wash. Change the PBS on the parafilm, and wash for 3 min; repeat.
4. Pipet 100 μL of the 50 mM glycine/PBS solution onto a sheet of parafilm. Then carefully transfer the grid onto the solution and incubate for 3 min. Repeat with fresh solution for a total of four washes (*see* **Note 10**).
5. Pipet 100 μL of the blocking buffer onto a sheet of parafilm. Then carefully transfer the grid onto the buffer and incubate for 10 min (*see* **Note 11**).
6. Pipet 5 μL of the appropriate diluted primary antibody onto a sheet of parafilm. Then carefully transfer the grid onto this solution and incubate for 30 min (*see* **Note 12**).
7. Pipet 100 μL of the wash buffer onto a sheet of parafilm. Then carefully transfer the grid onto the buffer for 3 min. Repeat with fresh wash buffer for a total of six washes. Do not let samples to dry out to avoid high-background or nonspecific staining.
8. (Optional) If a secondary antibody is necessary, repeat **steps 7** and **8** using the appropriately diluted secondary antibody.
9. Pipet 5 μL of the appropriate diluted protein A-gold conjugate onto a sheet of parafilm. Then carefully transfer the grid onto this solution and incubate for 20 min (*see* **Note 13**).
10. Pipet 100 μL PBS onto a sheet of parafilm. Carefully transfer the EM grid to PBS and wash for 3 min. Repeat using fresh PBS for a total of eight washes.
11. Pipet 50 μL of the 1% glutaraldehyde onto a sheet of parafilm. Then carefully transfer the grid onto the solution and incubate for 5 min to stabilize the immunoreaction.
12. Pipet 100 μL distilled water onto a sheet of parafilm. Then carefully transfer the grid onto the water and wash for 3 min. Repeat using fresh drops of water for a total of eight washes (*see* **Note 14**).
13. Contrast and embed the grids as described in Subheading 3.4, **steps 6** through **10**.
14. Examine the prepared grids under the TEM at 80 kV (Fig. 1c).

3.6 Characterization of Exosomes by Nanoparticle Tracking Analysis (NTA)

The nanoparticle tracking analysis (NTA) is designed to measure the size distribution of the exosome sample for quick validation of isolated particles. It tracks each particle's Brownian motion and calculates the particle's diameter by assuming it is perfectly spherical in the solution. This method can be valuable for quantifying exosomes, potentially reducing the bias measurement and making

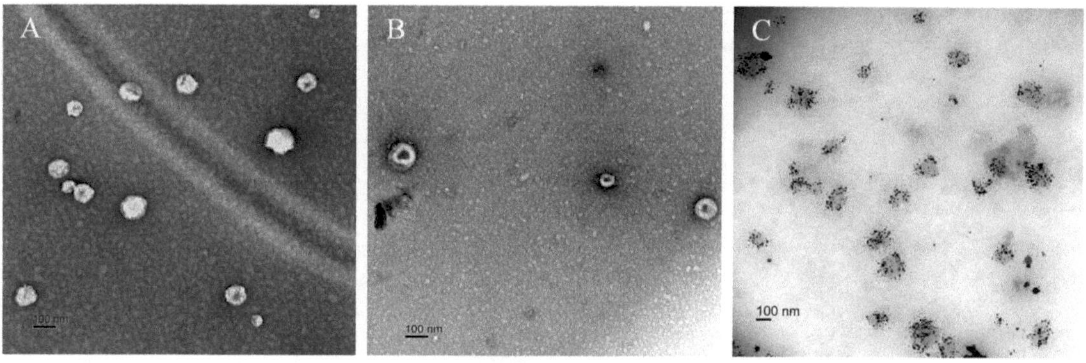

Fig. 1 The characteristics of exosomes with transmission electron microscopy. (**a**) Round-shaped exosomes. (**b**) Cup-shaped exosomes. (**c**) Immunogold labeling of CD171 molecules (10 nm gold particles). Scale bar = 100 nm

results more repeatable. Two major pieces of equipment are used in research: Nanosight and Zetaview [10, 11]. Even with the same equipment, each lab may have its preference of parameters based on its targets and experiences. Here are the experimental steps with a ZetaView PMX120 system.

1. Turn on the machine and start the software on the connected computer.
2. Follow the instruction to load 5 mL distilled water for cell check. If the result is not good, clean the cell before use.
3. Dilute 35 μL Nanosphere size standards in 10 mL distilled water to make standard #1. Invert the 15 mL tube to mix thoroughly.
4. Further dilute 10 μL of standard #1 in 10 mL distilled water to make standard #2. Invert the 15 mL tube to mix thoroughly.
5. Load 2 mL standard #2 into the cell. Input the dilution factor 285,700 in the software. Check the drift speed. If the particle number is below the green level, add more Nanosphere in standard #1. If the number is too high, reduce Nanosphere in standard #1 (*see* **Note 15**).
6. Once the drift speed is within the range, optimize the camera focus. If the focus optimization fails, then run an autoalignment to calibrate the camera and laser locations.
7. Use the preferred parameters to run a standard. The size should be about 100 ± 10 nm. If the size standard is out of range, repeat focus optimization or auto-alignment.
8. Flush the cell with PBS until the background particles ≤10. If large microparticles are detected in the PBS, filter through a 0.22um filter to clear the solution. If many small particles are still in the PBS after filtration, the authors suggest using commercially filtered PBS (*see* **Note 16**).

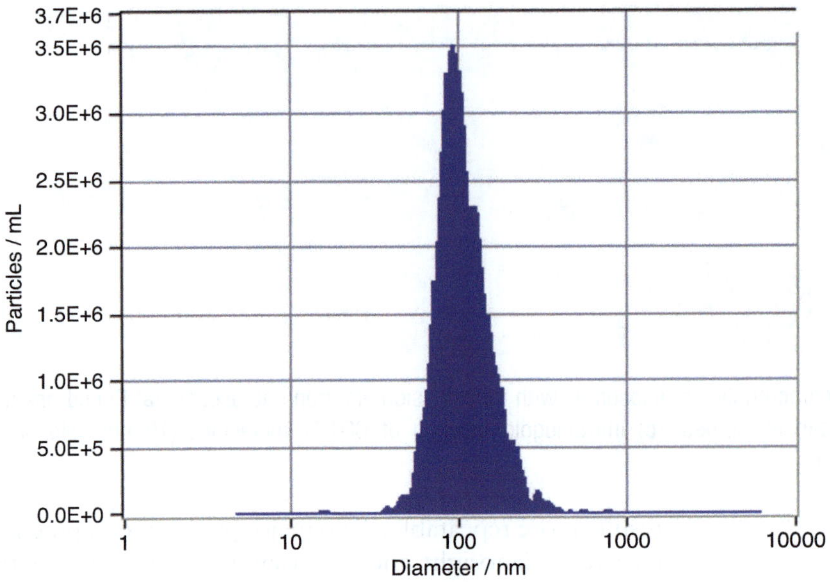

Fig. 2 The size distribution of an exosome sample reported by Zetaview software. Majority of particles detected by Zetaview distribute in the size range 70–170 nm. The peak is 93 nm

9. Dilute exosome suspension in PBS to make 1 mL solution and load it into the ZetaView cell. Input the dilution factor in the software.
10. If the first dilution was in the upper recommendation limit, dilute a smaller portion of the exosome in PBS. If the first dilution was close to the lower limit for an accurate particle count, dilute a larger portion of the exosome solution in PBS.
11. Flush the cell with PBS and load the newly diluted sample. Change the dilution factor in the software.
12. Once the drift speed is within the range, use the preferred parameters to run the sample (Fig. 2). If the sample is too concentrated, either dilute the original exosomes or use serial dilution to avoid pipetting bias. At least 2 μL exosome suspension should be taken for measurement.

3.7 Characterization of Exosomes by Immunoblotting

Exosome samples can be sent to a proteomics core facility to profile and analyze protein components. Several proteins were consistently identified in exosomes from various cell sources [12]. The identification of these common proteins can characterize isolated vesicles as exosomes. Immunoblotting is a convenient method to validate the expression of these proteins (Fig. 3).

1. Resuspend exosome pellet in ice-cold RIPA buffer with protease inhibitor.
2. Transfer the suspension to a 1.5 mL Eppendorf tube. Exosomal lysate can be stored for up to 4 weeks at −80 °C for future analysis.

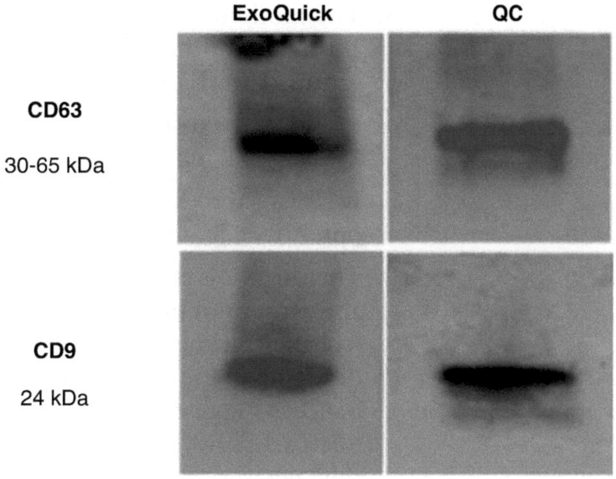

Fig. 3 Western blot analysis [adapted from Helwa et al. (2017) [11]] of CD63 and CD9 expression in exosome samples derived from human serum

3. Quantify the total protein concentration in exosome samples.
4. Prepare 10 μg total protein in the tube.
5. Add PBS to adjust the final volume to 18 μL.
6. Add 6 μL of 4 × Laemmli buffer. Vortex to mix.
7. Heat tubes at 95 °C for 8 min.
8. Load samples onto a 10% or 12% SDS-PAGE gel.
9. Run the gel, transfer proteins to a nylon membrane, and analyze exosome marker proteins using the specific antibody following standard Western blotting techniques.

4 Notes

1. The loop can be handmade by wrapping a stainless-steel wire around a P1000 pipette tip. The inner diameter of the loop should be slightly larger than the outer diameter of the EM grid.
2. Do not deplete FBS directly. Due to the high viscosity, depletion will eliminate many proteins and factors in the aggregated pellets, making the media lack nutrients.
3. For example, to prepare a 10% complete media, mix exosome-depleted 20% FBS media and serum-free media 1:1.
4. For example, if the rotor can load six samples, then sample 1 is directly opposite to sample 4. All tubes should be three-fourths full for this high-speed centrifugation.

5. The biofluid sample collected from the eye is usually less than 1 mL. For other large volumes of viscous biofluids, such as serum, 15 mL or 50 mL centrifuge tubes can be applied.
6. The mixed exosome/2% PFA solution can be stored for up to 1 week at 4 °C.
7. It is crucial to keep the membrane side of the grid wet but the opposite side dry.
8. The thickness of methyl cellulose film impacts the final contrast and structural preservation. The speed of absorption can control the thickness. If the no. 1 filter paper does not work well, different grade Whatman filter paper with a different absorbance is suggested. The thickness can be assessed under a stereo microscope. A blue-gold color is indicative of an optimum thickness.
9. The cup-shaped morphology is currently considered an artifact during the EM preparation process. The advanced technique of cryoelectron microscopy reveals round membrane vesicles (Fig. 1). EM can be used to measure the size of isolated particles. However, it takes a lot of effort and introduces bias to characterize the size and concentration distribution of the entire sample. EM is recommended as a quality control for particle isolation.
10. This solution quenches free aldehyde groups. 50 mM ammonium chloride (NH_4Cl) in PBS can be an alternative.
11. For all remaining immunolabeling steps, all diluents and washing buffers should contain the same proteins chosen for the blocking buffer.
12. Each antibody has different characteristics. Generally, test the antibody range between 2 and 20 μg/mL. All buffers should be freshly prepared, and antibody dilutions can be kept from 1 week to 1 month.
13. 10-nm gold particles are generally used for single labeling.
14. Double or triple labeling can be accomplished by repeating **steps 3** through **13**. A different size gold particle must be used (i.e., 10 nm and then 15 nm and then 25 nm) to distinguish the stained proteins.
15. It usually takes less than 5 min to equilibrate in the cell. However, if the sample temperature is too high (e.g., 37 °C), the Brownian motion will be vigorous and challenging to calibrate. Therefore, the authors suggest measuring exosome samples at 23–25 °C.
16. Since there are electrolytes in PBS, nanoparticles may aggregate over time. The authors suggest changing to a new bottle for exosome experiments after one month of opening.

Acknowledgments

The authors and the research have been supported by NIH grants P30EY031631, R01EY023242, R01EY032960, R21EY033961, and R21EY028671 and the Glaucoma Foundation, the Glaucoma Research Foundation, and the BrightFocus Foundation.

References

1. Colombo M, Raposo G, Thery C (2014) Biogenesis, secretion, and intercellular interactions of exosomes and other extracellular vesicles. Annu Rev Cell Dev Biol 30:255–289
2. Yanez-Mo M et al (2015) Biological properties of extracellular vesicles and their physiological functions. J Extracell Vesicles 4:27066
3. Raposo G, Stoorvogel W (2013) Extracellular vesicles: exosomes, microvesicles, and friends. J Cell Biol 200(4):373–383
4. van Niel G, D'Angelo G, Raposo G (2018) Shedding light on the cell biology of extracellular vesicles. Nat Rev Mol Cell Biol 19(4): 213–228
5. Tricarico C, Clancy J, D'Souza-Schorey C (2017) Biology and biogenesis of shed microvesicles. Small GTPases 8(4):220–232
6. Thery C, Zitvogel L, Amigorena S (2002) Exosomes: composition, biogenesis and function. Nat Rev Immunol 2(8):569–579
7. Dismuke WM et al (2015) Human aqueous humor exosomes. Exp Eye Res 132:73–77
8. Zhao Y et al (2018) Liquid biopsy of vitreous reveals an abundant vesicle population consistent with the size and morphology of exosomes. Transl Vis Sci Technol 7(3):6
9. Rider MA, Hurwitz SN, Meckes DG Jr (2016) ExtraPEG: a polyethylene glycol-based method for enrichment of extracellular vesicles. Sci Rep 6:23978
10. Bachurski D et al (2019) Extracellular vesicle measurements with nanoparticle tracking analysis – an accuracy and repeatability comparison between NanoSight NS300 and ZetaView. J Extracell Vesicles 8(1):1596016
11. Helwa I et al (2017) A comparative study of serum exosome isolation using differential ultracentrifugation and three commercial reagents. PLoS One 12(1):e0170628
12. Thery C et al (2018) Minimal information for studies of extracellular vesicles 2018 (MISEV2018): a position statement of the International Society for Extracellular Vesicles and update of the MISEV2014 guidelines. J Extracell Vesicles 7(1):1535750

Chapter 7

Time-Lapse Live-Cell Imaging Using Fluorescent Protein Sensors in Outflow Pathway Cells Under Fluid Flow Conditions

Myoung Sup Shim and Paloma B. Liton

Abstract

The role of shear stress in regulating aqueous humor (AH) outflow and intraocular pressure (IOP) in the trabecular meshwork (TM) and Schlemm's canal (SC) of the eye is an emerging field. Shear stress has been shown to activate mechanosensitive ion channels in TM cells and induce nitric oxide production in SC cells, which can affect outflow resistance and lower IOP. Live-cell imaging using fluorescent protein sensors has provided real-time data to investigate the physiological relationship between fluid flow and shear stress in the outflow pathway cells. The successful application of time-lapse live-cell imaging in primary cultured cells has led to the identification of key cellular and molecular mechanisms involved in regulating AH outflow and IOP, including the role of autophagy and primary cilia as mechanosensors. This chapter presents a detailed protocol for conducting time-lapse live-cell imaging under fluid flow conditions in the outflow pathway cells.

Key words Conventional outflow pathway, Fluorescent protein sensor, Schlemm's canal, Time-lapse live-cell imaging, Trabecular meshwork, Fluid flow, Shear stress

1 Introduction

The trabecular meshwork (TM) and Schlemm's canal (SC) are critical structures in the eye responsible for regulating the outflow of aqueous humor (AH) and maintaining intraocular pressure (IOP). As aqueous humor flows through the TM and SC, it exerts a force on the surrounding cells and extracellular matrix, generating shear stress, defined as the force that is parallel to a surface exerted by a fluid as it flows over that surface. In the TM, shear stress has been shown to activate mechanosensitive ion channels, which can modulate cellular signaling and affect outflow resistance. The flow of AH through the SC generates shear stress on the endothelial cells lining the inner wall of the vessel, which is intensified with increasing IOP and collapse of the SC lumen. Localized regions of high

Tatjana Jakobs and Paloma B. Liton (eds.), *Glaucoma: Methods and Protocols*, Methods in Molecular Biology, vol. 2858, https://doi.org/10.1007/978-1-0716-4140-8_7,

shear stress are also observed in the areas near the collector channels downstream of the SC. SC cells respond to shear stress by rearranging the actin architecture and producing nitric oxide (NO), which has been shown to increase AH outflow and lower IOP in mouse and human eyes. However, the physiological relationship between fluid flow and shear stress in the TM and SC is an emerging field. Recently, we have successfully applied time-lapse real-time live-cell imaging analysis to fluid flow studies.

Live-cell imaging technique has been an invaluable tool for current biological and biomedical science. Since green fluorescent protein (GFP) is firstly used to monitor gene expression and protein localization in living organisms [1], which enabled GFP to win the Nobel prize in 2008 in Chemistry [2], GFP and its derivatives have been intensively used for the live-cell imaging system, resolving cellular and molecular process spatiotemporally in more detail [3]. Currently, this technique has been applied for investigating not only gene expression and subcellular localization but also signaling pathway and metabolic activities [4]. The successful application of time-lapse live-cell imaging to our studies has provided valuable real-time data in the primary cultured cells from the conventional outflow pathway. So far, this technique has led us to demonstrate the role of nuclear localization of LC3, autophagy marker proteins [5], and autophagy as regulator of transforming growth factor (TGF)β/SMAD-induced fibrogenesis in TM cells [6] as well as the role of primary cilia, a nonmotile cell protrusion from cell surface, as a mechanosensor responsible for mechanical stress-induced autophagy in TM cells [7]. In this chapter, we introduce our technique and provide more detailed protocol to monitor to conduct time-lapse live-cell imaging in outflow pathway cells under fluid flow conditions using fluorescent protein sensors.

2 Materials

2.1 Cell Culture Materials

1. Primary cultures of human TM and/or SC cells: isolated from human donor cadaver eyes, cultured, and characterized as previously described [8–12].
2. Cell culture media: Low-glucose Dulbecco's modified Eagle's medium (DMEM) supplemented with 10% fetal bovine serum (FBS), 1% Penicillin-streptomycin, 1% nonessential amino acids, and 50 μg/mL Gentamycin.
3. Phosphate-buffered saline (PBS).
4. Hank's Balanced Salt Solution (HBSS).
5. Tissue culture dishes/plates or cell culture flasks.
6. μ-Slide VI $^{0.4}$ and μ-slides I $^{0.6}$ Luer,

7. Optical Bottom 96-Well Cell Culture Microplate.
8. Conventional CO_2 incubator set at 37 °C for cell culture and CO_2 gas.

2.2 Transfection and Transduction Materials

1. Fluorescence probe: expressed in either plasmid constructs or recombinant virus (*see* **Note 1**).
2. 1 M HEPES (pH 7.0 ~ 7.6)
3. 0.3 M $CaCl_2$
4. 2X HBS: 280 mM NaCl, 1.5 mM Na_2HPO_4, and 50 mM HEPES
5. NanoDrop ™ spectrophotometer or a comparable device.
6. TC-20™ automated cell counter or a comparable device.

2.3 Real-Time Fluid Flow Imaging System

1. CELENA® X High Content Imaging System equipped with high-power light-emitting diode (LED) filters (*see* **Note 2**).
2. Ibidi Stage Top Incubation System, Universal Fit, for 1 Chamber, CO_2/O_2—Blue Line (10722, ibidi) or Heating System, Multi-Well Plates, K-Frame—Blue Line (10929, ibidi).
3. Ibidi Pump System.
4. Transfer tubing.
5. BriskHeat INSUL78 INSUL-LOCK DS Flexible Pipe Insulation, Closed Cell, For 1/2″ diameter pipe, 6 ft. long.
6. Air Jacketed CO_2 Incubator, Mini.
7. CO_2 gas.
8. FIJI.

3 Methods

All procedures with human TM and SC cells should be carried out under sterile conditions in a biological safety cabinet before being placed within the stage incubator.

3.1 Expression of Fluorescent Probe in TM and/or SC Cultured Cells

3.1.1 Plasmid Transfection Using Calcium/Phosphate (See Note 3)

1. Plate primary human TM and SC cells and culture at 80% confluence on the one well of 6-well plate in 2 mL volume of the growth medium in the day of transfection.
2. Dissolve 5 μg plasmid expressing the fluorescence protein in 167 μL of 0.3 M $CaCl_2$ using 1.5 mL tube and mix well by pipetting.
3. Add the DNA/$CaCl_2$ mixtures dropwise to equal volume of 2xHBS and mix gently by repeated pipetting (*see* **Note 4**).
4. Add DNA/$CaCl_2$/HBS suspensions immediately to the plate containing cells in a dropwise fashion and swirl the plate gently.

5. Incubate the cells at 37 °C, 5% CO_2 for 6 h. Meanwhile, equilibrate 5 mL of cell growth medium at 10% CO_2, 37 °C (*see* **Note 5**).
6. Remove the cell culture medium from transfected cells and wash with PBS one time.
7. Add 2 mL preequilibrated medium in a 10% CO_2 to the cells and incubate the cells at 37 °C, 10% CO_2 for 30 min to remove the DNA-calcium-phosphate precipitates from the cell surface (*see* **Note 6**). Repeat the process if DNA-calcium-phosphate precipitates were not properly removed.
8. Replace the cells with original growth medium and incubate at 37 °C, 5% CO_2 for 24 ~ 72 h to allow transgene expression.

3.1.2 Adenovirus Transduction

Follow the biohazard procedures in accordance with the standard operating procedure (SOP) for the use of adenoviral vectors. Viral particles are kept at −80 °C and always keep viral particles on ice when use. Do not freeze and thaw the virus repeatedly to keep viral titer consistently (*see* **Note** 7).

1. Harvest cells grown in a culture dish.
2. Count cell number and resuspend ~2 x 10^5 cells in 400 μL of culture medium in a 15 mL centrifuge tube.
3. Calculate the viral volume required to achieve the desired multiplicity of infection (m.o.i.), and dilute the viral stock accordingly in 100 μL of culture medium (*see* **Note 8**).
4. Add 100 μL of diluted virus into the 15 mL centrifuge tube containing cells. Gently mix by repeating pipetting.
5. Let viral particles attach to the cell surface homogeneously for 2–5 min.
6. Add 1.5 mL of culture medium into the tube containing cells, mix by pipetting up and down, and transfer the cells into one well of a 6-well plate.
7. Incubate the cells at 37 °C, 5% CO_2 for 24–72 h.

3.1.3 Enhanced Adenovirus Transduction with Calcium-Phosphate (See Note 9)

1. Plate primary cultures of SC cells at 80% confluence onto one well of a 6-well plate in 2 mL culture medium and incubate at 37 °C, 5% CO_2 for 2 days.
2. Add 1 μL adenoviral particle (~1x10^{10} pfu/mL) to 167 μL of 0.3 M $CaCl_2$ in 1.5 mL tube and mix well by pipetting (*see* **Note 10**).
3. Add the adenovirus/$CaCl_2$ mixtures dropwise to equal volume and gently mix by pipetting up and down.

4. Immediately, add adenovirus/$CaCl_2$/HBS suspensions to the plate containing cells in a dropwise fashion, gently swirling the plate for even distribution.
5. Perform **steps 5–8** described in Subheading 3.1.1 and 3.2.

3.2 Setting Up the Live-Cell Fluid Flow Imaging System

The schematic diagram of whole system for long-term time-lapse live-cell imaging during shear stress is described in Fig. 1.

1. Set up the modified perfusion set, which contains an extended transfer tubing (100 cm) below a branched tubes for insertion in pinch valves, into the fluidic unit in a biological safety cabinet (*see* **Note 11**).
2. Set up the stage-top incubation station (37 °C, 5% CO_2) on the CELENA® X High Content Imaging System follows:
   2.1 Put the universal frame which contains single slider holder on microscope stage and adjust its position tightly.
   2.2 Connect it to an ibidi Gas Mixer CO_2/O_2 and an ibidi Temperature Controller, respectively.
   2.3 Open the CO_2 gas valve. Turn on air pressure generator and adjust pressure approximately 1.2 bar.
   2.4 Turn on the gas mixer and temperature controller. Then, set the flow rate, CO_2 concentration, humidity (Flow:10, CO_2%: 5, Hum%:80), and temperature for universal frame (Lid: 42 °C and Plate: 37 °C), respectively.

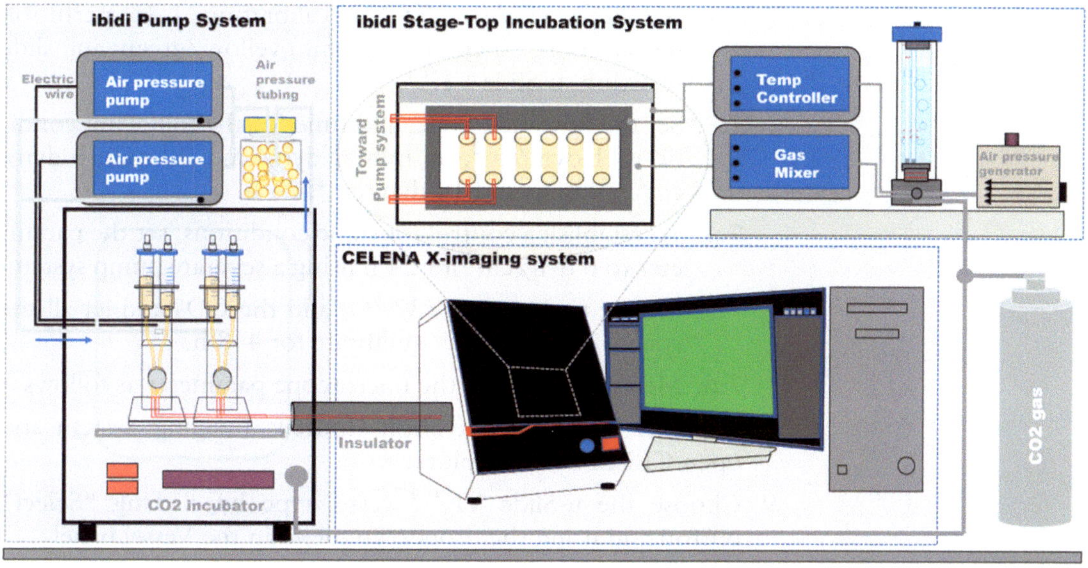

Fig. 1 Schematic diagram for long-term time-lapse live-cell imaging system during shear stress application

3.3 Realtime Image Acquisition Using Live-Cell Imaging System During Shear Stress

1. Plate 2×10^4 cells expressing the fluorescence probe onto one channel of a μ-Slide VI $^{0.4}$ in 30 μL of volume and incubate at 37 °C, 5% CO_2 for additional 72 h ~ 7 days until reaching 100% confluency (*see* **Note 12**).
2. Add 14 mL of culture medium to one of the syringes and allow to gravitationally flow through the tube being careful of not introducing any air bubble. When the medium reaches an opposite syringe and the volume of the medium is equilibrated in both syringes, place up the syringe to a higher level, and allow the medium to go back through the tube by gravity force. Repeat until no air bubbles are observed (*see* **Note 13**).
3. Within a biological safety cabinet, put the μ-Slide VI $^{0.4}$ containing cells into the slider holder, which is included in the ibidi Heating System, Universal Fit, and connect the extended transfer tubes from the fluidic unit into the slide.
4. Put the fluidic unit into the 37 °C, 5% CO_2 incubator, and the slider holder on a preequilibrated stage-top incubation station (37 °C, 5% CO_2).
5. Insulate the transfer tubing between the CO_2 incubator and the stage-top incubation station using insul-lock Ds flexible closed cell pipe insulation.
6. Connect the fluidic unit to the computer-controlled pump system.
7. Follow the steps below to set up the parameters in the ibidi PumpControl® software:
   - 7.1. Open the ibidi PumpControl® software.
   - 7.2. Set the parameters of the fluid unit to the following values as follows: viscosity, 0.0072; calibration, 1.36; perfusion set selection, 50 cm; ID, 1.6 mm yellow/green; and slide selection, μ-Slide VI $^{0.4}$.
   - 7.3. Set the flow rate, cycle, and time for the following conditions: 1 dyn/cm^2, 30 min; 2 dyn/cm^2, 30 min; 5 dyn/cm^2, 30 min; and 10 dyn/cm^2, 24 h.
   - 7.4. To establish a control for static conditions, set the parameter to 0 dyn/cm^2 for 24 h using a separate pump system.
   - 7.5. Set the temperature (37 °C) and the CO_2 and let all the system components equilibrate for 4–8 h.
   - 7.6. Meanwhile, set up the microscope parameter as follows.
8. Turn on CELENA® X High Content Imaging System and open CELENA® X Explore.
9. Choose the μ-Slide VI $^{0.4}$ vessel type by clicking "Select" button and using the dropdown menu in the Vessel panel.

10. Select well positions and fields of interest in the slide, using map for Vessel and Well in the Vessel panel.
11. Select Objective (40X), channel, and adjust the values of Gain (25 ~ 30), Light (200 ~ 600), and Exposure (200–600) in the CHANNEL panel (*see* **Note 14**).
12. Select a field of interest and adjust the fine focus in the Focus Sub-panel, click Multiscan AF, and select autofocus frequency to Every Field. Check Laser AF and click Prescan button. If the focus is good, click OK.
13. Designate an appropriate total time and interval for live imaging (i.e., total time, 1 h, and interval, 5 s) in the TimeLaps subpanel.
14. Apply all parameters by clicking "Add" button in the CHANNEL panel. And click +Create project button to make a project file. Designate file path, name, and save (*see* **Note 15**).
15. Click "Start" button in the ibidi PumpControl® software to initiate the flow experiment.
16. Click "Run" button in the CELENA® X Explore to start live-cell imaging.

3.4 Image Analysis by Using Fiji

1. Import the image sequence obtained in Subheading 3.3. into the Fiji software by clicking File-Image-Image sequence.
2. Designate pseudocolor to the image sequence by clicking Image-Lookup Table-Color (i.e., cyan).
3. Select the image portion that contains your area of interest (i.e., the primary cilium in our example in Fig. 2) using select tools, and crop the portion by clicking Image-Crop.
4. Set the image scale by clicking Analyze-Set Scale (Distance in pixel: 1, known distance, 0.1465; pixel distance ratio, 1; unit of length, um) (*see* **Note 16**).
5. Add scale bar and time information by clicking Analyze-Tools-Scale bar and Images-Stacks-Label, respectively (*see* **Note 17**).
6. Save the file by clicking File-Save as-Tiff for the analysis of individual photo and -AVI for making video file.

4 Notes

1. Although not described here, fluorescence dyes can be additionally used.
2. Here we describe our fluid flow imaging system setup, which was built based on the compatibility between Celena imaging system, Ibidi pump, and Ibidi stage Incubator. Similar systems can be used.

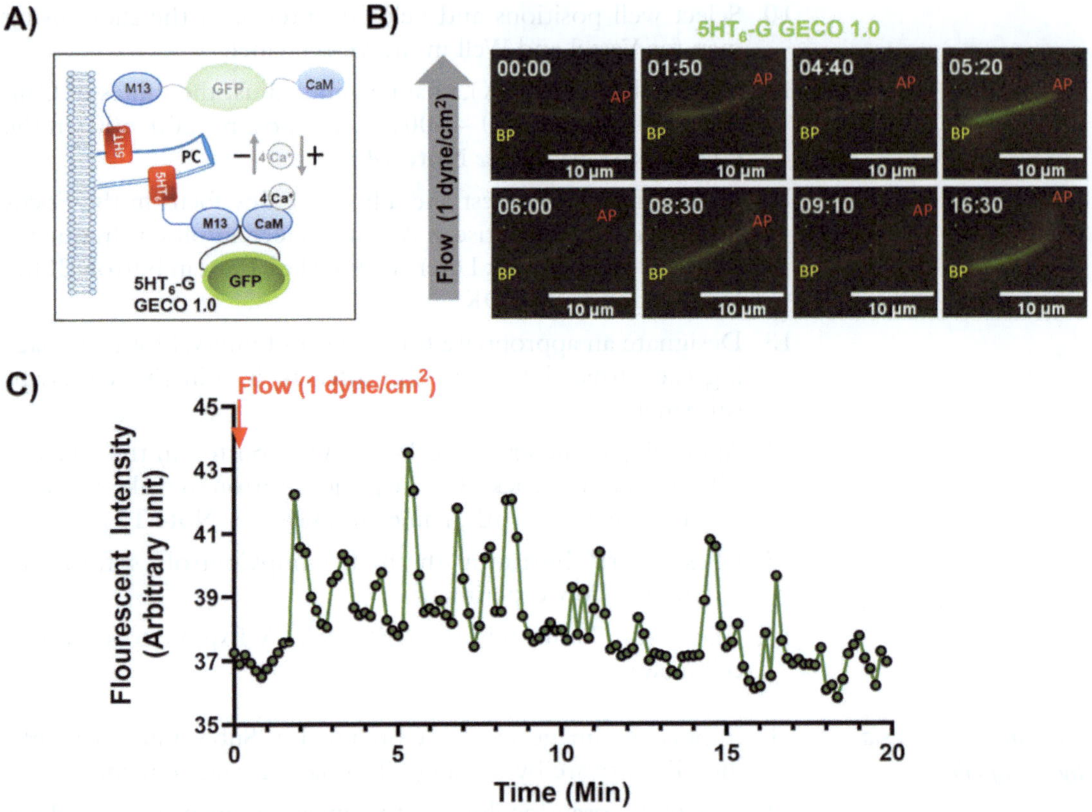

Fig. 2 Real-time live-cell imaging for Ca^{2+} signaling pathway in PC of TM. (**a**) Schematic diagram of $5HT_6$-G GECO 1.0 (**a**) gift from Dr. Takanari Inoue, Addgene plasmid no. 47499; www.addgene.org/ 47499/; RRID: Addgene_47499). Representative images (**b**) and quantitative graph (**c**) for intracellular Ca^{2+} amount in PC upon shear stress. *AP, BP*: apical, basal process. Scale bars:10 μm. min:sec

3. Plasmid transfection efficiency is extremely low in primary human TM and SC cells compared to viral transduction.
4. It is critical to mix gently the DNA/$CaCl_2$ solution with HBS buffer to produce a homogeneous snow-like precipitate (optimal particle size 1–3 μm) [13]. Rapid mixing the whole volume of the mixture makes nonhomogenous mixture containing the large size of DNA-calcium-phosphate precipitates.
5. Monitor the size of the DNA-calcium-phosphate precipitates attached to cell surface using microscope during this time; large precipitates reduce the transection efficiency.
6. The slight acidic conditions of 10% CO_2-equilibriated medium help to dissolve the excessive DNA-calcium-phosphate precipitates which causes cytotoxicity to the cells [13].
7. The efficiency of adenoviral transduction into TM cells is high and lower for SC cells. In this latter, the methods can be adapted for the transduction of lentiviruses.

8. The optimal m.o.i. of adenovirus for live-cell imaging in TM cells is 5–10 pfu/cell.
9. The authors recommend this method for adenoviral transduction of SC cells, which are more resilient to productive adenoviral infection.
10. The volume of virus particle is dependent on the original virus titer.
11. Refer the instruction manual of ibidi pump system for the detailed procedure.
12. Incubation periods are dependent on the purpose of the experiments. For the shear stress experiment, usually, long incubation periods are recommended [14].
13. To avoid forming air bubbles, first clip the middle part of both branched tube and allow the medium to go through the extended transfer tubing and reach to an opposite syringe. When the whole part of extended transfer tubing is filled up with the medium, remove the clip and fill up the remaining part with same way.
14. These are the parameters used, for example, in Fig. 2. The optimum values of Light, Gain, and Exposure are dependent on the fluorescence signal intensity of the probe expressed in the cells. Generally, for the long-time live-cell imaging, high Gain, low Light, and low Exposure values are recommended.
15. The project file and whole images taken during live-cell imaging will be saved in the folder.
16. The length of 1 pixel is 5.86 μm and the image size is 1600X1200 for the CELENA X Imaging System. When different magnification objectives are used, calculate the length of 1 pixel accordingly (i.e., 4X, 1.465; 20X, 0.293 μm; etc.).
17. The parameters are dependent on each experiment (i.e., time format, 00:00:00-hh: mm: ss; starting value, 0; time interval, 5).

Acknowledgments

Funding was provided by the National Institutes of Health, Eye Institute (EY026885, EY033600, EY005722), Glaucoma Research Foundation (2022 Shaffer Grant), BrightFocus Foundation (G2022010S), and Unrestricted Research to Prevent Blindness Grant.

References

1. Chalfie M, Tu Y, Euskirchen G, Ward WW, Prasher DC (1994) Green fluorescent protein as a marker for gene expression. Science 263(5148):802–805. https://doi.org/10.1126/science.8303295
2. Swaminathan S (2009) GFP: the green revolution. Nat Cell Biol 11(S1):S20–S20. https://doi.org/10.1038/ncb1953
3. Rodriguez EA, Campbell RE, Lin JY, Lin MZ, Miyawaki A, Palmer AE, Shu X, Zhang J, Tsien RY (2017) The growing and glowing toolbox of fluorescent and photoactive proteins. Trends Biochem Sci 42(2):111–129. https://doi.org/10.1016/j.tibs.2016.09.010
4. Depaoli MR, Bischof H, Eroglu E, Burgstaller S, Ramadani-Muja J, Rauter T, Schinagl M, Waldeck-Weiermair M, Hay JC, Graier WF, Malli R (2019) Live cell imaging of signaling and metabolic activities. Pharmacol Ther 202:98–119. https://doi.org/10.1016/j.pharmthera.2019.06.003
5. Shim MS, Nettesheim A, Hirt J, Liton PB (2020) The autophagic protein LC3 translocates to the nucleus and localizes in the nucleolus associated to NUFIP1 in response to cyclic mechanical stress. Autophagy 16(7): 1248–1261. https://doi.org/10.1080/15548627.2019.1662584
6. Nettesheim A, Shim MS, Hirt J, Liton PB (2019) Transcriptome analysis reveals autophagy as regulator of TGFbeta/Smad-induced fibrogenesis in trabecular meshwork cells. Sci Rep 9(1):16092. https://doi.org/10.1038/s41598-019-52627-2
7. Shim MS, Nettesheim A, Dixon A, Liton PB (2021) Primary cilia and the reciprocal activation of AKT and SMAD2/3 regulate stretch-induced autophagy in trabecular meshwork cells. Proc Natl Acad Sci USA 118(13). https://doi.org/10.1073/pnas.2021942118
8. Stamer WD, Roberts BC, Howell DN, Epstein DL (1998) Isolation, culture, and characterization of endothelial cells from Schlemm's canal. Invest Ophthalmol Vis Sci 39(10):1804–1812
9. Perkumas KM, Stamer WD (2012) Protein markers and differentiation in culture for Schlemm's canal endothelial cells. Exp Eye Res 96(1):82–87. https://doi.org/10.1016/j.exer.2011.12.017
10. Stamer WD, Seftor RE, Williams SK, Samaha HA, Snyder RW (1995) Isolation and culture of human trabecular meshwork cells by extracellular matrix digestion. Curr Eye Res 14(7): 611–617
11. Stamer WD, Clark AF (2017) The many faces of the trabecular meshwork cell. Exp Eye Res 158:112–123. https://doi.org/10.1016/j.exer.2016.07.009
12. Keller KE, Bhattacharya SK, Borras T, Brunner TM, Chansangpetch S, Clark AF, Dismuke WM, Du Y, Elliott MH, Ethier CR, Faralli JA, Freddo TF, Fuchshofer R, Giovingo M, Gong H, Gonzalez P, Huang A, Johnstone MA, Kaufman PL, Kelley MJ, Knepper PA, Kopczynski CC, Kuchtey JG, Kuchtey RW, Kuehn MH, Lieberman RL, Lin SC, Liton P, Liu Y, Lutjen-Drecoll E, Mao W, Masis-Solano M, McDonnell F, McDowell CM, Overby DR, Pattabiraman PP, Raghunathan VK, Rao PV, Rhee DJ, Chowdhury UR, Russell P, Samples JR, Schwartz D, Stubbs EB, Tamm ER, Tan JC, Toris CB, Torrejon KY, Vranka JA, Wirtz MK, Yorio T, Zhang J, Zode GS, Fautsch MP, Peters DM, Acott TS, Stamer WD (2018) Consensus recommendations for trabecular meshwork cell isolation, characterization and culture. Exp Eye Res 171:164–173. https://doi.org/10.1016/j.exer.2018.03.001
13. Jiang M, Chen G (2006) High Ca2+-phosphate transfection efficiency in low-density neuronal cultures. Nat Protoc 1(2):695–700. https://doi.org/10.1038/nprot.2006.86
14. Ashpole NE, Overby DR, Ethier CR, Stamer WD (2014) Shear stress-triggered nitric oxide release from Schlemm's canal cells. Invest Ophthalmol Vis Sci 55(12):8067–8076. https://doi.org/10.1167/iovs.14-14722

Chapter 8

Human Anterior Segment Perfusion Organ Culture

Uttio Roy Chowdhury and Michael P. Fautsch

Abstract

The human anterior segment perfusion organ culture is an ex vivo model system for studying the human conventional outflow pathway with reference to pressure regulation. In this model, anterior segments dissected from human donor eyes can be fixed to a modified petri dish and perfused with media along with various study agents at the physiological flow rate of 2.5 μL/min. The model mimics the one-way flow of aqueous humor in human eyes and can be used to evaluate the effects of various drugs on eye pressure in real time. Using this model, cells and tissues of the anterior segment can be maintained for up to 28 days, enabling histological and molecular evaluations.

Key words Anterior segment perfusion culture, Ex vivo eye culture, Perfusion organ culture, Trabecular meshwork, Conventional outflow, Distal outflow

1 Introduction

Glaucoma is a progressive neurodegenerative eye disorder that affects nearly 80 million people worldwide [1–4]. While family history, advanced age, and diabetes are linked to the disease, the most prevalent risk factor is elevated intraocular pressure (IOP). All therapeutic modalities for treating glaucoma are aimed at lowering IOP, even in subtypes of the disease where IOP is normal. Understanding how IOP is generated and defining the mechanisms associated with its regulation are important for future development of novel and more effective treatment modalities.

IOP is generated by the balance between formation of aqueous humor from the ciliary body and removal through either the uveoscleral or the conventional outflow pathway. The uveoscleral pathway is nonpressure dependent in that aqueous humor moves passively by diffusion through the supraciliary and suprachoroidal space and enters the venous circulation in the ciliary muscle, choroidal vessels, emissarial canals, sclera, and lymphatic vessels. In contrast, the conventional outflow pathway is pressure-dependent with the proximal region containing the trabecular meshwork and

Tatjana Jakobs and Paloma B. Liton (eds.), *Glaucoma: Methods and Protocols*, Methods in Molecular Biology, vol. 2858, https://doi.org/10.1007/978-1-0716-4140-8_8,

the inner wall of Schlemm's canal and the distal region consisting of the outer wall of Schlemm's canal, collector channels, and the episcleral vasculature. Due to its increased association with glaucoma, the conventional outflow pathway has received much attention [5–7]. Both the proximal and distal regions of the conventional outflow pathway have important roles in generating resistance to aqueous humor removal from the anterior chamber [5, 8–11].

Prior to 1873, aqueous humor was believed to be a stagnant fluid until Theodor Leber injected a dye into the anterior chamber and recognized that the dye moved slowly through the anterior chamber and into surrounding vessels [12, 13], which were later defined as aqueous veins by Carl Asher in 1942 [14]. Since the discovery that aqueous humor is secreted into and removed from the anterior chamber, investigators have been trying to understand how this process is regulated. Some of the prominent research in the field was performed by Morton Grant in the 1960s by perfusing 0.9% sodium chloride into normal and glaucoma whole human donor eyes to evaluate fluid flow at various pressures [10]. In more advanced models, Dr. Grant incorporated fritted glass discs that were calibrated and used as flowmeters and a potentiometer to record electrical pressure signals [10, 15]. These models were successful in establishing some of the foundations that support current-day understanding that in glaucoma, elevated IOP is due to a decrease in aqueous humor removal from the anterior chamber, that is, decreased outflow facility.

While these early model systems provided valuable information to understand how aqueous humor moved through the anterior segment, they utilized the whole eye, making it difficult to study the structural and functional aspects of the conventional outflow pathway and the specific contribution from associated tissues and cells. To overcome this issue, several groups in the late 1980s initiated studies to determine if an ex vivo model system could be developed that utilized human anterior segments [16–18]. In 1987, Tschumper and Johnson published a seminal paper showing that anterior segments dissected from human eyes could be successfully maintained in culture and that data recording systems could be utilized to measure the pressure in the closed system (*see* Fig. 1) [18]. Known as the ex vivo human anterior segment perfusion organ culture model, it is the only human model used to examine the effects of various agents on pressure related to the conventional outflow pathway. Here we describe the step-by-step method of preparing and culturing human anterior segments for experimental analysis. We discuss how the data obtained can be analyzed and highlight the technical requirements and limitations to consider when designing and performing experiments with this model. The human anterior segment perfusion culture model is a powerful ex vivo system that can produce accurate data and contribute to our

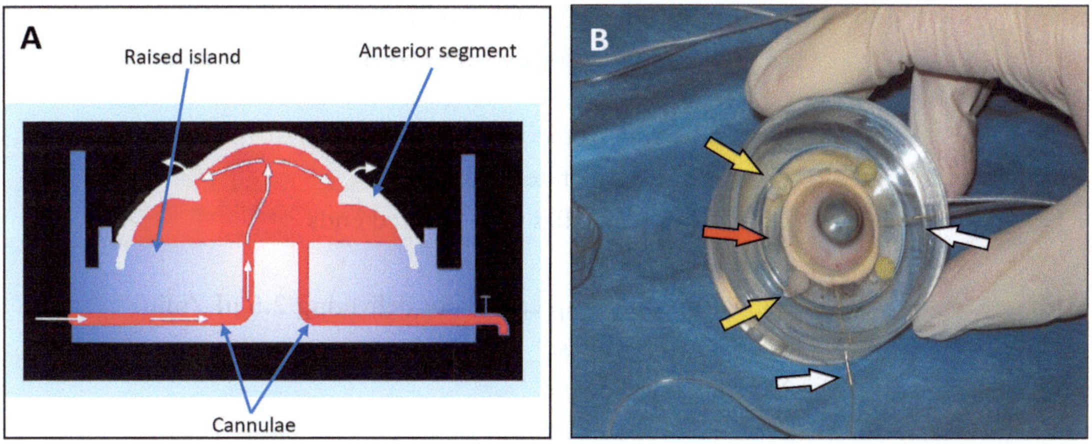

Fig. 1 The human anterior segment perfusion organ culture model used by the Fautsch lab at the Mayo Clinic, Rochester, MN, USA. (**a**) Schematic of the modified petri dish with a clamped anterior segment showing directional flow of media through one cannula and outflow through the conventional outflow area (white arrows). The second cannula is connected to the pressure transducer. (**b**) Dissected and prepped anterior segment clamped on the central island of a modified petri dish using a fitted ring (red arrow) and plastic screws (yellow arrows). DMEM with or without experimental agents are perfused through one cannula while the second cannula is connected to a pressure transducer (white arrows)

understanding of the conventional outflow pathway in normal and glaucomatous eyes.

2 Materials (*See* Note 1)

1. Human donor eyes procured from eye banks or mortuaries.
2. Povidone-iodine solution.
3. Sterile phosphate-buffered saline (PBS).
4. 100 mL specimen containers.
5. Fine forceps (2–3 pairs).
6. Curved surgical scissors.
7. Scalpel blades #15.
8. Lens hook.
9. Sterile gauze pads.
10. Perfusion media: high-glucose DMEM supplemented 1% v/v with antibiotic/antimycotic.
11. Sterile tissue culture hood.
12. Custom-designed petri dishes with raised center island, rings, and screws (*see* Fig. 1).
13. Tissue culture incubator capable of maintaining 37 °C and a 5% CO_2 concentration in a nonhumidified environment.

14. Intravenous (IV) pressure transducers.
15. Computer software to record data generated by pressure transducers.
16. Three-way stop cocks.
17. 0.2 μm sterile filter
18. 21-gauge needles with blunted ends
19. PE60 tubing.
20. Perfusion pump capable of delivering 2.5 μL/min.
21. 12 mL syringes.
22. 1 mL syringes.

3 Methods

The human anterior segment perfusion organ culture model described below is based on the original perfusion culture system designed by Dr. Douglas Johnson [18]. The human anterior segment perfusion organ culture model enables investigators to study the importance of various cells and its associated extracellular matrix on aqueous humor fluid flow. Keeping the tissues and extracellular matrix in a native environment allows for investigators to study the various interactions in normal eyes and to compare these findings to diseased eyes, particularly glaucoma, where IOP is generally elevated. This chapter will describe the eye dissection, setup, and data retrieval methods. Note that all dissection procedures are performed in a sterile tissue culture hood.

3.1 Preparation of Human Eyes

1. Human donor eyes, procured from eye banks or hospital mortuaries, are dissected as described below (*see* **Notes 2** and **3**).
2. Using three 100 mL specimen containers, fill one with 50 mL of povidone-iodine and the other two containers with sterile PBS. Place eyes in the container with povidone-iodine for 3 min and then rinse in PBS for 1 min by subsequent transfer from one container to the next.
3. Remove eyes from PBS and place on sterile gauze. Gently remove excess liquid (*see* Fig. 2a). Using curved surgical scissors, carefully remove the conjunctiva and any excess muscle and orbital fat from the exterior eye. Do not puncture the eye wall.
4. Make a superficial incision with a #15 scalpel blade around the limbus being careful to not fully penetrate the eye. This step releases the vascular resistance created by aqueous and episcleral veins (*see* Fig. 2b).

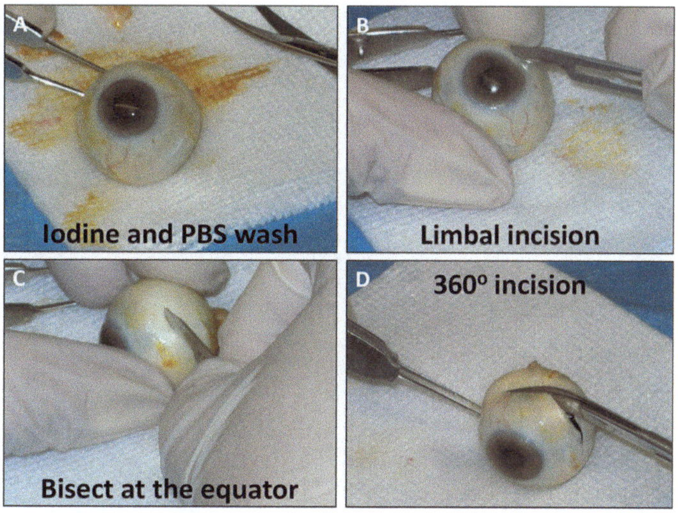

Fig. 2 Preparation of human eyes for ex vivo culture. (**a**) Prior to dissection, human donor eyes are incubated in povidone-iodine solution and rinsed in PBS. Excess solution is removed by a sterile gauze pad. (**b**) A superficial incision is made around limbus to reduce resistance in episcleral veins. (**c**) A small incision is made at the equator and (**d**) a curved surgical scissors is used to dissect the eye in half

5. Place the eye on its side so that the cornea and optic nerve are on opposite sides. Holding the eye in place with your fingertips, make a small incision at the equator of the eye with a #15 scalpel blade (*see* Fig. 2c).
6. Insert one end of a curved surgical scissors into the opening and carefully make a straight cut around the circumference of the eye, essentially cutting the eye in half (*see* Fig. 2d). It is important to leave at least 8 mm of tissue below the limbus so that enough of the sclera is available for setup (*see* Fig. 2d). Use posterior end for further experimentation or discard.

3.2 Dissection of Anterior Segment

1. Remove remnants of vitreous humor from the anterior segment. Vitreous humor is generally gel-like and can be teased out of the anterior segment using fine forceps. If in a liquid state, the vitreous humor can be slowly drained by tipping the anterior segment on its side and blotting with sterile gauze (*see* Fig. 3a).
2. Extract lens nucleus and cortical debris by placing a lens hook between the iris and lens and slowly lift up to remove (*see* Fig. 3b).
3. Following lens removal, use a forceps to grab hold of the iris and remove by gently pulling (*see* **Note 4**). Continue around the circumference of the anterior segment until iris is free. Alternatively, use a forceps to grab the iris and use scissors to

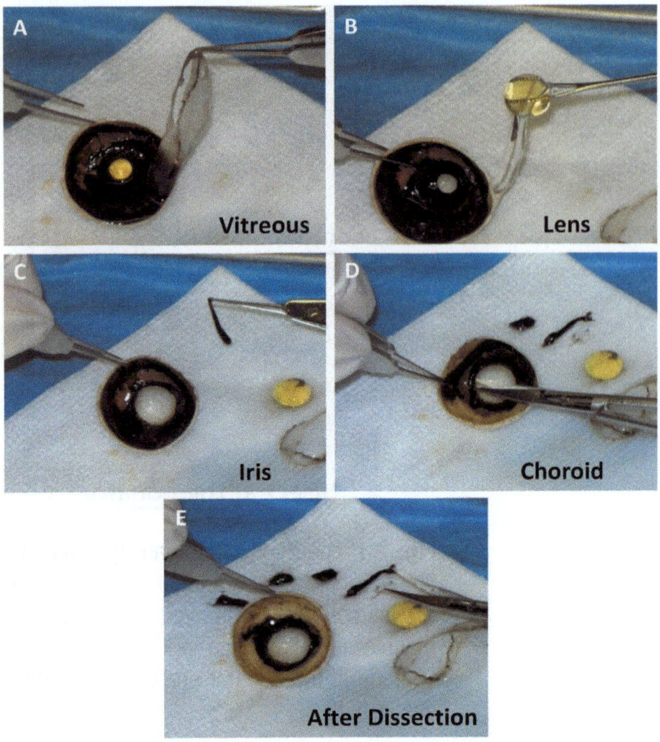

Fig. 3 Dissection of the human anterior segment before placement into culture. (**a**) Vitreous humor is gently teased out with fine forceps. (**b**) Lens is removed using a lens hook. (**c**) Iris is teased out with fine forceps. (**d**) Choroid and pars plana of ciliary body are removed with curved surgical scissors. (**e**) Dissected anterior segment is carefully rinsed with sterile PBS

cut and remove the tissue. Iris can be discarded following removal (*see* Fig. 3c) (*see* **Note 5**).

4. Remove remnants of the choroid and pars plana of the ciliary body by grabbing with a forceps and carefully cutting with a scissors while not disturbing the pars plicata (*see* Fig. 3d).
5. Wash the anterior segment several times with sterile PBS to remove any loose tissue and debris. Figure 3e shows the final dissected anterior chamber.

3.3 Culture Setup

1. To place the dissected anterior segments in culture, the investigator will need a specialized culture dish that contains a raised central island (*see* Fig. 1a, b). The island should contain two small cannulae that open to the outside to allow for media perfusion and pressure monitoring.
2. Place the dissected anterior segment over the central island of the modified petri dish (*see* Fig. 4a).
3. Carefully lower a circular ring around the anterior segment so that the ring pushes the tissue evenly against the central island.

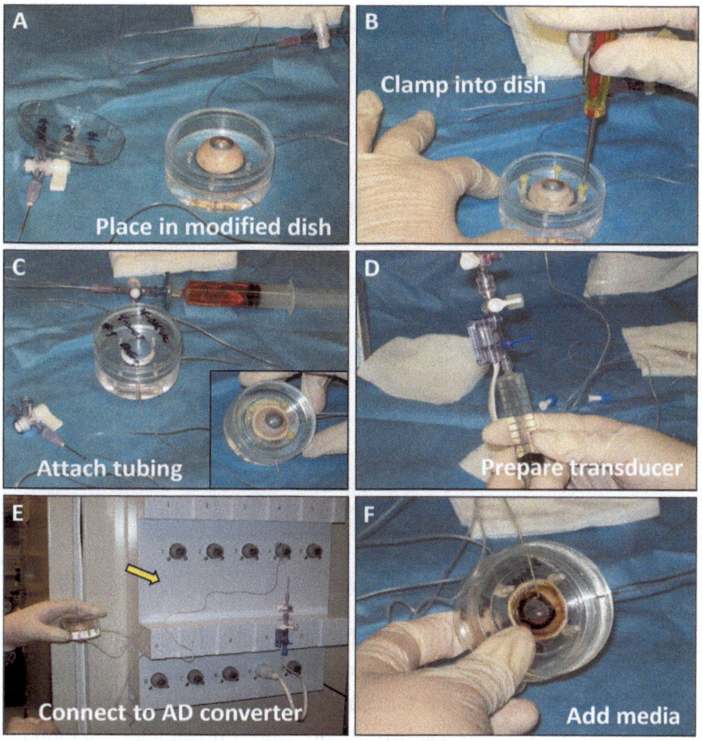

Fig. 4 Placing eyes in culture dish and initiating perfusion. (**a**) The dissected and prepped anterior segments are placed in a modified petri dish over the central island. (**b**) Eyes are clamped using a circular ring and plastic screws. (**c**) PE60 tubing, three-way stopcock, 0.2 μm sterile filter, and 12 mL syringe are attached to the cannulae of the petri dish. Inset shows a cultured eye with PE60 tubing attached to the cannulae. (**d**) Pressure transducers are prepared by injecting sterile PBS by inserting a 12 mL syringe into the flush line. The pressure transducer is attached to a 21 gauge needle and PE60 tubing leading from the second cannula. (**e**) The transducer is plugged into an analogue to digital (AD) converter box (yellow arrow) affixed to the side of the tissue culture incubator. (**f**) Media is perfused into the anterior chamber via one cannula, making sure there are no trapped air bubbles

4. Fasten the ring to the petri dish with four plastic screws, creating an airtight seal between the tissue and the central island (*see* Fig. 4b) (*see* **Note 6**).
5. Attach PE60 tubing to one of the canulae ports leading from the central island to the outside (*see* Fig. 4c). The other end of the PE60 tubing is attached to a 21-gauge blunt end needle. Attach a three-way stopcock, a 0.2 μm disc sterile filter, and a 12 mL syringe containing perfusion media to the needle head.
6. To the second cannula originating from the central island, attach PE60 tubing. Connect the other end of the tubing to

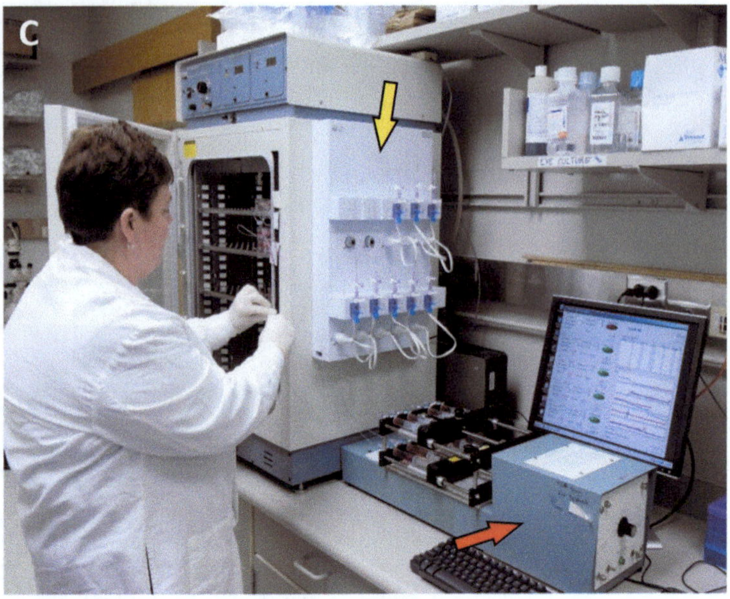

Fig. 5 Perfusion organ culture system. A perfusion pump (red arrow) is set at the physiological flow rate of 2.5 μL/min and used to perfuse media through one of the two cannulae of the petri dish that is placed in a 37 °C incubator containing 5% CO_2. All pressure transducers are plugged into an analog to digital converter (yellow arrow) that feeds data into custom-designed software. The software records pressure at 1-min intervals in real time and averages 60 reads to plot hourly pressures throughout the duration of culture

a 21-gauge blunt end needle that is attached to a three-way stopcock and a pressure transducer (*see* Fig. 4d).

7. Prepare pressure transducers by connecting a 12 mL syringe containing PBS to the flush line. Inject PBS into the transducer using the 12 mL syringe. Clear all air bubbles from the transducer.
8. Attach the transducer to the computer system capable of recording pressure data (*see* Fig. 4e).
9. Once anterior segment has been secured to the petri dish, open the three-way stopcock near the 12 mL syringe to the anterior segment. At the same time, open up the three-way stopcock near the pressure transducer to the outside. Slowly inject perfusion media into the PE60 tubing and start to fill the anterior segment (*see* Fig. 4f). At this point, turn the culture dish upside down, so you can monitor the anterior chamber filling with media and can see that all air bubbles have been removed. Continue to inject media so that all air bubbles are removed from the anterior segment and that media runs through the PE60 tubing connected to the second cannula. Once media starts to come out of the three-way stopcock, check PE60

tubing to make sure all air bubbles have been removed. If air bubbles are present, continue to inject media until they have been removed. The presence of air bubbles in the tubing can affect pressure readings. Once all air bubbles have been removed, close the stopcock by the pressure transducer to the outside.

10. Connect 12-mL syringe containing media to perfusion pump. Start perfusion pump so that fluid is flowing at 2.5 μL/ min (*see* **Note 7**). Place the anterior segments in a 37 °C incubator containing 5% CO_2 and attach pressure transducer to the side of the incubator level with the cultured anterior segments (*see* Fig. 5).
11. There should now be continuous one-way fluid movement from the 12 mL syringe containing culture media through the anterior segment and to the pressure transducer, with computer software recording pressure in the closed setup. After the pressure transducers have been plugged in for at least 30 min, they should be zeroed. Open the stopcock near the transducer to air and reset to zero by pressing the corresponding number of the transducer on the computer keypad.
12. If continuous cultures are being used, new media will need to be added to the 12 mL syringe every third day (*see* **Note 8**). To do this, stop media flow to the anterior segment by closing off the three-way stopcock by the 12 mL syringe. Disconnect the 12 mL syringe from the 0.2 μm sterile filter attached to the three-way stopcock. Discard any remaining media and refill syringe with fresh media. Remove air bubbles from the syringe. Reattach syringe to the 0.2 μm sterile filter, place syringe unit on perfusion pump, and open system to media flow while closing system to the outside using the three-way stopcock.
13. After replenishing media, waste media should also be removed from the culture dish using a sterile pipette. Waste media can be collected for analysis or discarded.

3.4 Data Acquisition

1. Pressure data from the anterior segment is collected in real time using either commercially available or custom designed software. For our studies, we use customized software that collects pressure data at different time intervals and averages the time points to provide a one-hour readout. In general, we collect one-minute data that uses 60 consecutive timepoints to calculate one-hour pressure data.
2. Data can be viewed as pressure over time by taking the hourly pressure data and graphing pressure on the Y axis and time on the X axis. Figure 6 shows an example of a pressure graph from

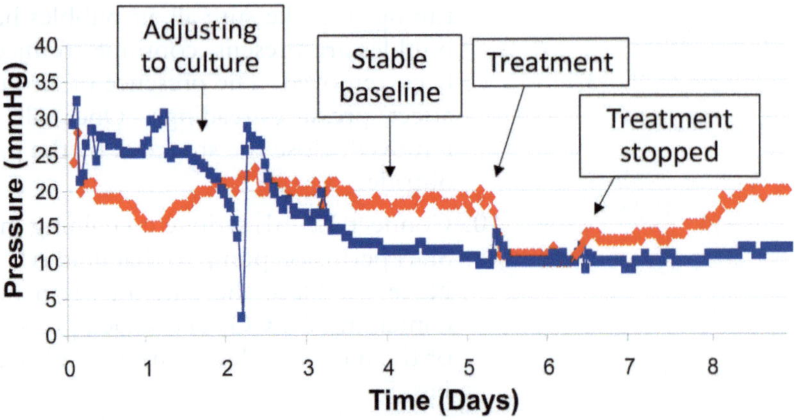

Fig. 6 Representative pressure graph. A pressure vs. time graph is generated by the custom-designed software used in conjunction with the human anterior segment eye culture model. Cultured anterior segments take 2–4 days to acquire a stable baseline. Once a pressure is maintained for 24–48 h, anterior segments can be used for experimental purposes. Note that each point on the graph represents the mean value from 60 consecutive 1-min readings, averaged to plot an hourly pressure value

initial placement in culture to treatment with an experimental drug.

3. Data can also be graphed as outflow facility. Since the model does not contain episcleral venous pressure and does not have a functional uveoscleral outflow pathway, the pressure data can be substituted in a modified Goldman equation of C=F/P (C, outflow facility; F, flow rate; P, Pressure) to calculate outflow facility for each time point. Because we use a constant flow rate of 2.5 μL/min, the recorded pressure data can be inserted into the modified Goldman's equation to calculate outflow facility (*see* **Note 9**).

3.5 Experimental Design

The human anterior segment perfusion organ culture model has been used to address a number of basic science questions. This includes novel insights into the functioning of the conventional outflow pathway in normal and glaucomatous eyes, analysis of endogenous molecules and their impact on conventional outflow pathway tissue function, and examining the importance of the proximal and distal portion of the pathway regarding pressure regulation. It also has been extensively used to examine small molecules to identify more effective pharmacological agents for treating elevated IOP. Below we describe the steps involved in treating human anterior segments with a small molecule or protein (referred to as drug).

1. Dissolve drug in the anterior segment culture media at the desired concentration.

2. Once eyes have reached stable baseline pressure, the entire volume of media in the anterior segment is removed and simultaneously replaced with media containing drug. To do this, disconnect the three-way stopcock from the 21-gauge needle. Attach a 1 mL syringe to the 21-gauge needle and tape the needle to the side of the incubator about 15 cm above the anterior segments.
3. Fill the 1 mL syringe with media containing drug using a transfer pipette, making sure to not introduce any air bubbles.
4. Open the three-way stopcock attached to the pressure transducer to the outside. This should enable gravity-driven media exchange within the tubing and anterior segment, which lasts 1–3 min. Close off three-way stopcock by the pressure transducer just before all the drug containing media in the 1 mL pipette has been transferred. This will reduce the chance of introducing air bubbles into the culture setup.
5. If the goal is to perfuse media containing drug continuously, replace media in the 12 mL syringe with drug containing media, and reattach the 21-gauge needle to the 0.2 μm sterile filter, three-way stopcock, and 12 mL syringe. Alternatively, if no continuous drug is required, reattach the 12 mL syringe containing culture media to the 0.2 μm sterile filter/three-way stopcock, and open the stopcock so that there is continuous, one-way fluid flow through the anterior segment.

3.6 Confirmation of Tissue Integrity

All cultured human anterior segments utilized in experiments need to undergo a thorough histological analysis of at least two small tissue sections 180° apart to verify the cultures were healthy. For data to be considered valid, anterior segments must have a trabecular meshwork with healthy cells and beams and intact inner and outer walls of Schlemm's canal with cells containing healthy appearing nuclei (*see* Fig. 7).

4 Notes

1. In order to minimize variability across experiments and maximize the viability of each anterior segment in culture, custom petri dishes, clamps, screws, tubing, needles, and stopcocks need to be sterilized before initiating culture process.
2. Note that eye retrieval will not be discussed here but can be reviewed in a recent ARVO best practice statement (https://www.arvo.org/globalassets/arvo/journals-and-publications/eye-bank/best-practices-for-using-human-eye-tissue-in-research.pdf).

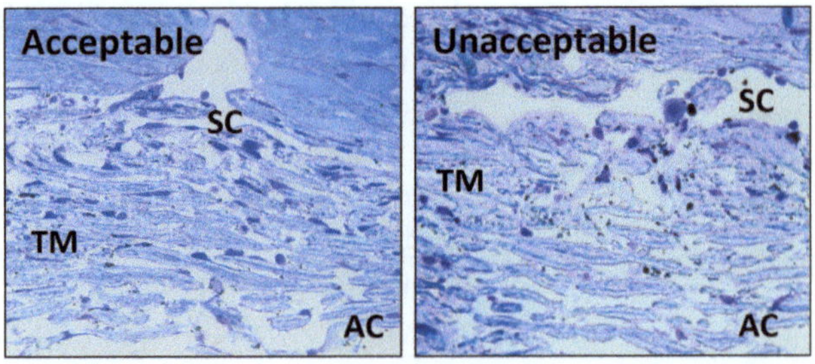

Fig. 7 Conventional outflow histology following human anterior segment perfusion organ culture. For results obtained from a cultured anterior segment to be considered acceptable for use in data collection, they require appropriate histology. The image on the left is taken from an acceptable cultured human anterior segment. This culture contains a trabecular meshwork with healthy appearing cells and beams. The inner and outer walls of Schlemm's canal are intact and contain healthy appearing nuclei. In contrast, the image on the right shows an unacceptable human anterior segment culture. There are no healthy trabecular meshwork cells present. Only a few nuclei can be seen, and they appear rounded and swollen, suggestive of dying cells. The trabecular beams also appear swollen. The inner and outer walls of Schlemm's canal appear somewhat intact although disruptions can be noted on the outer wall. No healthy appearing Schlemm's canal cells are present

3. The investigator should obtain past ocular history to ensure the human donor eyes meet the criteria of the study for which they will be used. Also, document time of death, time of enucleation, and time to culture. Eyes that are dissected and cultured within 24 h of death from donors <80 years of age tend to have a high success rate, although eyes up to 48-hr old have been successfully reported in the literature.
4. When removing the vitreous, iris, lens, and pars plana of the ciliary body, care should be taken so that the trabecular meshwork is not disrupted.
5. The human anterior segment perfusion organ culture model can be modified to study the distal portion of the conventional outflow pathway simply by removing the trabecular meshwork and the inner wall of Schlemm's canal. Anterior segments put into culture with these modifications will show a residual pressure representing the resistance generated by the episcleral vasculature. Using the model in this manner, you can identify changes that affect the distal region of the conventional outflow pathway. Roy Chowdhury et al. showed that treatment of anterior segments lacking the trabecular meshwork and inner wall of Schlemm's canal with ATP-sensitive potassium channel openers lowered pressure, indicating that the agents were directly targeting the distal outflow pathway [19].

6. It is important to create a closed chamber while securing the anterior segment on the central island of the petri dish. Even a small leak may cause the system to record erroneous pressure, in such cases check screws and tubing. Sometimes tightening the screws will help. It is also possible to remove the anterior segment from the petri dish, trim the edges, and reattach it to the central island. However, it should be noted that repeat handling of the tissue can increase chances of infection and diminish the chances of establishing a stable baseline pressure and successful culture.
7. The human anterior segment perfusion organ culture model is excellent for defining the role of the conventional outflow pathway. However, it is an ex vivo model and therefore lacks the impact of innervation, blood pressure, and muscle contraction and relaxation. Because of this, there is no episcleral venous pressure, no uveoscleral outflow pathway, and no ocular pulse, and the flow rate is artificially generated.
8. The human anterior segment perfusion organ culture model is an acute model that can be maintained for up to 28 days. It can be used to study biochemical, molecular, physiologic, and morphologic data from the same experiment. Outside of living humans, it is the only model system to study effects of pressure change and to document changes in normal and glaucoma human eyes.
9. Initial pressures in culture may appear high at first but generally fall within a range of 8–25 mmHg (outflow facility of 0.1–0.3 mL/min/mmHg). To ensure the quality of the data obtained from the culture model, it is important to use eyes with stable baseline pressures within this range.

Acknowledgments

This study is supported by NIH grant EY21727 (MPF), the Mayo Clinic Department of Ophthalmology grant (URC), and Mayo Foundation (MPF).

References

1. Quigley HA (1996) Number of people with glaucoma worldwide. Br J Ophthalmol 80(5): 389–393
2. Quigley HA (2011) Glaucoma. Lancet 377(9774):1367–1377. https://doi.org/10.1016/S0140-6736(10)61423-7
3. Quigley HA, Broman AT (2006) The number of people with glaucoma worldwide in 2010 and 2020. Br J Ophthalmol 90(3):262–267
4. Weinreb RN, Khaw PT (2004) Primary open-angle glaucoma. Lancet 363(9422): 1711–1720. https://doi.org/10.1016/S0140-6736(04)16257-0
5. Andres-Guerrero V, Garcia-Feijoo J, Konstas AG (2017) Targeting Schlemm's canal in the medical therapy of glaucoma: current and future considerations. Adv Ther 34(5):

1049–1069. https://doi.org/10.1007/s12325-017-0513-z

6. Goldberg JL, Wax M, Clark A, Civan MM (2019) Ophthalmology. In: Yanoff M, Duker JS (eds) Ophthalmology, 5th edn. Elsevier, pp 1018–1023
7. Weinreb RN, Aung T, Medeiros FA (2014) The pathophysiology and treatment of glaucoma: a review. JAMA 311(18):1901–1911. https://doi.org/10.1001/jama.2014.3192
8. Carreon T, van der Merwe E, Fellman RL, Johnstone M, Bhattacharya SK (2017) Aqueous outflow – a continuum from trabecular meshwork to episcleral veins. Prog Retin Eye Res 57:108–133. https://doi.org/10.1016/j.preteyeres.2016.12.004
9. Grant WM (1955) Facility of flow through the trabecular meshwork. AMA Arch Ophthalmol 54(2):245–248. https://doi.org/10.1001/archopht.1955.00930020251012
10. Grant WM (1963) Experimental aqueous perfusion in enucleated human eyes. Arch Ophthalmol 69:783–801
11. McDonnell F, Dismuke WM, Overby DR, Stamer WD (2018) Pharmacological regulation of outflow resistance distal to Schlemm's canal. Am J Physiol Cell Physiol 315(1):C44–C51. https://doi.org/10.1152/ajpcell.00024.2018
12. Leber TPA (1906) New researches on the fluid interchange in the eye. Arch F OPhthal Bd. LXIV
13. Blum M, Hykin PG, Sanders M, Volcker HE (1992) Theodor Leber: a founder of ophthalmic research. Surv Ophthalmol 37(1): 63–68. https://doi.org/10.1016/0039-6257(92)90006-f
14. Ascher KW (1946) Further observations on aqueous veins. Am J Ophthalmol 29(11): 1373–1387. https://doi.org/10.1016/0002-9394(46)92033-8
15. Johnstone MA, Grant WG (1973) Pressure-dependent changes in structures of the aqueous outflow system of human and monkey eyes. Am J Ophthalmol 75(3):365–383
16. Erickson-Lamy K (1992) The perfused human ocular anterior segment as a model for aqueous outflow physiology. J Glaucoma 1:44
17. Erickson-Lamy K, Rohen JW, Grant WM (1988) Outflow facility studies in the perfused bovine aqueous outflow pathways. Curr Eye Res 7(8):799–807. https://doi.org/10.3109/02713688809033211
18. Johnson DH, Tschumper RC (1987) Human trabecular meshwork organ culture. A new method. Invest Ophthalmol Vis Sci 28(6): 945–953
19. Roy Chowdhury U, Rinkoski TA, Bahler CK, Millar JC, Bertrand JA, Holman BH, Sherwood JM, Overby DR, Stoltz KL, Dosa PI, Fautsch MP (2017) Effect of Cromakalim prodrug 1 (CKLP1) on aqueous humor dynamics and feasibility of combination therapy with existing ocular hypotensive agents. Invest Ophthalmol Vis Sci 58(13):5731–5742. https://doi.org/10.1167/iovs.17-22538

Chapter 9

Segmental Aqueous Humor Outflow

Mary J. Kelley, Mini Aga, and Ted S. Acott

Abstract

Of the known risk factors for glaucoma, elevated intraocular pressure (IOP), is the primary one. The conventional aqueous humor outflow pathway contains the key source of IOP regulation, which is predominantly the trabecular meshwork (TM). Studies of outflow have demonstrated that the outflow pathway is not uniform around the circumference of the eye but highly segmental with regions of relative high flow (HF) and intermediate or medium flow (IF) and regions of low or no flow (LF). Herein we present protocols that we use to study outflow segmentation through the conventional outflow pathway, mostly focusing on human eyes. These methods are quite similar for nonhuman primates and other species. These studies are mostly conducted using ex vivo intact globes or perfused anterior segment organ culture. One potential therapy for IOP reduction in those with elevated IOP to reduce progression of glaucomatous optic nerve damage would be to increase HF or IF and reduce LF proportions.

Key words Outflow segmentation, Aqueous humor outflow, Intraocular pressure regulation, High and low flow regions, Perfused anterior segment

1 Introduction

The trabecular meshwork (TM) and Schlemm's canal inner wall endothelium (SCE) are the primary pathway of aqueous humor outflow and of IOP regulation [1]. Sustained IOP elevations are sensed by these outflow pathway tissues, and they respond by adjusting the resistance to outflow, which resides primarily within them, to restore IOP to appropriate levels [2, 3]. In much of glaucoma, this IOP homeostatic response has been lost and sustained elevations remain, culminating in glaucomatous optic nerve damage and specific patterns of vision loss [4].

The aqueous humor outflow pathway includes (1) TM outer trabecular beams covered with a monolayer of TM cells, which are attached to extracellular matrix (ECM) with embedded elastin and collagen fibers; (2) the juxtacanalicular region or JCT, which contains stellate-shaped JCT cells interspersed with ECM; and (3) the closely associated inner wall SCE which forms a monolayer lining of

Tatjana Jakobs and Paloma B. Liton (eds.), *Glaucoma: Methods and Protocols*, Methods in Molecular Biology, vol. 2858, https://doi.org/10.1007/978-1-0716-4140-8_9,

Schlemm's canal. This is the conventional outflow pathway. The adjustable outflow resistance is thought to reside in the deepest portion of the JCT and SCE inner wall cell basement membrane [1].

1.1 Segmental Outflow

Segmental outflow refers to the nonuniform pattern of flow of aqueous humor around the circumference of the conventional outflow pathway [5–10]. In the anterior segment of human and other species, some areas exhibit relatively high flow (HF), some low flow (LF), and some intermediate flow (IF) [6, 7, 10–14]. In normal humans, these areas are approximately equal in proportions around the TM. In glaucomatous eyes, there is relatively more LF than in normal eyes [4]. These differences do not appear to be reflected in the cellularity of these regions in normal or glaucomatous eyes, as this number does not show significant differences between regions [15].

The segmentation patterns exist at two levels, a macroscale level of segmentation measured in millimeters and within it microscale level segmentation patterns that measure around 100 microns [8, 16]. Figure 1 shows a typical macroscale labeling pattern for a normal human eye with HF, IF, and LF regions [7]. Figure 2 shows a magnification of part of a macroscale HF region of a normal human eye exhibiting microscale segmentation [16]. Interestingly, these segmentation patterns can change over time in each eye

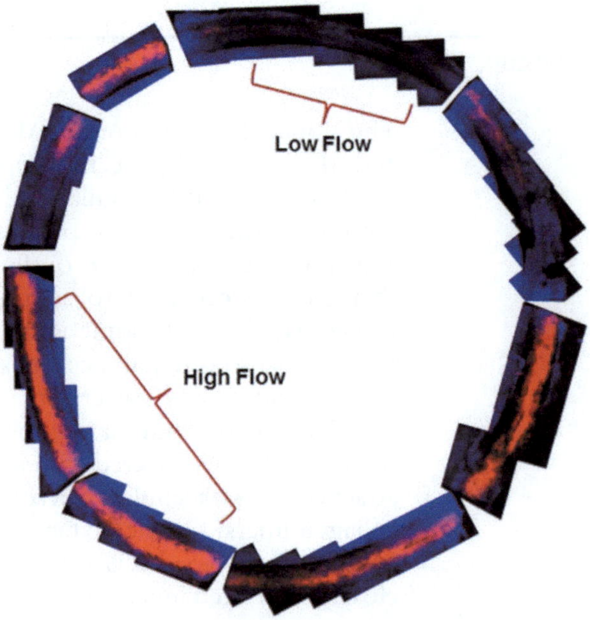

Fig. 1 *En face* view of TM macroscale outflow segmentation patterns of perfused red (Qtracker-655) Qdots showing relative high flow, intermediate flow, and low flow regions [7]

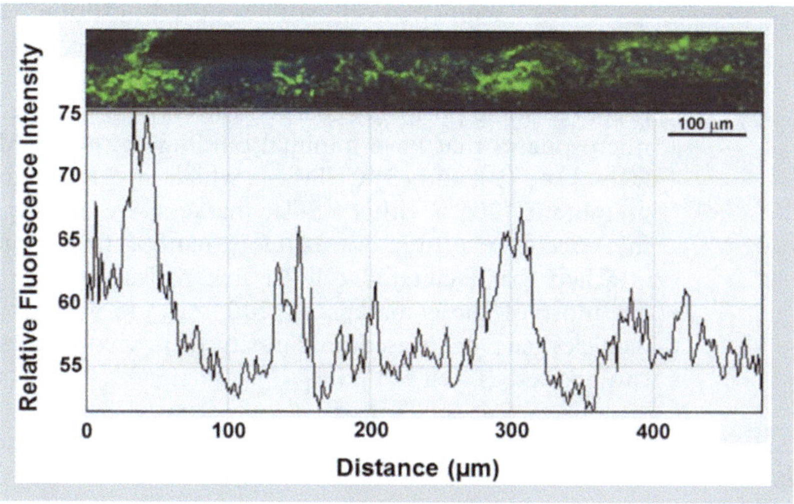

Fig. 2 Microscale outflow segmentation patterns within a macroscale high flow region labeled with 200 nm diameter green FluoSpheres [16]. Relative fluorescence intensity from FIJI or Image J quantitation of an image of a small segment from a high flow region is plotted against that region's length. The distance bar indicates 100 µm

[14, 16]. In young mice, the pattern of segmentation in vivo was determined to move markedly over a period of 1 week [14]. In the microscale flow regions viewed at relatively high resolution, most of flow markers had moved significantly and had lost their positional correlations [14]. It seems likely from these data that the movements were small distances, although the movement is probably just closure of a microscale flow region and opening of another, not necessarily related, region [1]. The pattern of changes in older mice was less pronounced, with the proportion of movements in positions lessened considerably compared to that noted in the young mice [14]. In an ex vivo perfusion culture system, aged human eyes perfused for 1 week at 1x pressure showed only a trend of reduced HF and LF regions with increased IF regions [17]. When the paired eyes were perfused at 2× pressure for 1 week, larger decreases in HF and LF regions were observed associated with statistically significant increases in IF regions [17].

1.2 Approaches Used for Marking Segmental Outflow Patterns

In early segmentation studies, cationic ferritin, which binds to negatively charged residues in the extracellular matrix and cell surfaces, was perfused, and segmental patterns were noted in the TM [12]. This study also noted segmentation pattern differences between normal and glaucomatous eyes. When repeated at somewhat higher concentrations, the cationic ferritin reduced outflow facility (simplified for these studies as C = Flow/Pressure) [18]. The outflow facility reduction with cationic ferritin is presumably due to binding to the numerous negatively charged sites in the outflow pathway and obstructing flow [18].

Other segmentation studies used cationic ferritin [5]: (1) amino-derivatized FluoSpheres (see Materials) which bind tightly to the vast field of negative charges on cells and in ECM [16], (2) some positively charged carboxylate-attached fluorescent microspheres that have minimal binding to the ECM or cell surfaces, [14, 19], and (3) CellMask, which integrates into the plasma membrane [20] or other similar markers. We initially used 10 nm fluorescent quantum dot (QDot) nanoparticles with a peptide attached that facilitated cellular internalization [7]. A good size for most of these markers is 200 nm and a variety of colored particles have been used. For in situ or in vivo studies, fluorescein can be used as well [21].

2 Materials

1. Paired human cadaver eyes: whole eye, obtained within 48 h of death from a local eye bank (*see* **Note 1**).
2. Scalpel or single edge razor blade.
3. Nitrile or latex disposable gloves.
4. Laminar flow biosafety cabinet: sterilized with 70% ethanol and/or UV light for 10 min.
5. Autoclaved paper towels: To securely hold the globe for dissection (*see* **Note 2**).
6. Perfusion media: Dulbecco's Modified Eagle's Medium (DMEM), high glucose: low glucose mix (1:1), supplemented with 1% Penicillin/Streptomycin/Fungizone.
7. Sterile CO_2 incubator: Set at 37 °C, 5% CO_2, and 100% humidity (*see* **Note 3**).
8. Anterior segment perfusion system: including PVC-machined flow cells with mounting pedestal, clamping ring, and four perfusion ports [22–24]. (*see* Fig. 3) (*see* **Note 4**).
9. Small gauge Tygon or polyethylene tubing: Diameter should fit the perfusion ports of the anterior segment perfusion flow cell.
10. Sterile 100 mL glass bottle or 50 mL plastic conical tube: To be used as a perfusion reservoir for the DMEM medium.
11. Micro balance: less than 0.001 gram sensitivity.
12. Pen and lined paper for direct readings of balances or *see* **Note 5** for continuous readings.
13. Meterstick to measure perfusion pressure head.
14. Tracer beads: FluoSpheres [fluorescently labeled amine-modified 200 nm diluted 1:500 in phosphate-buffered saline (PBS)] (*see* **Note 6**), CellMask (diluted 1:500 in PBS) (*see*

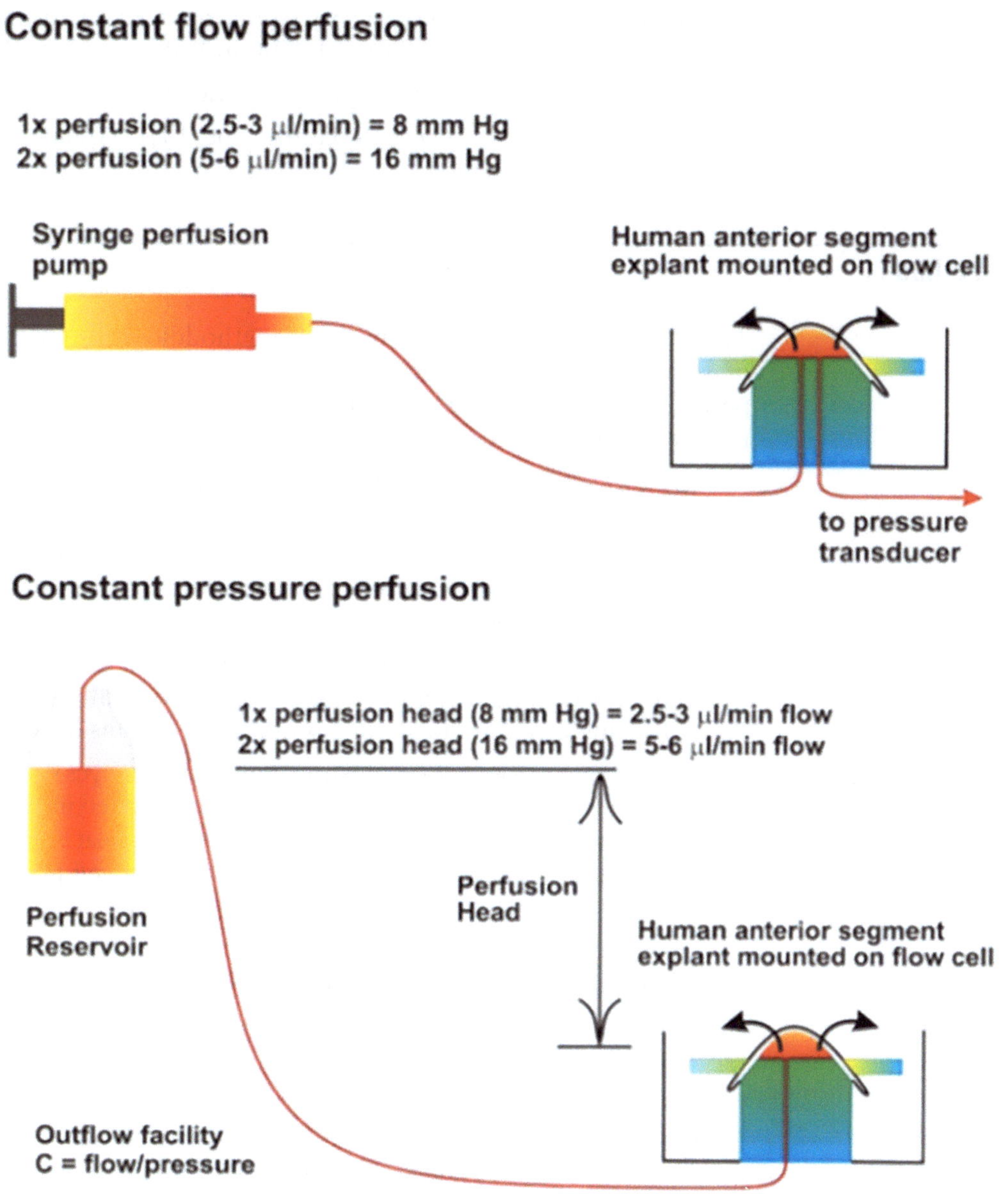

Fig. 3 Perfused anterior segment organ culture may utilize one of two approaches. A constant flow approach with a pressure transducer can be set up to monitor resultant pressure, or the other approach is to use constant pressure with gravimetric measurement of the resultant flow rate. The scleral rim of the anterior segment is clamped on a tapered pedestal with a matching clamping ring. Perfusion fluid enters through a port on the flow cell, enters the anterior chamber, and flows out through the TM, across Schlemm's canal inner wall endothelium, into collector channels, and out through the aqueous plexus. Typical 1× flow rates average around 2.75 mL/min and typical pressure differentials between the anterior chamber and Schlemm's Canal are 8 or 8.8 mm Hg. For an intraocular (IOP) homeostatic 2× pressure challenge, these values are doubled [1–3, 22–24]

Note 7), or Polystyrene basic black uniform dyed microspheres (200 nm, 5% solution, diluted 1/500 in PBS) (*see* **Note 8**).

15. Fluorescent microscope equipped with camera.
16. Image J (https://imagej.NIH.gov) or FIJI (ImageJ.net/software/fiji/download).

3 Methods

This chapter focuses on describing the methodology for the study of segmental outflow using FluoSpheres in a constant pressure perfusion system (*see* Fig. 3). The protocol can be easily adapted for the use of alternative tracers (*see* **Notes** 7 and **8**).

1. In a biosafety laminar flow hood, bisect the whole globes at the equator of the eye. A sufficient rim of sclera (~10 mm) should be left on the anterior half of the eye to allow for clamping in the perfusion device. The anterior half of the eye is retained for the perfusion studies.
2. Using a forceps, gently remove the ciliary body, iris, and lens. Frequent rinsing in sterile media or phosphate-buffered saline (PBS) and attention to sterility is necessary for this dissection.
3. To facilitate recovery from postmortem effects in eyes obtained after 24 h postmortem, anterior segments are placed in stationary organ culture for 5–7 days [25]. For this, place anterior segments concave side up in wells of a sterile 6-well plate and completely cover with perfusion media (*see* **Note 9**).
4. Incubate the 6-well plate containing the anterior segments at 37 °C in a 5% CO_2 incubator at 100% humidity.
5. Replace the medium every 2–3 days under sterile conditions in a laminar flow biosafety cabinet.
6. After 5–7 days, clamp the scleral rim of the anterior segment onto an engineered PVC flow cell using a clamping ring with the cornea facing up [22, 24]. Maintain sterility.
7. Attach Tygon tubing to the flow cell port with the tubing from a reservoir placed at 8.8 mm Hg above for 1× (physiological pressure) or 17.6 mmHg above for 2× pressure, with 2× being a pressure challenge (*see* Fig. 1, **Note 10**) [1–3].
8. Attach the other end of the tubing to the underside of the flow cell to flow the perfusion medium into the anterior chamber and out through the TM and Schlemm's canal.
9. Fill the reservoir with perfusion media and perfuse at a constant pressure of 8.8 mm Hg (1× pressure) for approximately 24 h to establish stable normal flow conditions [23].

10. Add a 300 μL bolus of diluted FluoSpheres to the perfusion media for both the experimental and control eyes whenever it is experimentally advantageous to do so.
11. Label the anterior segments with the FluoSpheres for 1 h. If a different flow rate is observed between the experimental and control eye or different flow rates are used, perfuse the exact same volume into each anterior segment for proper comparison (*see* **Note 11**).
12. [**Optional**] To examine changes in segmental regions after different treatments or experimental conditions, conduct the appropriate treatment in the experimental and paired-eye sham control. After the appropriate time interval, repeat **steps 10** and **11** by pursuing a second colored FluoSphere (*see* **Notes 12–14**).
13. Check FluoSphere distribution in the TM by fluorescence microscopy viewing the tissue *en face*.
14. Photograph the 360° circumference of the TM tissue, again *en face*, using the appropriate excitation and emission wavelengths, and capturing multiple overlapping images.
15. Stitch images together in Photoshop forming a continuous circular collage of overlapping segments to obtain a macroscale segmentation pattern (*see* Fig. 1) [7].
16. This circular image can be straightened to a linear image using Image J or FIJI software. Either stitched circular or linear images can then be quantified in Image J or FIJI.
17. Identifying regions of HF, IF, or LF can be achieved from the scanned region quantitation. First establish the maximum brightness of the segments, and then list everything above 50% of the maximum as high flow. Intermediate flow may be identified as everything below the 50% maximum, except for the last 2–3%, which can be labeled as low flow. This is also done for the microscale segmentation distributions (Fig. 2) [16].
18. [**Optional**] Use Pearson's correlation coefficient to compare the positional overlap if two different colors of FluoSpheres were perfused before and after treatments [14, 17].

4 Notes

1. Retain information supplied by the eye bank on race, age, sex, and known ocular history. This information is recorded for future reference, as it will frequently be required for publication. Avoid eyes from donors with a complicating ocular disease history or surgeries that would compromise the outcome.

2. Sterile gauze can be used alternatively.
3. Addition of sterile disinfectant to the water tray helps to prevent contamination.
4. A constant flow perfusion system can be used.
5. If weighing continuously, a USB connection from the micron balance can be routed through a GaugeMux or other convertors and into a laptop for capture at 10-min interval readings in Excel (other time intervals can be used).
6. The 200 nm FluoSpheres are an appropriate size to avoid them getting stuck and obstructing outflow.
7. CellMask can be used instead of FluoSpheres when the particles interfere with the method of measurement, that is, when performing atomic force microscopy.
8. PolyStyrene Basic Black Uniform Dyed Microspheres (200 nm) may be used if light microscopy rather than fluorescence microscopy is used for flow region identification. The black beads permit the HF and LF regions to be identified by light microscopy.
9. If eyes are obtained within less than 24 h postmortem, stationary culture may be omitted, as postmortem effects on the tissue are minimal at this time [25].
10. To investigate IOP homeostasis, use 1× pressure or 2× pressure perfusion [1–3], and follow the simplified modified Goldmann's equation that outflow facility, C = flow/pressure. This may be studied by constant flow perfusion, where the resultant pressure is measured with a pressure transducer, or by constant pressure perfusion, where the flow rate is measured gravimetrically with a balance [23, 26]. In the latter case, the weight decrease of the bottle of fluid per time is converted into a volume of fluid that flowed per minute.
11. To validate that the markers are marking flow and not just regional marker-tissue interactions, the marker is "soaked in" instead of "flowed in." When the FluoSpheres are soaked in with no flow overnight, the pattern will be uniform with no segmentation. This verification protocol should be run once with each different flow marker type used.
12. It is important that wavelengths of the first and second FluoSpheres do not overlap. Green and/or red are often good choices although others are possible.
13. A two-color control experiment must be done. For this, flow in the same amount of marker for both colors. Flow in first color marker, and then immediately afterward flow in second color (same amount) with no changes in conditions, that is, flow them back-to-back. When this is done for the control, the

beads should be highly coincident with a Pearson's correlation coefficient = +1. For treatments, flow in the first color marker, perform the treatment, and flow in the second color marker. The degree of difference between first and last marker positions caused by the treatment is indicated by the Pearson' correlation coefficient being less than +1. For assessing temporal pattern movements, the amount of time elapsed is the treatment and the process is the same. To see whether the markers moved rather than the flow area moving, the marker is flowed in and imaged. The treatment or elapsed time is completed. The position of the marker is imaged again. The degree that the marker moved will be reflected in the *loss of coincidence* of the same marker in the before and after images with Pearson's correlation coefficient declining below +1. Totally noncoincident would be −1. For overlapping the two readings, one can be false colored.

14. A series of overlapping fluorescence microscope images of the TM are taken around the circumference from the anterior chamber view, *en face*. These are then stitched together in Photoshop. Image J or Fiji can be used to quantify fluorescence.

Acknowledgments

Support NIH/NEI grants EY031071 (MJK), EY021800 (MJK), EY008274 (TSA), EY003279 (TSA), EY025721 (TSA), EY030238 (TSA), EY010572 (TSA); Lewis Rudin Glaucoma Prize (MJK), Glaucoma Research Foundation Shaffer Award (MJK), and an unrestricted grant to the Casey Eye Institute, Oregon Health & Science University from Research to Prevent Blindness Foundation.

Thanks We wish to also acknowledge Lions' VisionGift of Portland, Oregon, and the donors and their families for supplying the human eyes for this work.

References

1. Acott TS, Vranka JA, Keller KE, Raghunathan V, Kelley MJ (2021) Normal and glaucomatous outflow regulation. Prog Retin Eye Res 82:100897. https://doi.org/10.1016/j.preteyeres.2020.100897
2. Acott TS, Kelley MJ, Keller KE, Vranka JA, Abu-Hassan DW, Li X, Aga M, Bradley JM (2014) Intraocular pressure homeostasis: maintaining balance in a high-pressure environment. J Ocul Pharmacol Ther 30(2–3): 94–101. https://doi.org/10.1089/jop.2013.0185
3. Acott TS, Kelley MJ, Keller KE, Vranka JA, Abu-Hassan DW, Li X, Aga M, Bradley JM

(2016) IOP Homeostasis—why most people do not ever develop glaucoma. In: Knepper PA, Samples JR (eds) Glaucoma research and clinical advances 2016–2018. Kugler Publications, Amsterdam, pp 87–98

4. Raghunathan VK, Benoit J, Kasetti R, Zode G, Salemi M, Phinney BS, Keller KE, Staverosky JA, Murphy CJ, Acott T, Vranka J (2018) Glaucomatous cell derived matrices differentially modulate non-glaucomatous trabecular meshwork cellular behavior. Acta Biomater 71:444–459. https://doi.org/10.1016/j.actbio.2018.02.037
5. Hann CR, Bahler CK, Johnson DH (2005) Cationic ferritin and segmental flow through the trabecular meshwork. Invest Ophthalmol Vis Sci 46(1):1–7
6. Hann CR, Fautsch MP (2009) Preferential fluid flow in the human trabecular meshwork near collector channels. Invest Ophthalmol Vis Sci 50(4):1692–1697. https://doi.org/10.1167/iovs.08-2375
7. Keller KE, Bradley JM, Vranka JA, Acott TS (2011) Segmental versican expression in the trabecular meshwork and involvement in outflow facility. Invest Ophthalmol Vis Sci 52(8):5049–5057. https://doi.org/10.1167/iovs.10-6948
8. Chang JY, Folz SJ, Laryea SN, Overby DR (2014) Multi-scale analysis of segmental outflow patterns in human trabecular meshwork with changing intraocular pressure. J Ocul Pharmacol Ther 30(2–3):213–223. https://doi.org/10.1089/jop.2013.0182
9. Swaminathan SS, Oh DJ, Kang MH, Rhee DJ (2014) Aqueous outflow: segmental and distal flow. J Cataract Refract Surg 40(8):1263–1272. https://doi.org/10.1016/j.jcrs.2014.06.020
10. Cha ED, Xu J, Gong L, Gong H (2016) Variations in active outflow along the trabecular outflow pathway. Exp Eye Res 146:354–360. https://doi.org/10.1016/j.exer.2016.01.008
11. Hann CR, Johnson DH (2007) Trabecular meshwork pigmentation and collector channels—areas of higher flow? Invest Ophthalmol Vis Sci 48:2053
12. de Kater AW, Melamed S, Epstein DL (1989) Patterns of aqueous humor outflow in glaucomatous and nonglaucomatous human eyes. A tracer study using cationized ferritin. Arch Ophthalmol 107(4):572–576
13. Carreon TA, Edwards G, Wang H, Bhattacharya SK (2017) Segmental outflow of aqueous humor in mouse and human. Exp Eye Res 158:59–66. https://doi.org/10.1016/j.exer.2016.08.001
14. Reina-Torres E, Baptiste TMG, Overby DR (2022) Segmental outflow dynamics in the trabecular meshwork of living mice. Exp Eye Res 225:109285. https://doi.org/10.1016/j.exer.2022.109285
15. Kuehn MH, Vranka JA, Wadkins D, Jackson T, Cheng L, Ledolter J (2021) Circumferential trabecular meshwork cell density in the human eye. Exp Eye Res 205:108494. https://doi.org/10.1016/j.exer.2021.108494
16. Vranka JA, Bradley JM, Yang YF, Keller KE, Acott TS (2015) Mapping molecular differences and extracellular matrix gene expression in segmental outflow pathways of the human ocular trabecular meshwork. PLoS One 10(3):e0122483. https://doi.org/10.1371/journal.pone.0122483
17. Vranka JA, Staverosky JA, Raghunathan V, Acott TS (2020) Elevated pressure influences relative distribution of segmental regions of the trabecular meshwork. Exp Eye Res 190:107888. https://doi.org/10.1016/j.exer.2019.107888
18. Ethier CR, Chan D-H (2001) Cationic ferritin changes outflow facility in human eyes whereas anionic ferritin does not. Invest Ophthalmol Vis Sci 42:1795–1802
19. Battista SA, Lu Z, Hofmann S, Freddo T, Overby DR, Gong H (2008) Reduction of the available area for aqueous humor outflow and increase in meshwork herniations into collector channels following acute IOP elevation in bovine eyes. Invest Ophthalmol Vis Sci 49(12):5346–5352. https://doi.org/10.1167/iovs.08-1707
20. Vranka JA, Staverosky JA, Reddy AP, Wilmarth PA, David LL, Acott TS, Russell P, Raghunathan VK (2018) Biomechanical rigidity and quantitative proteomics analysis of segmental regions of the trabecular meshwork at physiologic and elevated pressures. Invest Ophthalmol Vis Sci 59(1):246–259. https://doi.org/10.1167/iovs.17-22759
21. Saraswathy S, Bogarin T, Barron E, Francis BA, Tan JCH, Weinreb RN, Huang AS (2020) Segmental differences found in aqueous angiographic-determined high—and low-flow regions of human trabecular meshwork. Exp Eye Res 196:108064. https://doi.org/10.1016/j.exer.2020.108064
22. Johnson DH, Tschumper RC (1987) Human trabecular meshwork organ culture. Invest Ophthalmol Vis Sci 28:945–953
23. Bradley JMB, Kelley MJ, Zhu XH, Anderssohn AM, Alexander JP, Acott TS (2001) Effects of mechanical stretching on trabecular matrix

metalloproteinases. Invest Ophthalmol Vis Sci 42:1505–1513

24. Bradley JMB, Vranka JA, Colvis CM, Conger DM, Alexander JP, Fisk AS, Samples JR, Acott TS (1998) Effects of matrix metalloproteinase activity on outflow in perfused human organ culture. Invest Ophthalmol Vis Sci 39:2649–2658
25. Acott TS, Kingsley PD, Samples JR, Van Buskirk EM (1988) Human trabecular meshwork organ culture: Morphology and glycosaminoglycan synthesis. Invest Ophthalmol Vis Sci 29: 90–100
26. Johnson DH (1996) Human trabecular meshwork cell survival is dependent on perfusion rate. Invest Ophthalmol Vis Sci 37:1204–1208

Chapter 10

Human Corneal Rim Perfusion Culture

Weiming Mao

Abstract

Human anterior segment perfusion cultures are frequently used for trabecular meshwork research. However, this model requires the use of whole eye globes which are expensive. Here, we describe a method using human corneal rims as an alternative to anterior segments for perfusion culture. In this method, the human corneal rim is glued to a three-dimensional-printed perfusion plates instead of using mechanical compression in traditional perfusion culture setup. The corneal rim and perfusion plate are placed onto a special holder for perfusion culture. This method is affordable and easy to set up. The instruments for traditional perfusion culture studies can be used for this model without modification.

Key words Corneal rim perfusion culture, Intraocular pressure, Outflow facility

1 Introduction

There are three classes of models for trabecular meshwork (TM) research: TM cell cultures (in vitro), lab animals (in vivo), and perfusion-cultured tissues (ex vivo). Trabecular meshwork cells can be passaged up to ten times without noticeable changes in their morphology or biology [1]. They are the most widely used for TM research and often serve as the "first-line" model. However, they do not provide the data of intraocular pressure (IOP) or outflow facility. In contrast, lab animals provide all required physiology data. The disadvantage of animal models includes high cost, time consuming, and difference in ocular anatomy and physiology compared to human eyes (except for nonhuman primates), as well as ethical concerns/restrictions. Perfusion-cultured tissue models have a good balance between the pros and cons of the in vitro and in vivo models: they are easy to set up and can provide IOP and outflow facility data [2]. More importantly, they are the closet models (if human donor eyes are used) to in vivo conditions of human eyes in preclinical research.

Human, bovine, and porcine eyes have been used for perfusion culture for many years [3–6]. Although whole eye globes can be

Tatjana Jakobs and Paloma B. Liton (eds.), *Glaucoma: Methods and Protocols*, Methods in Molecular Biology, vol. 2858,
https://doi.org/10.1007/978-1-0716-4140-8_10,

perfused directly [7], this method is only suitable for short-term studies because the retina and uveal tract cannot be maintained in perfusion medium, and the dead tissue may clog the trabecular meshwork outflow pathway. Instead, the anterior segments are frequently used for short- and long-term studies. The first anterior segment perfusion culture model was developed by Johnson and Tschumper [3] (refer to Chap. 8 in this volume). In this model, the whole eye globe is bisected at the equator. The retina, choroid, vitreous, and lens are removed from the anterior segment so that the anterior segment contains the anterior sclera, cornea, TM, iris, and ciliary body. The posterior segment is discarded. In some modified methods, the iris and ciliary body are also removed [5, 6]. The anterior segment is mounted on a specially designed plexi-glass dish, and the peripheral sclera is clamped onto the dish using a rigid plexi-glass ring, forming a water-tight artificial anterior chamber. There are two predrilled channels communicating the anterior chamber to the outside: one channel is for medium infusion to mimic aqueous humor production (inflow) while the other channel is for IOP measurement.

As described previously, the anterior segment perfusion culture model requires whole eye globes. Due to the high cost and limited availability of whole eye globes, it is challenging to conduct such experiments with large sample sizes. In contrast, human corneal rims are readily available at eye banks with much lower costs. These rims contain the cornea, sclera, and TM, which are ideal for perfusion culture studies. The only disadvantage of corneal rims is the lack of sufficient amount of sclera for clamping since these rims are prepared using trephine and they are cut more anteriorly. Several groups, including our group, tried to reduce the perfusion culture dish to fit corneal rims. However, such modifications almost always result in high IOP (our unpublished observations). We postulate that this high IOP is due to the lack of spacing between the TM and the perfusion dish which blocks medium outflow.

Recently, we published a new method for corneal rim perfusion cultures [8]. The key difference between this new method and the traditional method is that chemical glues are used to secure and seal the corneal rim to the perfusion plate instead of using mechanical clamping. In this chapter, the experimental procedure of this corneal rim perfusion culture model will be reviewed and explained in detail.

2 Materials

1. A computer equipped with a signal acquisition systems such as the Powerlab 35 series, Octal Bridge Amplifier, or LabChart Pro software.

2. Human corneal rims from Eye Banks.
3. Phosphate-buffered saline (PBS), pH 7.4, sterile.
4. Opti-MEM culture medium or DMEM culture medium supplemented with antibiotics (*see* **Note 1**).
5. Perfusion culture plates: These plates can be three-dimensional printed. Three-dimensional print files can be downloaded by accessing Supplement Data of our published paper [8] (*see* **Note 2**).
6. Perfusion culture holders: The top part of the holder can be three-dimensional printed. Three-dimensional print files can be downloaded by accessing Supplement Data of our published paper [8]. The bottom part of the holder can be prepared using 3/4 inch diameter PVC pipes. Cut the pipe to about 2-inch (about 5 cm) pieces, and then cut a slot about 0.5 inch (about 1.25 cm) on the side of each piece. Glue the pipe to the bottom of the top part using a suitable glue such as epoxy glue. Make sure the slot on the top part and the slot on the bottom part align with each other. The slot is used to run plastic tubing.
7. Twenty-gauge stainless steel hypodermic tubing. We recommend cutting the tubing into about 2 or 3 cm in length using a rotary tool and a cutting wheel, and then glue them into the two channels of the perfusion culture plate. Be careful not to clog the stainless-steel tubing with glue.
8. A dissection microscope.
9. Dissection tools including forceps, ophthalmic scissors, surgical blades, and a diamond knife (optional but recommended).
10. 100 mm Petri dishes.
11. Gauze Pads.
12. Cotton swabs.
13. Gluture topical tissue adhesive.
14. Loctite Superglue Ultra Gel Control.
15. Contact lens.
16. Lab tape.
17. Pressure transducers with stopcocks.
18. Pressure gauge kit for calibration.
19. Plastic tubing with 0.03 inch inner diameter.
20. Luer-stub adapter 20-gauge.
21. Two-way stopcocks.
22. Nonvented plugs for stopcocks.
23. Syringe filters (optional).
24. Plastic syringes (20 or 30 mL; other sizes can also be used).

25. A cell culture incubator with CO_2 supply.
26. Syringe pumps such as PHD2000 or F200× with syringe racks.

3 Methods

3.1 Equipment Setup

1. Wire and connect the bridge amplifier, Powerlab, computer, and power source.
2. Connect the pressure transducer to the bridge amplifier using the supplied cable.
3. Turn on the main power on the Powerlab.
4. Let the equipment warm up for at least 15 min.

3.2 Tissue Preparation

All tissue preparation is conducted according to BSL2 standard such as within a biosafety hood or outside the hood but with necessary PPE (e.g., N-95 masks), depending on individual lab's approved biosafety protocols. Our experience is that this model is not sensitive to contamination and it is not necessary to conduct all procedures in a biosafety hood or even in a lamina flow room unless there are special concerns.

1. Before opening the tissue vial, check the serological test report (if supplied) of the donor and make sure that the donor is negative for blood borne pathogens such as HIV, hepatitis B/hepatitis C, etc.
2. Place a 100 mm Petri dish on the bench and remove the lid.
3. Place a piece of sterile gauze pad on the dish.
4. Carefully, open the tissue vial and transfer the corneal rim onto the gauze pad with the corneal epithelial layer facing down.
5. Working under a dissection microscope, use a sterile surgical blade to carefully scrape off remaining uveal tract tissues without damaging the TM.
6. Rinse the tissue with PBS.
7. Score the sclera 360° using a surgical blade or a diamond knife 1–2 mm from the TM at both inner and outer sides.
8. Dry both sides of the part of the sclera to be glued to the perfusion plate using cotton applicators. Do not dry the TM or cornea.

3.3 Corneal Rim Mount

1. Place the perfusion plate onto the holder.
2. Do a test fit of the corneal rim to the perfusion plate (*see* **Note 3**). If it fits well, dry the plate and apply a thin layer of Gluture into the groove of the plate.

3. Quickly but carefully place the corneal rim on the plate and make sure the edge of the corneal rim sits in the groove. Make slight adjustment if needed.
4. Place the entire set (holder + plate + corneal rim) in the cell culture incubator and let the glue cure for about 5 min (*see* **Note 4**).
5. After Gluture cures completely, take the entire set out of the incubator and place it on the bench.
6. Cover the cornea with a piece of contact lens to protect the cornea from glue contamination and from drying.
7. Apply a thin bead (as little as possible!) of Superglue Ultra Gel Control glue at the base of the corneal rim. Make sure the bead of glue contacts both the sclera and the perfusion plate (*see* **Note 5**). Resist the temptation to apply more glue than necessary.
8. Place the entire set back in the cell culture incubator and let the glue to cure for a few hours.
9. In the meantime, calibrate the pressure transducer (*see* **Note 6**).

3.4 Connect the Perfusion System to the Pressure Transducer

A wiring diagram and images of equipment setup are summarized in Fig. 1.

1. Fill one syringe with perfusion medium (Opti-MEM or DMEM).

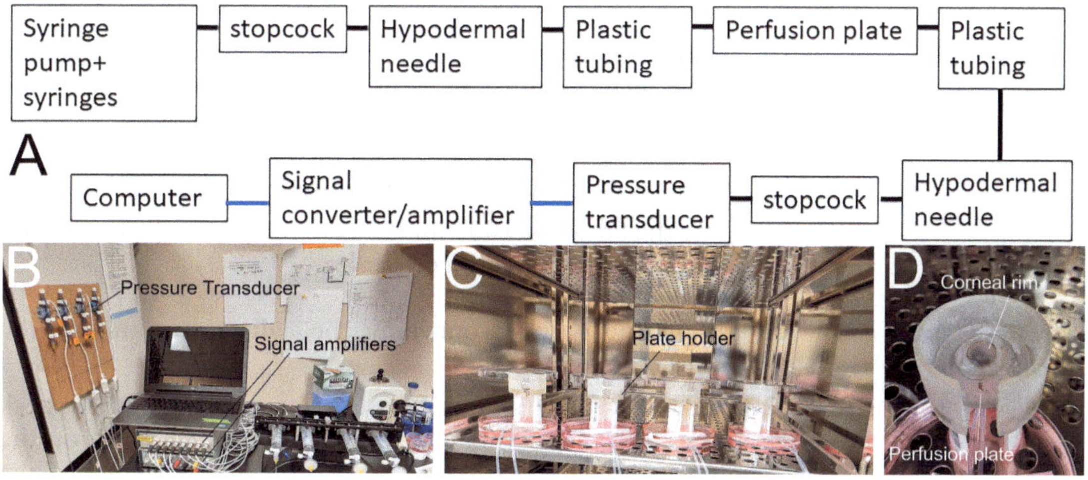

Fig. 1 Experimental setup. (**a**) Wiring diagram of perfusion culture setup. (**b**) An overview of the equipment setup. (**c**) A side view of the plate holder with the perfusion plate and corneal rim inside a cell culture incubator. A Petri dish was used to collect perfusate, and another dish was used as a lid. (**d**) A perfusion plate containing a corneal rim was placed in a plate holder. Note the cornea was not very cloudy after 1 month of perfusion

2. Connect the syringe containing the culture medium to the stainless-steel tubing in the center, using plastic tubing, a Luer-stub adapter, and two-way stopcocks.
3. Connect an empty syringe to the stainless-steel tubing off the center in a similar way. We use the following setup: perfusion plate—plastic tubing—stub adapter—stopcock—syringe filter (optional for the infusion side; do not add filter to the pressure monitoring side)—syringe (*see* **Note 7**).
4. Turn the perfusion plate upside down (the cornea faces down) and place it on the holder.
5. Replace the air in the anterior chamber with culture medium. To do so, gently push the plunger of the syringe containing the culture media and pull the plunger of the empty syringe. To effectively eliminate any smaller air bubbles, tilt the plate in a manner where the stainless-steel tubing positioned off-center is at the highest point (12 o'clock).
6. Fill the stopcock of the pressure transducer with distilled water or medium using a syringe and remove any air bubbles by pushing the syringe.
7. Remove the empty syringe and connect the stopcock that is connected to the empty syringe to the stopcock connected to the pressure transducer. Then, remove any air bubble that may form by pushing the plunger of the syringe containing the culture medium (*see* **Note 8**).
8. Cap all stopcocks' open ends with plugs.
9. Place the perfusion set in the CO_2 cell culture incubator and close the incubator door (*see* **Note 9**).
10. Mount the pressure transducer on a rack or tape it on the side of the incubator. We attach a cork board to the side of the incubator and securely pin the pressure transducer onto it. Make sure the pressure transducer is at the same level as the corneal rim to eliminate hydrostatic pressure difference.
11. Place the lid of the 100 mm Petri dish on top of the holder and place the holder on the Petri dish.

3.5 Preperfusion and Establishment of Baseline IOP

1. Mount the syringe containing the culture medium on the perfusion pump.
2. Prime the syringe(s). For this, turn the switch on the stopcock toward the plastic tubing, remove the plug, and turn on the pump at a high perfusion rate (i.e., 1 mL per min). When medium starts to drip from all syringes, turn off the pump, recap the stopcock, and turn the switch toward the plug. Culture medium should now flow to the plastic tubing.
3. Reset the perfusion rate at 2.5 μL/min and turn on the pump.

4. Click the start button in the software to initiate IOP recording. We usually record IOP once per minute.
5. The next day, carefully remove the contact lens using forceps. The contact lens should look cloudy due to polymerized glue vapor, while the cornea should look clear. We recommend leaving the contact lens on the cornea overnight since early removal will likely result in glue polymerization on the cornea which is almost impossible to remove.
6. Resume perfusion and allow IOP to stabilize for 16–24 h.

3.6 Treatment Application

Once stable baseline IOP is reached, treatment of your choice (i.e., *compounds) can be applied, either topically (eyedrops),* via *injection through the cornea (paracentesis), or by perfusion. Here, we will describe perfused treatment application.*

1. Prepare culture medium containing the desired treatment or vehicle control.
2. Load culture medium into a new syringe.
3. Stop the pump; turn the switch of the stopcock toward the old syringe, to prevent air bubbles from entering the stopcock; and replace the old syringe with the new one containing treatment.
4. Prime the new syringes as described earlier (Subheading 3.5, **step 2**) and restart the pump (*see* **Note 10**).

3.7 Data Analysis

IOP data can be averaged every hour/half day/day, depending on the experiment. The IOP after treatment minus the baseline IOP is plotted over time to show IOP changes (ΔIOP-time curve) (*see* **Note 11**).

3.8 Sample Collection During and After Perfusion

During perfusion, perfusates (conditioned medium) can be collected for studies such as ELISA and/or Western immunoblotting. At the end of perfusion study, the cornea rim can be carefully separated from the perfusion plate using a surgical blade (*see* **Note 12**). The corneal rim can be used for histology studies, immunostaining, PCR, and/or Western immunoblotting.

4 Notes

1. Make sure fetal bovine serum (FBS) is not added to the culture media. Addition of FBS may clog the perfusion system.
2. There are many three-dimensional printing technologies available. We recommend resin-based three-dimesional printing methods such as liquid crystal display (LCD) and Stereolithography (SLA). It is important to use a transparent or translucent resin so that air bubbles can be visualized through the

perfusion plate. Although the TM tissue does not contact the three-dimensional print directly, using clear biocompatible resins, for example, Acura ClearVue (three-dimensional systems, Rock Hill, SC, USA) and BioClear resin (Formlabs, Somerville, MA, USA), may avoid potential toxicity.

3. The corneal rim is prepared using a trephine by technicians at the eye bank. However, sometimes the edge of the corneal rim is uneven and therefore must be trimmed using ophthalmic scissors. It does not need to be perfect but should be flat enough to fit into the groove of the perfusion plate without leaving visible gaps. The gaps caused by uneven edges need to be filled with a large amount of glue, which increases the chance of clogging the TM by glue, and very high IOP will be observed.
4. The two types of glue work by polymerization in the presence of moisture. Therefore, placing the whole set in the cell culture incubator accelerates glue polymerization.
5. The first thin fluid Gluture provides initial attachment, while the thick Superglue Ultra Gel Control glue seals the corneal rim to the perfusion plate.
6. Pressure transducer calibration varies on the equipment used and should be done following the manufacturer's suggestions.
7. The stainless tubing in the center is designed for medium infusion, and the one off the center is used for pressure monitoring.
8. It is crucial to ensure the complete removal of all air bubbles from the anterior chamber, plastic tubing, and stopcocks. This is a critical step.
9. The plastic tubing is usually rigid enough to withstand the door seal.
10. We advise readers who utilize the AdInstrument data acquisition system to avoid pausing data recording through the software during the syringe change process. The duration of this procedure typically lasts around 5–10 min, which is considered to be a relatively short timeframe that should not significantly impact the results.
11. Theoretically, outflow facility can be calculated as follows: 2.5 μL/min (inflow) ÷ IOP. However, the IOP measured is likely not the "true" IOP inside the corneal rim. The system is very sensitive, and IOP readings can be affected by numerous factors such as calibration, tubing length, temperature, etc. Although theoretically the IOP of paired eyes should be very close to each other, several mmHg differences in baseline IOP even between paired eyes are very common, due to these errors. Assuming that measured baseline IOP is 7 mmHg,

while the actual IOP inside the corneal rim is 10 mmHg, using 2.5uL/min perfusion rate, calculated outflow facility (2.5÷7) will be 44% higher than actual outflow facility (2.5÷10). If accurate outflow facility data are needed, the author recommends to perfuse the corneal rim at multiple (at least 5–7) perfusion rates (i.e., 1, 2, 3, 4, 5, 6, 7 uL/min), plot a perfusion rate-IOP graph, and conduct a linear regression analysis. The slope of the linear function represents more accurate outflow facility. However, for most of the studies in which an agent is tested, knowing the absolute outflow facility is not important since ΔIOP represents the change in outflow facility.

12. Do not try to "tear/peel" the cornea rim from the plate due to strong glue bonding.

Acknowledgments

R01EY026962 (WM), R01EY031700 (WM), R21EY033929 (WM), BrightFocus Foundation G2023009S (WM), and a challenge grant from the Research to Prevent Blindness (Department of Ophthalmology, Indiana University School of Medicine).

References

1. McDowell CM, Kizhatil K, Elliott MH, Overby DR, van Batenburg-Sherwood J, Millar JC, Kuehn MH, Zode G, Acott TS, Anderson MG, Bhattacharya SK, Bertrand JA, Borras T, Bovenkamp DE, Cheng L, Danias J, De Ieso ML, Du Y, Faralli JA, Fuchshofer R, Ganapathy PS, Gong H, Herberg S, Hernandez H, Humphries P, John SWM, Kaufman PL, Keller KE, Kelley MJ, Kelly RA, Krizaj D, Kumar A, Leonard BC, Lieberman RL, Liton P, Liu Y, Liu KC, Lopez NN, Mao W, Mavlyutov T, McDonnell F, McLellan GJ, Mzyk P, Nartey A, Pasquale LR, Patel GC, Pattabiraman PP, Peters DM, Raghunathan V, Rao PV, Rayana N, Raychaudhuri U, Reina-Torres E, Ren R, Rhee D, Chowdhury UR, Samples JR, Samples EG, Sharif N, Schuman JS, Sheffield VC, Stevenson CH, Soundararajan A, Subramanian P, Sugali CK, Sun Y, Toris CB, Torrejon KY, Vahabikashi A, Vranka JA, Wang T, Willoughby CE, Xin C, Yun H, Zhang HF, Fautsch MP, Tamm ER, Clark AF, Ethier CR, Stamer WD (2022) Consensus recommendation for mouse models of ocular hypertension to study aqueous humor outflow and its mechanisms. Invest Ophthalmol Vis Sci 63(2):12. https://doi.org/10.1167/iovs.63.2.12
2. Pang IH, McCartney MD, Steely HT, Clark AF (2000) Human ocular perfusion organ culture: a versatile ex vivo model for glaucoma research. J Glaucoma 9(6):468–479. https://doi.org/10.1097/00061198-200012000-00009
3. Johnson DH, Tschumper RC (1987) Human trabecular meshwork organ culture. A new method. Invest Ophthalmol Vis Sci 28(6):945–953
4. Loewen RT, Roy P, Park DB, Jensen A, Scott G, Cohen-Karni D, Fautsch MP, Schuman JS, Loewen NA (2016) A porcine anterior segment perfusion and transduction model with direct visualization of the trabecular meshwork. Invest Ophthalmol Vis Sci 57(3):1338–1344. https://doi.org/10.1167/iovs.15-18125
5. Mao W, Tovar-Vidales T, Yorio T, Wordinger RJ, Clark AF (2011) Perfusion-cultured bovine anterior segments as an ex vivo model for studying glucocorticoid-induced ocular hypertension and glaucoma. Invest Ophthalmol Vis Sci 52(11):8068–8075. https://doi.org/10.1167/iovs.11-8133
6. Keller KE, Bradley JM, Kelley MJ, Acott TS (2008) Effects of modifiers of glycosaminoglycan biosynthesis on outflow facility in perfusion culture. Invest Ophthalmol Vis Sci 49(6):2495–2505. https://doi.org/10.1167/iovs.07-0903

7. Grant WM, Trotter RR (1955) Tonographic measurements in enucleated eyes. AMA Arch Ophthalmol 53(2):191–200. https://doi.org/10.1001/archopht.1955.00930010193003
8. Peng M, Margetts TJ, Sugali CK, Rayana NP, Dai J, Sharma TP, Raghunathan VK, Mao W (2022) An ex vivo model of human corneal rim perfusion organ culture. Exp Eye Res 214:108891. https://doi.org/10.1016/j.exer.2021.108891

Chapter 11

The Inducible TGFβ2 Ocular Hypertension Mouse Model

Colleen M. McDowell

Abstract

There is a great need for the development of mouse models of ocular hypertension. Here, we describe an inducible mouse model of ocular hypertension that produces a homogeneous intraocular pressure (IOP) response and can be induced in any mouse strain of choice without the need for extensive breeding. The procedure utilizes an ocular hypertension and glaucoma-relevant transgene, bioactivated TGFβ2, and an adenovirus 5 virus with select tropism for the trabecular meshwork (TM).

Key words TGFβ2, Ocular hypertension, Inducible model, IOP

1 Introduction

It is well established that aqueous humor levels of TGFβ2 are elevated in POAG patients [1–4]. TGFβ2 treatment of TM cells alters the ECM composition [5–8] and induces ECM cross-linking [9–11], and it is well known that TGFβ2 signals through the canonical SMAD and non-SMAD pathways to alter the ECM in human TM cells [9, 10, 12]. In addition, TGFβ2 has been shown to elevate IOP in anterior segment perfusion organ culture (POC) models [5, 13, 14]. The advent of an inducible model of ocular hypertension has shown that overexpression of a bioactivated form of TGFβ2 in mouse eyes causes ocular hypertension [8, 15] and TGFβ2 signaling through the canonical SMAD pathway is essential for TGFβ2-induced ocular hypertension in mice [16]. These data suggest that TGFβ2 regulates the expression of ECM proteins in the TM and effects of TGFβ2 signaling are a major component in the development of ocular hypertension.

Here we describe in detail the protocol utilizing adenovirus 5 to transduce the trabecular meshwork and overexpress human bioactivated TGFβ2 containing two-point mutations incorporated into the LAP-binding portion (C226S, C228S), referred to throughout as Ad5.TGFβ2, to induce ocular hypertension in mice

Tatjana Jakobs and Paloma B. Liton (eds.), *Glaucoma: Methods and Protocols*, Methods in Molecular Biology, vol. 2858,
https://doi.org/10.1007/978-1-0716-4140-8_11,

[15]. Transduction of the TM with adenoviruses has previously been shown to exhibit relatively strong transgene expression as well as select tropism to the TM tissue with some transduction to the ciliary body, cornea endothelium, and iris [17–21]. Shepard et al. first reported the use of Ad5.TGFβ2 to elevate IOP [15], and the method has been extensively used since. It has also been demonstrated that Ad5.null, Ad5.GFP, and transgenes not associated with glaucomatous phenotypes have no effect on ocular hypertension [15, 17, 22, 23].

2 Materials

All experiments using adenoviruses should be conducted following BSL2 practices. Adenoviruses should be stored at −80 degrees Fahrenheit and multiple freeze-thaws should be avoided. Diligently follow all waste disposal regulations according to BSL2 practices.

1. Replication-incompetent recombinant adenovirus expressing constitutively active TGFβ2 (Ad5.TGFβ2): prepared as in vivo grade purified adenovirus in phosphate-buffered saline (PBS)/ 3% sucrose.
2. Replication-deficient recombinant adenovirus control (Ad5. Null) (*see* **Note 1**).
3. Sterile 1×PBS.
4. Sterile 1.5 mL microcentrifuge tubes.
5. Sterile 33 gauge needle: point style 4, 1 inch length, and 12 degrees angle.
6. Sterile blunted 27G needle: cut to 1.5 cm length using a dremel rotary-tool.
7. 10 mL Hamilton syringe
8. Surgical tape.
9. Dissecting microscope.
10. Proparacaine HCl (0.5%) or other numbing eye drops.
11. Antibiotic ointment.
12. Sterile artificial tears.
13. Sterile cotton swab.
14. Anesthesia: Final concentration 100 mg/kg ketamine and 10 mg/kg xylazine.
15. Analgesic: Final concentration 0.1 mg/kg Buprenorphine.
16. Heating pad.
17. Mice: mouse strain of choice (*see* **Note 2**).

18. Slit-lamp microscope or ophthalmoscope.
19. TonoLab tonometer.

3 Methods

3.1 Preparation of Adenovirus

1. Thaw a vial of Ad5.TGFβ2 and control virus on ice. Adenoviruses must remain on ice at all times. Do not thaw with your fingers or on the benchtop.
2. Prepare the Ad5.TGFβ2 working stock in a sterile 1.5 mL microcentrifuge tube. Concentration is prepared so each animal receives a total of 2.5×10^7 particle forming units (pfu) in a volume of 2 μL (working concentration 1.25×10^7 pfu/μL) (*see* **Note 3**). Sterile PBS is the vehicle solution used. All pipette tips and tubes should be disposed according to BSL2 guidelines.

3.2 Assembly of Needle and Syringe

1. Carefully take the 33-gauge needle from its case without removing the thin wire inside the needle.
2. Place the 33-gauge needle onto the 10 μL Hamilton syringe by unscrewing the end of the syringe head and placing the rubber end of the needle into the syringe. Feed the syringe head back over the thin wire sticking out of the needle and then the needle itself, screwing the syringe head tight on the syringe base. Do not touch the needle tip with the metal syringe head during this process. The dissecting microscope can be used to facilitate this process if needed.
3. Feed the blunted 27-gauge needle over the thin wire sticking out of the needle and then the needle itself. Do not touch the needle tip during this process. The dissecting microscope can be used to facilitate this process if needed. Secure the blunted needle to the syringe base with a small piece of surgical tape (wrapped around about two times). Do not use too much tape or the syringe will not fit into the microcentrifuge tube. The blunted 27-gauge needle provides support for the 33-gauge needle, so it does not bend during the injection procedure.

3.3 Intravitreal Injection Procedure (See Note 4)

1. Anesthetize mice by intraperitoneal injection of a ketamine and xylazine cocktail resulting in a final dose of 100 mg/kg of ketamine/body weight and 10 mg/kg of xylazine/body weight (*see* **Note 5**). After induction, wait 15 min. Assess the plane of anesthesia by application of a painful toe-pinch (hind limb) to determine if the flexor withdrawal response is still present. No response indicates that animal is deeply anesthetized.

2. Move the animal to the dissecting microscope and apply one drop of a solution of proparacaine HCl (0.5%) topically on the eye for corneal anesthesia, and wait for a further 5 min.
3. Whisk away the proparacaine HCl drop with a cotton swab.
4. For right-handed persons, place the animal on its side facing to the left. Gently place your left pointer finger and thumb on the mouse head near the eye for support. Avoid applying unnecessary pressure or covering the nose/mouth area. Gently protrude the eye slightly from its socket to expose the limbus. The right hand will push the needle into the eye. Inject the left eye of the mouse on the inferior side, 1–2 mm behind the limbus. The needle should be at a 45-degree angle to the eye to avoid penetrating or touching the lens. Insert the needle until the needle head is completely inside the eye. It is helpful to have the needle head facing up. Once inside, carefully lift your left hand to the syringe plunger, and slowly inject 2 μL of virus (over the course of 10–15 s) into the eye. Left hand can return to gently supporting the head while the right hand continues to hold the needle inside of the eye for an additional 30 s to 1 min. Slowly remove needle from eye (*see* **Note 6**).
5. Apply antibiotic ointment to the eye using a sterile cotton swab. If only one eye was injected, apply artificial tears to the contralateral eye using a sterile cotton swab.
6. If both eyes are injected, repeat **steps 2–5** for the other eye, right-handed persons will inject right eye on the superior side. Left-handed persons will inject opposite as described.
7. Inject animal subcutaneously with 0.1 mg/kg body weight of buprenorphine.
8. Return animal to cage placed on a heating pad until the animal is fully awake.

3.4 Clinical and Histological Assessment

1. Monitor the eyes of each animal by slit-lamp or ophthalmoscope examination throughout the experimental time course. Evidence of cataracts (due to hitting lens with needle) will appear as white spots on the lens. Evidence of inflammation (due to virus or infection) will appear as iris hyperemia or cloudy cornea.
2. Intraocular pressure should be measured prior to injection and weekly throughout the experimental time course to confirm significant intraocular pressure elevation above baseline for each eye as well as compared to uninjected and Ad5.null-injected eyes. Intraocular pressure should be measured as previously described [24]. All measurements should be taken at the same time of day and under the same conditions (i.e., with similar anesthesia).

3. Immunohistochemical analysis should be performed to confirm overexpression of TGFβ2 as well as histological changes to the TM as previously described [24].

4 Notes

1. An empty adenovirus 5 (commonly referred to as Ad5.null) should be used as a control for all experiments.
2. Strain, sex, and age differences have previously been documented [8, 25]. Always use proper strain, sex, and age-matched controls.
3. Appropriate titers for adenoviral vectors for delivery and expression in the TM are between 1×10^7 and 1×10^8 pfu [23]. Care must be taken to note levels of inflammation with each titer of virus, which can be dependent on the age and strain of mice. Immunomodulation of animals has significantly lowered the inflammatory response as well as enhanced the duration and expression of the transgenes by intraperitoneal injection of anti-CD40L antibody 1 day prior to intraocular delivery of the adenovirus [23] or by desensitization to adenovirus by a subcutaneous injection of 3 μL of the adenovirus with a titer of 3×10^6 pfu into the lower back of newborn pups and subsequent intraocular injection of the adenovirus at 2 months of age [26].
4. Intracameral injections have previously been used although the IOP effect and duration have been shown to be less [15, 17, 22, 23]; therefore, intravitreal injection is the preferred method of delivery [23]. For intravitreal injections, the vitreous serves as a depot for the virus allowing it to slowly percolate to the anterior chamber and transduce the TM.
5. Isoflurane anesthesia can also be used instead of ketamine/xylazine. Care must be taken to ensure the animal receives continued isoflurane exposure and remains in an appropriate depth of anesthesia throughout the procedure. Hand placement may vary using isoflurane to avoid the anesthesia tubing/placement on the mouse nose.
6. Some investigators prefer using a micromanipulator to hold the needle and inject into the eye. Caution must be made to ensure the needle tip does not touch the lens.

Acknowledgments

This work was supported by the National Institute of Health grants R01EY02652 (CMM) and R21EY034295 (CMM). This work was also supported in part by the Unrestricted Grants from Research to Prevent Blindness to the UW-Madison Department of Ophthalmology and Visual Sciences.

References

1. Inatani M, Tanihara H, Katsuta H, Honjo M, Kido N, Honda Y (2001) Transforming growth factor-beta 2 levels in aqueous humor of glaucomatous eyes. Graefes Arch Clin Exp Ophthalmol 239(2):109–113. https://doi.org/10.1007/s004170000241
2. Ochiai Y, Ochiai H (2002) Higher concentration of transforming growth factor-beta in aqueous humor of glaucomatous eyes and diabetic eyes. Jpn J Ophthalmol 46(3):249–253
3. Ozcan AA, Ozdemir N, Canataroglu A (2004) The aqueous levels of TGF-beta2 in patients with glaucoma. Int Ophthalmol 25(1):19–22. https://doi.org/10.1023/b:inte.0000018524.48581.79
4. Tripathi RC, Li J, Chan WF, Tripathi BJ (1994) Aqueous humor in glaucomatous eyes contains an increased level of TGF-beta 2. Exp Eye Res 59(6):723–727. https://doi.org/10.1006/exer.1994.1158
5. Fleenor DL, Shepard AR, Hellberg PE, Jacobson N, Pang IH, Clark AF (2006) TGFbeta2-induced changes in human trabecular meshwork: implications for intraocular pressure. Invest Ophthalmol Vis Sci 47(1): 226–234. https://doi.org/10.1167/iovs.05-1060
6. Wordinger RJ, Fleenor DL, Hellberg PE, Pang IH, Tovar TO, Zode GS, Fuller JA, Clark AF (2007) Effects of TGF-beta2, BMP-4, and gremlin in the trabecular meshwork: implications for glaucoma. Invest Ophthalmol Vis Sci 48(3):1191–1200. https://doi.org/10.1167/iovs.06-0296
7. Fuchshofer R, Yu AH, Welge-Lussen U, Tamm ER (2007) Bone morphogenetic protein-7 is an antagonist of transforming growth factor-beta2 in human trabecular meshwork cells. Invest Ophthalmol Vis Sci 48(2):715–726. https://doi.org/10.1167/iovs.06-0226
8. Hernandez H, Medina-Ortiz WE, Luan T, Clark AF, McDowell CM (2017) Crosstalk between transforming growth factor beta-2 and toll-like receptor 4 in the trabecular meshwork. Invest Ophthalmol Vis Sci 58(3): 1811–1823. https://doi.org/10.1167/iovs.16-21331
9. Tovar-Vidales T, Clark AF, Wordinger RJ (2011) Transforming growth factor-beta2 utilizes the canonical Smad-signaling pathway to regulate tissue transglutaminase expression in human trabecular meshwork cells. Exp Eye Res 93(4):442–451. https://doi.org/10.1016/j.exer.2011.06.011
10. Sethi A, Jain A, Zode GS, Wordinger RJ, Clark AF (2011) Role of TGFbeta/Smad signaling in gremlin induction of human trabecular meshwork extracellular matrix proteins. Invest Ophthalmol Vis Sci 52(8):5251–5259. https://doi.org/10.1167/iovs.11-7587
11. Welge-Lussen U, May CA, Eichhorn M, Bloemendal H, Lutjen-Drecoll E (1999) AlphaB-crystallin in the trabecular meshwork is inducible by transforming growth factor-beta. Invest Ophthalmol Vis Sci 40(10):2235–2241
12. Zode GS, Sethi A, Brun-Zinkernagel AM, Chang IF, Clark AF, Wordinger RJ (2011) Transforming growth factor-beta2 increases extracellular matrix proteins in optic nerve head cells via activation of the Smad signaling pathway. Mol Vis 17:1745–1758
13. Gottanka J, Chan D, Eichhorn M, Lutjen-Drecoll E, Ethier CR (2004) Effects of TGF-beta2 in perfused human eyes. Invest Ophthalmol Vis Sci 45(1):153–158. https://doi.org/10.1167/iovs.03-0796
14. Sharma TP, Curry S, McDowell CM (2020) Effects of toll-like receptor 4 inhibition on transforming growth factor-beta2 signaling in the human trabecular meshwork. J Ocul Pharmacol Ther 36(3):170–178. https://doi.org/10.1089/jop.2019.0076
15. Shepard AR, Millar JC, Pang IH, Jacobson N, Wang WH, Clark AF (2010) Adenoviral gene transfer of active human transforming growth factor-{beta}2 elevates intraocular pressure and reduces outflow facility in rodent eyes. Invest Ophthalmol Vis Sci 51(4):2067–2076. https://doi.org/10.1167/iovs.09-4567
16. McDowell CM, Tebow HE, Wordinger RJ, Clark AF (2013) Smad3 is necessary for transforming growth factor-beta2 induced ocular hypertension in mice. Exp Eye Res 116:419–423. https://doi.org/10.1016/j.exer.2013.10.017
17. Shepard AR, Jacobson N, Millar JC, Pang IH, Steely HT, Searby CC, Sheffield VC, Stone EM, Clark AF (2007) Glaucoma-causing myocilin mutants require the Peroxisomal targeting

signal-1 receptor (PTS1R) to elevate intraocular pressure. Hum Mol Genet 16(6):609–617. https://doi.org/10.1093/hmg/ddm001

18. Borras T, Bryant PA, Chisolm SS (2006) First look at the effect of overexpression of TIGR/MYOC on the transcriptome of the human trabecular meshwork. Exp Eye Res 82(6):1002–1010. https://doi.org/10.1016/j.exer.2005.11.005
19. Borras T, Rowlette LL, Erzurum SC, Epstein DL (1999) Adenoviral reporter gene transfer to the human trabecular meshwork does not alter aqueous humor outflow. Relevance for potential gene therapy of glaucoma. Gene Ther 6(4):515–524. https://doi.org/10.1038/sj.gt.3300860
20. Budenz DL, Bennett J, Alonso L, Maguire A (1995) In vivo gene transfer into murine corneal endothelial and trabecular meshwork cells. Invest Ophthalmol Vis Sci 36(11):2211–2215
21. Hoffman LM, Maguire AM, Bennett J (1997) Cell-mediated immune response and stability of intraocular transgene expression after adenovirus-mediated delivery. Invest Ophthalmol Vis Sci 38(11):2224–2233
22. McDowell CM, Luan T, Zhang Z, Putliwala T, Wordinger RJ, Millar JC, John SW, Pang IH, Clark AF (2012) Mutant human myocilin induces strain specific differences in ocular hypertension and optic nerve damage in mice. Exp Eye Res 100:65–72
23. Millar JC, Pang IH, Wang WH, Wang Y, Clark AF (2008) Effect of immunomodulation with anti-CD40L antibody on adenoviral-mediated transgene expression in mouse anterior segment. Mol Vis 14:10–19
24. McDowell CM, Kizhatil K, Elliott MH, Overby DR, van Batenburg-Sherwood J, Millar JC, Kuehn MH, Zode G, Acott TS, Anderson MG, Bhattacharya SK, Bertrand JA, Borras T, Bovenkamp DE, Cheng L, Danias J, De Ieso ML, Du Y, Faralli JA, Fuchshofer R, Ganapathy PS, Gong H, Herberg S, Hernandez H, Humphries P, John SWM, Kaufman PL, Keller KE, Kelley MJ, Kelly RA, Krizaj D, Kumar A, Leonard BC, Lieberman RL, Liton P, Liu Y, Liu KC, Lopez NN, Mao W, Mavlyutov T, McDonnell F, McLellan GJ, Mzyk P, Nartey A, Pasquale LR, Patel GC, Pattabiraman PP, Peters DM, Raghunathan V, Rao PV, Rayana N, Raychaudhuri U, Reina-Torres E, Ren R, Rhee D, Chowdhury UR, Samples JR, Samples EG, Sharif N, Schuman JS, Sheffield VC, Stevenson CH, Soundararajan A, Subramanian P, Sugali CK, Sun Y, Toris CB, Torrejon KY, Vahabikashi A, Vranka JA, Wang T, Willoughby CE, Xin C, Yun H, Zhang HF, Fautsch MP, Tamm ER, Clark AF, Ethier CR, Stamer WD (2022) Consensus recommendation for mouse models of ocular hypertension to study aqueous humor outflow and its mechanisms. Invest Ophthalmol Vis Sci 63(2):12. https://doi.org/10.1167/iovs.63.2.12
25. Sugali CK, Rayana NP, Dai J, Peng M, Mao W (2022) Age and sex affect TGFbeta2-induced ocular hypertension in C57BL/6J mice. Exp Eye Res 219:109055. https://doi.org/10.1016/j.exer.2022.109055
26. Gramlich OW, Godwin CR, Wadkins D, Elwood BW, Kuehn MH (2021) Early functional impairment in experimental glaucoma is accompanied by disruption of the GABAergic system and inceptive neuroinflammation. Int J Mol Sci 22(14). https://doi.org/10.3390/ijms22147581

Chapter 12

Mouse Model of Glucocorticoid-Induced Glaucoma

Prabhavathi Maddineni, Yogapriya Sundaresan, and Gulab Zode

Abstract

Extended glucocorticoid (GC) treatment can lead to ocular hypertension and induce iatrogenic open-angle glaucoma. GC-induced glaucoma mimics many clinical and pathological features of primary open-angle glaucoma (POAG), and therefore mouse models of GC-induced glaucoma are utilized to study pathophysiology of glaucoma. We have recently demonstrated that weekly periocular injections of dexamethasone-21-acetate (Dex-Ac) lead to robust and significant intraocular pressure (IOP) elevation, retinal ganglion cell (RGC) loss, and optic nerve degeneration in mice. Our mouse model exhibits signature features of POAG including significant IOP elevation due to reduced outflow facility, progressive optic nerve degeneration, and structural and functional loss of RGCs. Dex-induced IOP elevation is associated with increased aqueous outflow resistance due to trabecular meshwork (TM) dysfunction including excessive extracellular matrix deposition and induction of endoplasmic reticulum stress. Mouse model of Dex-induced glaucoma represents an ideal animal model to investigate both glaucomatous damage to the TM and RGC axons and to develop novel therapies. Here, we present a detailed protocol for developing this model in laboratory settings.

Key words Glucocorticoids, Trabecular meshwork, Mouse model of glaucoma, Ocular hypertension, Outflow facility, Pattern electroretinogram, Neurodegeneration

1 Introduction

Glaucoma is a chronic neurodegenerative disease of the eye. It is associated with progressive loss of retinal ganglion cells (RGCs) and optic nerve degeneration leading to visual field defects and permanent vision loss. To date, glaucoma is the second leading cause of blindness, affecting about 80 million people worldwide, which is expected to reach 111 million by 2040 [1, 2]. Glaucoma is a multifactorial disease, and the underlying pathophysiological mechanisms causing the disease are not completely understood [3]. Hence, there is a great necessity to develop an appropriate animal model which will faithfully replicate the disease phenotype to study the etiology of human glaucoma. Since the mouse eyes share similar anatomical and developmental characteristics of the

Tatjana Jakobs and Paloma B. Liton (eds.), *Glaucoma: Methods and Protocols*, Methods in Molecular Biology, vol. 2858, https://doi.org/10.1007/978-1-0716-4140-8_12,

anterior chamber and dynamics of trabecular outflow pathway with humans, mice are believed to be the most attractive animal models to study many aspects of glaucoma [4]. Also, mouse model is a useful tool for identifying and testing potential therapeutic targets for glaucomatous neurodegeneration.

Elevated intraocular pressure (IOP) due to trabecular meshwork (TM) dysfunction is the major causative and the only known modifiable risk factor for primary open-angle glaucoma (POAG), the most common form of glaucoma [5, 6]. Most of the available glaucoma treatment strategies including medical and surgical interventions are targeted toward IOP reduction [7–9]. Like POAG, prolonged glucocorticoid (GC) therapy can cause IOP elevation and subsequent iatrogenic open-angle glaucoma [4, 10, 11]. If untreated, GC-induced IOP elevation can lead to vision loss [12]. The degree of GC-induced IOP elevation depends on the potency of GCs, duration of GC therapy, and the route of administration [4]. Interestingly, GC-induced glaucoma shares many clinical and morphological features of POAG including IOP elevation due to TM dysfunction, characteristic optic neuropathy, and permanent vision loss [13]. Several mouse models of GC-induced glaucoma have been developed to investigate the pathophysiology of glaucoma [14–16]. Unfortunately, most of these studies have focused only on outflow pathway and IOP elevation. There are limited studies that examined glaucomatous neurodegeneration due to chronic GC therapy.

Recently, we have developed a mouse model of GC-induced glaucoma using weekly periocular injections of Dexamethasone-21-Acetate (Dex-Ac) [13, 17]. We demonstrated that weekly periocular injections of Dex-Ac cause sustained and significant IOP elevation, which is associated with reduced aqueous humor outflow facility [13, 17]. We have also observed an increased synthesis and deposition of extra cellular matrix (ECM) proteins (like fibronectin, collagen, laminin, etc.) [13] and induction of chronic endoplasmic reticulum (ER) stress in the TM of mouse model of Dex-induced glaucoma [18–20]. In this mouse model, optic nerve degeneration is preceded by structural and functional loss of the RGC soma [13]. Axonal degeneration involves initial insult at the optic nerve as early as 5 weeks, which gradually progresses and worsens at 8 and 10 weeks. Functional and structural loss of RGCs (soma) is not evident until 8 weeks of Dex-Ac treatment (Fig. 1) [13]. Moreover, Dex-induced glaucomatous neurodegeneration is IOP-dependent. Reduction in IOP either by topical ocular IOP lowering drugs or by withdrawing Dex-Ac-during the early stages of disease onset can prevent the progression of glaucomatous neurodegeneration [13]. Like human glaucoma, IOP-induced axonal damage initially occurs at the optic nerve head and rapidly progresses toward the distal ends of the optic nerve, following Wallerian axonal degeneration [13]. The axonal degeneration in this mouse model is

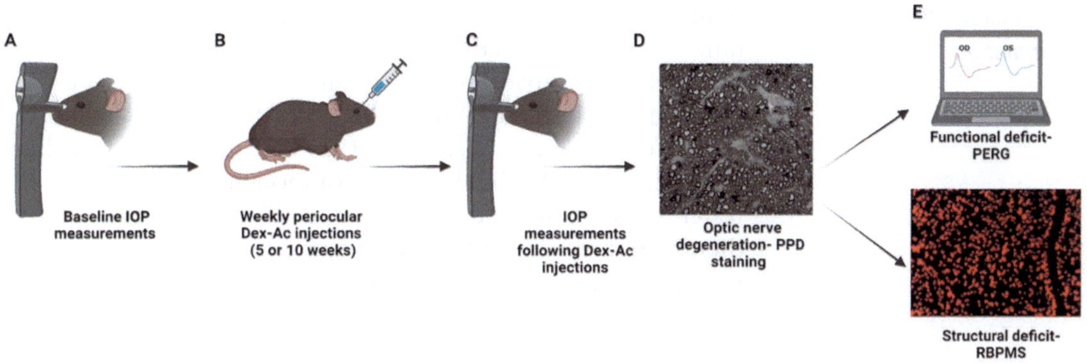

Fig. 1 Schematic showing timeline for glaucoma phenotypes in mouse model of Dex-induced glaucoma: (**a**) Measurement of baseline IOP in three-month-old C57BL/6 mice before Dex-Ac injection; (**b**) weekly periocular injection of Dex-Ac; (**c**) IOP elevation starting from the first week of Dex-Ac treatment and reduced outflow facility at 5 weeks of Dex-Ac treatment; (**d**) optic nerve axonal degeneration initiating at 5 weeks, which further worsens at weeks 8 and 10; and (**e**) functional (PERG) and structural (RBPMS) loss of RGCs is evident at 8 and 10 weeks of Dex-Ac treatment

associated with reactivation of astrocytes, glial scar formation, and immune cell infiltration [13]. Therefore, Dex-induced mouse model of glaucoma is an ideal model to study several underlying pathological aspects of human glaucoma including TM tissue damage, RGC loss, and axonal degeneration. Here, we describe a detailed protocol to develop this mouse model.

2 Materials

2.1 In Vivo Studies

1. Three-month-old C57BL/6 J mice.
2. Anesthesia: isoflurane (2.5%) and oxygen (0.8 L/min). Ketamine and Xylazine (100 mg/kg and 10 mg/kg).
3. 25 μL glass syringes
4. 0.375 inch 32GA needle
5. Tonolab rebound iCare tonometer.
6. Topical ocular proparacaine HCl (0.5%) eye drops.
7. Pattern electroretinogram (PERG) stimulator system, including subcutaneous stainless steel needles, rectal probe, and light-emitting diode tablets.
8. 0.1% Cholera toxin B (CTB) conjugated with either Alexa fluor 555 or Alexa fluor 480
9. CO_2 unit for euthanization.

2.2 Dexamethasone Formulation

1. Vehicle: Sodium chloride (USP granular) 0.667 g/dL, creatinine NF 0.5 g/dL, edetate disodium USP dihydrate 0.05 g/dL, carboxymethylcellulose sodium USP (medium viscosity) 0.5 g/dL, polysorbate 80 NF 0.1 mL/dL, benzyl alcohol NF 0.9 g/dL, sodium bisulfite FCC 0.1 g/dL, and sodium hydroxide 1%. Each chemical component is added to the water sequentially and adjusted the pH to 7. Suspension is then stored at 4 °C until further use.
2. Dexamethasone-21-Acetate: Micronized.
3. 5 mm—stainless steel beads.
4. 2.0 mL microfuge tubes.
5. Aluminum foil.
6. TissueLyser LT.

2.3 Paraphenylene-diamine (PPD) Staining

1. 1% osmium tetroxide
2. Glutaraldehyde.
3. Sodium cacodylate buffer (pH 7.2).
4. Eponate-12.

2.4 Embedding and Sectioning

1. Paraformaldehyde (4%): To prepare 100 mL of 4% PFA, measure 75 mL of 1XPBS and add 25 mL of 16% PFA. Mix the solutions well.
2. Sucrose (30–10%): To prepare 100 mL of 30% sucrose solution, measure 30 gms of D-Sucrose, dissolve using 1× PBS, and make it up to 100 mL. Similarly, to prepare 100 mL of 20% and 10% sucrose solution, measure 20 and 10 gms of D-Sucrose into individual glass bottles, respectively. Dissolve sucrose with 1× PBS and make up the volume to 100 mL.
3. OCT compound.
4. Cryotome.

2.5 Immunostaining

1. Glass slides.
2. Blocking buffer is prepared by combining 10% Goat serum with 0.2% Triton ×-100 in 1×PBS.
3. Humidified incubation chamber. Fill the incubation chamber with water to maintain moisture and humidity before placing the slides treated with primary antibody for overnight incubation. Similarly, use the same water-filled chamber to incubate the slides after the addition of secondary antibody.
4. DAPI mounting.
5. Cover slips.
6. Primary and secondary antibodies (*see* Table 1).
7. Fluorescence microscope.

Table 1
List of antibodies used for immunostaining

	Antibody	Dilutions	Catalog	Manufacturer
Primary antibody	Fibronectin (FN)	1 in 200	sc-18,825	Santa Cruz biotechnology
	Collagen1 (ColI)	1 in 200	NB600–408	Novus biology
	Phalloidin 650	1 in 50	12956S	Cell signaling
	RBPMS	1 in 200	GTX118619	Gentex
	GFAP	1 in 100	ab10062	Abcam
Secondary antibody	Goat antirabbit 568	1 in 500	A11011	Invitrogen
	Goat antimouse 488	1 in 500	A11001	Invitrogen
	Goat antimouse 568	1 in 500	A11031	Life technologies
	Goat antirabbit 488	1 in 500	A11034	Invitrogen

3 Methods

3.1 Preparation of Dex-Ac Formulation

1. In a sterile 2 mL microcentrifuge tube, add 10 mg of micronized Dex-Ac to 1 mL of Veh solution (see **Note 1**).
2. To obtain uniform Dex-Ac formulation, add two stainless steel 5-mm beads to the tube, and mix in a TissueLyser LT for 5 min at 50 oscillations per second.
3. Wrap the microcentrifuge tube containing Dex-Ac suspension with aluminum foil to protect from light and rotate overnight at 4 °C or until further use (see **Note 2**).

3.2 Dex-Ac Periocular Injections

1. Fill 25 μL volume Hamilton glass microsyringe with a 32-gauge needle with 20 μL of Dex-Ac suspension (10 mg/mL) or vehicle solution (*see* **Note 3**).
2. Anaesthetize C57BL/6 mice using isoflurane (2.5%) and oxygen (0.8 L/min).
3. Under anesthesia, retract the lower eyelids and inject the needle (3–5 mm deep) into the periocular space or periocular conjunctival fornix of the eyes.
4. Over the course of 10–15 s, release the Dex-Ac formulation or vehicle solution (*see* **Note 4**).
5. Slowly withdraw the needle without touching any ocular tissues.
6. Repeat periocular injections once a week until the end of the study (see **Note 5**).

3.3 IOP Measurements

1. Measure IOPs during the daytime between 10 AM and 2 PM using a TonoLab rebound tonometer under conscious or isoflurane anesthetic conditions.
2. In a masked manner, take an average of six IOP readings per eye twice a week until the end of study period (*see* **Note 6**).

3.4 Outflow Facility Measurement

Aqueous humor conventional outflow facility is measured in vehicle and Dex-injected mice following 5 weeks of sustained IOP elevation (*see* **Note 7**). There are different outflow facility systems available. Here we describe the constant-flow infusion method.

1. Anesthetize the mice with ketamine/xylazine solution (100/10 mg/kg).
2. Maintain their body temperature at physiological levels by placing the mice on a 37 °C heating pad during the entire procedure (*see* **Note 8**).
3. Apply topical ocular proparacaine HCl (0.5%) eye drops on mouse eyes for corneal anesthesia.
4. Cannulate the anterior chamber of the mouse eye with a 30-gauge needle through the cornea without touching the iris, anterior lens capsule, or corneal endothelium.
5. Connect the cannulated needles to a precalibrated flow-through BLPR-2 pressure transducer, and maintain continuous pressure within the perfusion system.
6. Connect the opposing end of the transducer to a 1 mL syringe, loaded into a micro dialysis infusion pump.
7. Fill the perfusion system with sterile 1×PBS, and infuse the eyes at a flow rate of 0.1 μL/min to 0.5 μL/min (in 0.1 μL/min increments).
8. Record three stabilized pressures at 5 min intervals for each flow rate, and take an average of these three stabilized pressures as a mean stabilized pressure.
9. For calculating the aqueous humor outflow facility, take the reciprocal of the slope of a plot of mean stabilized pressure as the ordinate and flow rate as the abscissa.

3.5 Fixation of Ocular Tissues

1. At the end of study period, euthanize the mice through intracardiac perfusion of PBS followed by 4% paraformaldehyde (PFA) or carbon dioxide (CO_2) inhalation method followed by cervical dislocation.
2. Enucleate the eyes along with the optic nerves and further fix with 4% PFA for 2 h at room temperature.
3. Wash the fixed ocular tissues in 1× PBS for 15 min.

3.6 Immunostaining

1. Incubate the PFA fixed eyes in a gradient concentration of sucrose solution (10–30%) overnight at 4 °C in a rotating shaker.
2. Embed the sucrose-treated tissues in OCT.
3. Using a cryostat, take 12-micron tissue sections for immunostaining.

3.6.1 Paraphenylene-diamine (PPD) Staining

1. Fix the optic nerves in 1.5% PFA and 1.5% glutaraldehyde in 100 mM sodium cacodylate buffer (pH 7.2) for at least 24 h.
2. Later, process the optic nerves for PPD staining.

3.6.2 Analysis of Selected Markers by IHC

Like human POAG, TM dysfunction due to increased deposition of ECM proteins is observed in Dex-induced mouse model of glaucoma [18–20]. In addition, chronic IOP elevation in this mouse model is associated with reactivation of astrocytes at the optic nerve head [13]. In order to examine the TM pathology and reactive astrocytes in optic nerve head, we have analyzed the expression of ECM (FN & ColI) and Phalloidin in TM and GFAP expression (for reactive astrocytes) at optic nerve head by immunostaining.

1. Incubate the 12 micron tissue sections in blocking buffer for 2 h at room temperature.
2. Later, incubate the tissue sections overnight with specific primary antibody (diluted in blocking buffer) at 4 °C in a humidified chamber.
3. Wash the tissue sections with 1× PBS three times, and further incubate the sections with corresponding secondary antibodies (1:500 dilution in 1× PBS) at room temperature for 2 h.
4. Following 1× PBS wash (three times), mount the tissue sections with DAPI mounting solution.
5. Image the mounted sections using a fluorescence microscope.

3.7 Pattern Electroretinography

A noninvasive binocular snout PERG is used to analyze the function of RGCs in Dex-induced mouse model of glaucoma.

1. To carry out PERG, anesthetize the mice with ketamine/xylazine solution (100/10 mg/kg), and position them on a heated stage throughout the procedure.
2. Monitor the body temperature of mice using a rectal probe.
3. Obtain the PERG measurements concurrently from each eye of the animal by using subcutaneous stainless-steel electrodes placed at the snout (active), back of the head (reference), and tail (ground). The pattern stimuli are generated on two identical custom-made light-emitting diode tablets alternating at slightly different frequencies (OD, 0.984 Hz; OS, 0.992 Hz).
4. Obtain individual PERG signals from each eye using one-channel continuous acquisition and phase-locking average (OD, 369 epochs of 492 ms; OS, 372 epochs of 496 ms).
5. Calculate the average of the final PERG values of two consecutive measurements taken from each eye [13, 21].

3.8 Axonal Transport

The functional deficit of axons in terms of anterograde transport (movement of the cargo from cell body toward the axon tip) is investigated by cholera toxin B (CTB) labelling.

1. At the end of study period, anesthetize the mice and intravitreally inject 3 μL of 0.1% CTB conjugated with either Alexa fluor 555 or Alexa fluor 480 using a Hamilton syringe with a 33-gauge needle.
2. After 48 h of injection, euthanize the mice through intracardiac perfusion to enucleate the eyes and brain tissues.
3. Fix the tissues in 4% PFA for 12 h at 4 °C.
4. Wash the fixed eyes and brain tissue in 1× PBS, and treat them in a gradient concentrations of sucrose solution (10–30%) for 3 days.
5. Embed the sucrose-treated tissues in OCT compound.
6. Section the embedded eyes at 12-micron thickness.
7. To visualize the axonal anterograde transport of CTB in the superior colliculus, take serial frontal sections of the brain at 30-micron thickness.
8. Wash the sections with 1× PBS and mount with mounting medium containing nuclear stain DAPI.
9. Image the mounted slides using a fluorescence microscope [13].

3.9 RGC Staining

In Dex-induced mouse model of glaucoma, we have observed significant loss of RGC as early as at week 8 (see **Note 9**) [13]. We have used whole-mount retina stained with RBPMS antibody to examine the total number of surviving RGCs in Dex-mouse model of glaucoma.

1. Enucleate the eyes from Veh or Dex-injected mice and fix in 4% PFA for 12 h at 4 °C.
2. Rinse the eyeballs in 1x PBS and remove the retina from the posterior cup.
3. Incubate the isolated retinas in blocking buffer for 12 h at 4 °C.
4. Following this step, incubate the retinas with RBPMS antibody for 3 days at 4 °C.
5. Following incubation, wash the stained retinas for 2 h in 1× PBS.
6. After washing, retinas are treated with the corresponding secondary antibody (1:500 dilution in 1× PBS) for 2 h at room temperature.
7. Wash the retinas for 1 h in 1× PBS and mount them with mounting medium containing DAPI nuclear stain.

8. For counting RGCs, take at least 16 nonoverlapping images from the entire retina, captured at 20× magnification using a fluorescence microscope.
9. Use ImageJ software to count RBPMS-positive cells.

3.10 PPD Staining

We have used PPD staining to examine the optic nerve degeneration in Dex-induced mouse model of glaucoma. PPD stains the myelin sheath of healthy axons and darkly stains the axoplasm of damaged axons.

1. Treat the glutaraldehyde/paraformaldehyde fixed optic nerves overnight with 1% osmium tetroxide at 4 °C.
2. Following this step, rinse the optic nerves in 0.1 M phosphate buffer twice for 10 min and once in 0.1 M sodium acetate buffer.
3. Dehydrate the optic nerves in graded ethanol concentrations.
4. Embed the optic nerves in Eponate-12 resin and cut 1 micron sections.
5. Stain the sections with 1% PPD for 10 min.
6. To analyze Dex-induced optic nerve degeneration, take ten nonoverlapping images covering the entire optic nerve at a magnification of 63×, and count the axons in an area equal to 10% of the total nerve cross-sectional area.

4 Notes

1. In our laboratory, we have observed a similar trend in IOP elevation using either micronized Dex-Ac or dexamethasone. In our lab, we use micronized forms of Dex-Ac to obtain uniform formulations with small particle size.
2. Dex formulations form larger particles/clumps after 2 weeks, which can clog the syringe needle and result in variable amounts of drug being delivered with each injection. An important point to note is that Dex formulations containing large particles can lead to the death of mice following periocular injections. Therefore, we recommend using freshly prepared Dex formulation for weekly injections.
3. The optimum dosing concentration of Dex (either Dex-Ac or Dexamethasone) for periocular injection is 200 μg/eye. Administration of high doses of Dex may result in the death of mice (after approximately 5 weeks of weekly periocular injections).
4. In C57BL/6 mice, we performed bilateral injections (where each mouse was injected with either Dex or a Veh in both eyes) as well as unilateral injections (where each mouse was injected

with Dex in one eye and Veh in the other eye) for 10 weeks. With unilateral injections of Dex, we observed an increase in IOP in the contralateral eye after 8 weeks of injections. Considering this, we recommend avoiding unilateral injections of Dex for a prolonged duration.

5. To maintain sustained elevation of IOP, we perform weekly periocular injections of Dex (200 μg/eye). Dex-induced IOP elevation is reversible, and withdrawal of Dex injections can return IOP to its baseline.
6. Isoflurane could significantly decrease IOP in a very short period of time especially in eyes with elevated IOP [22]. It is therefore recommended to complete the IOP measurements within 4 min under isoflurane anesthetic conditions.
7. In Dex-induced glaucoma, morphological alterations (particularly an increased deposition of ECM proteins) in the TM are closely associated with outflow obstruction. We observed a significant ECM deposition in Dex-induced mouse model of glaucoma starting at week 4. Therefore, we recommend measuring aqueous humor outflow facility in this mouse model after 4 weeks of sustained IOP elevation.
8. In our mouse model, we have not observed any adverse effects of Dex, including a change in body weight. However, we noted a slight resistance to Ketamine/Xylazine anesthesia in Dex-injected mice as compared to vehicle-injected mice.
9. Our mouse model of Dex-induced glaucoma demonstrated significant IOP elevation from the first week of injection, and glaucomatous neurodegeneration at week 5, which further increased at weeks 8 and 10. It should be noted that we have characterized the effects of Dex on IOP elevation and neurodegeneration in three-month-old male mice. Depending on the age and gender of the mice, the timeline of glaucomatous neurodegeneration may differ.

References

1. Kingman S (2004) Glaucoma is second leading cause of blindness globally. Bull World Health Organ 82(11):887–888
2. Tham YC, Li X, Wong TY, Quigley HA, Aung T, Cheng CY (2014) Global prevalence of glaucoma and projections of glaucoma burden through 2040: a systematic review and meta-analysis. Ophthalmology 121(11): 2081–2090. https://doi.org/10.1016/j.ophtha.2014.05.013
3. Mantravadi AV, Vadhar N (2015) Glaucoma. Prim Care 42(3):437–449. https://doi.org/10.1016/j.pop.2015.05.008
4. Overby DR, Clark AF (2015) Animal models of glucocorticoid-induced glaucoma. Exp Eye Res 141:15–22. https://doi.org/10.1016/j.exer.2015.06.002
5. Kapetanakis VV, Chan MP, Foster PJ, Cook DG, Owen CG, Rudnicka AR (2016) Global variations and time trends in the prevalence of primary open angle glaucoma (POAG): a systematic review and meta-analysis. Br J Ophthalmol 100(1):86–93. https://doi.org/10.1136/bjophthalmol-2015-307223
6. Collaborative Normal-Tension Glaucoma Study Group (1998) Comparison of

glaucomatous progression between untreated patients with normal-tension glaucoma and patients with therapeutically reduced intraocular pressures. Am J Ophthalmol 126(4): 487–497. https://doi.org/10.1016/s0002-9394(98)00223-2

7. Collaborative Normal-Tension Glaucoma Study Group (1998) The effectiveness of intraocular pressure reduction in the treatment of normal-tension glaucoma. Am J Ophthalmol 126(4):498–505. https://doi.org/10.1016/s0002-9394(98)00272-4
8. Heijl A, Leske MC, Bengtsson B et al (2002) Reduction of intraocular pressure and glaucoma progression: results from the early manifest glaucoma trial. Arch Ophthalmol 120(10): 1268–1279. https://doi.org/10.1001/archopht.120.10.1268
9. Danias J, Podos SM (1999) Comparison of glaucomatous progression between untreated patients with normal-tension glaucoma and patients with therapeutically reduced intraocular pressures. The effectiveness of intraocular pressure reduction in the treatment of normal-tension glaucoma. Am J Ophthalmol 127(5):623–625. https://doi.org/10.1016/s0002-9394(99)00088-4
10. Bollinger K, Kim J, Lowder CY, Kaiser PK, Smith SD (2011) Intraocular pressure outcome of patients with fluocinolone acetonide intravitreal implant for noninfectious uveitis. Ophthalmology 118(10):1927–1931. https://doi.org/10.1016/j.ophtha.2011.02.042
11. Kiddee W, Trope GE, Sheng L et al (2013) Intraocular pressure monitoring post intravitreal steroids: a systematic review. Surv Ophthalmol 58(4):291–310. https://doi.org/10.1016/j.survophthal.2012.08.003
12. Becker B, Mills DW (1963) Corticosteroids and intraocular pressure. Arch Ophthalmol 70:500–507. https://doi.org/10.1001/archopht.1963.00960050502012
13. Maddineni P, Kasetti RB, Patel PD et al (2020) CNS axonal degeneration and transport deficits at the optic nerve head precede structural and functional loss of retinal ganglion cells in a mouse model of glaucoma. Mol Neurodegener 15(1):48. https://doi.org/10.1186/s13024-020-00400-9
14. Whitlock NA, McKnight B, Corcoran KN, Rodriguez LA, Rice DS (2010) Increased intraocular pressure in mice treated with dexamethasone. Invest Ophthalmol Vis Sci 51(12): 6496–6503. https://doi.org/10.1167/iovs.10-5430
15. Zode GS, Sharma AB, Lin X et al (2014) Ocular-specific ER stress reduction rescues glaucoma in murine glucocorticoid-induced glaucoma. J Clin Invest 124(5):1956–1965. https://doi.org/10.1172/JCI69774
16. Li G, Lee C, Agrahari V et al (2019) In vivo measurement of trabecular meshwork stiffness in a corticosteroid-induced ocular hypertensive mouse model. Proc Natl Acad Sci USA 116(5): 1714–1722. https://doi.org/10.1073/pnas.1814889116
17. Patel GC, Phan TN, Maddineni P et al (2017) Dexamethasone-induced ocular hypertension in mice: effects of Myocilin and route of administration. Am J Pathol 187(4):713–723. https://doi.org/10.1016/j.ajpath.2016.12.003
18. Maddineni P, Kasetti RB, Kodati B, Yacoub S, Zode GS (2021) Sodium 4-phenylbutyrate reduces ocular hypertension by degrading extracellular matrix deposition via activation of MMP9. Int J Mol Sci 22(18). https://doi.org/10.3390/ijms221810095
19. Kasetti RB, Maddineni P, Millar JC, Clark AF, Zode GS (2017) Increased synthesis and deposition of extracellular matrix proteins leads to endoplasmic reticulum stress in the trabecular meshwork. Sci Rep 7(1):14951. https://doi.org/10.1038/s41598-017-14938-0
20. Kasetti RB, Maddineni P, Patel PD, Searby C, Sheffield VC, Zode GS (2018) Transforming growth factor beta2 (TGFbeta2) signaling plays a key role in glucocorticoid-induced ocular hypertension. J Biol Chem 293(25): 9854–9868. https://doi.org/10.1074/jbc.RA118.002540
21. Chou TH, Bohorquez J, Toft-Nielsen J, Ozdamar O, Porciatti V (2014) Robust mouse pattern electroretinograms derived simultaneously from each eye using a common snout electrode. Invest Ophthalmol Vis Sci 55(4):2469–2475. https://doi.org/10.1167/iovs.14-13943
22. Ding C, Wang P, Tian N (2011) Effect of general anesthetics on IOP in elevated IOP mouse model. Exp Eye Res 92(6):512–520. https://doi.org/10.1016/j.exer.2011.03.016

Chapter 13

Trabecular Meshwork Stem Cells for Glaucoma Treatment

Yiqin Du, Sridhar Bammidi, and Enzhi Yang

Abstract

Elevated intraocular pressure (IOP) is the most important risk factor for primary open-angle glaucoma (POAG) and currently is the only effective treatment target for glaucoma to prevent vision loss. In POAG patients, the trabecular meshwork (TM) cellularity is reduced which might be the main pathologic reason for the conventional outflow pathway dysfunction leading to elevated IOP. Stem cell-based therapy has been shown promising to reduce IOP and preserve retinal ganglion cells and their function in animal models. In this chapter, we describe the method details on TM stem cell cultivation and identification; induction for differentiation into different cell types, including differentiation to TM cell responsiveness to dexamethasone treatment with phagocytic function; and transplantation into mouse anterior chamber for therapeutic purposes.

Key words Glaucoma, Trabecular meshwork, Stem cells, Culture, Identification, Differentiation, Intracameral injection

1 Introduction

Glaucoma is the second leading cause of irreversible blindness worldwide and affects 76 million people [1, 2]. Although the detailed pathophysiology of glaucoma is still unknown, elevated intraocular pressure (IOP) remains the most important risk factor for glaucoma. The main components of the conventional outflow pathway, the trabecular meshwork (TM) and the adjacent Schlemm's canal endothelium are the main resistant sites for aqueous humor outflow. When the resistance increases, it can cause the imbalance of aqueous humor inflow and outflow, resulting in accumulation of aqueous humor in the eye and elevation of IOP. Elevated IOP will damage the retinal ganglion cells (RGC) and optic nerve, leading to irreversible blindness. The effective treatment for glaucoma is to reduce the IOP via oral and/or topical medications, surgeries, and laser treatments. The pathophysiology of the outflow pathway has been partially discovered that the TM cellularity is reduced in primary open-angle glaucoma (POAG)

Tatjana Jakobs and Paloma B. Liton (eds.), *Glaucoma: Methods and Protocols*, Methods in Molecular Biology, vol. 2858,
https://doi.org/10.1007/978-1-0716-4140-8_13,

patients as compared to age-matched normal controls [3, 4]. The reduction of the TM cellularity could be associated with fused trabecular beams and naked trabecular beams without covering by the TM cells [5], which can cause TM dysfunction and elevated IOP, leading to RGC and optic nerve damage. Considering this pathological change in POAG, it has significant potential and feasibility to explore cell-based therapies as innovative approaches for treating glaucoma. Cell-based therapies can replenish the TM cellularity and reconstruct the TM extracellular matrix (ECM) that can recover the TM structure and function, hence decreasing the outflow resistance and reducing the elevated IOP to prevent vision loss.

Stem cells are self-renewal and multipotent that can differentiate into different functional cell types for function in vitro and in vivo. Theoretically, stem cells are the best candidate for cell-based therapies. Stem cells in the trabecular meshwork (TMSC) have been identified which are located in the insert region between the filtering TM region and the corneal endothelium [6–9]. We have successfully isolated and characterized human TMSC [2, 7, 10–14] and intracamerally injected human TMSC into mouse anterior chamber where the cells can home and integrate to the TM tissue [12, 13, 15–17], reconstructed laser-damaged TM tissue [13] and the TM tissue in transgenic mice with myocilin (MYOC) Y437H mutation [16]. TMSC homing to the TM tissue is associated with chemokine pair CXCR4/SDF1 [13], and their maintenance in the TM tissue is associated with integrin pair alpha5 beta1 integrin [17]. The results are promising toward clinical trials for treating POAG. In this chapter, we describe the detailed methods of TMSC cultivation; identification; and differentiation, including differentiation into TM cells characterized by dexamethasone responsiveness and phagocytosis; and transplantation into mouse anterior chamber.

2 Materials

2.1 TMSC Cultivation

1. Donated human corneal tissue including the limbus or corneal rims after removal of the central cornea for corneal transplant (*see* **Notes 1** and **2**). Corneal tissue should be preserved within 12 h after death and should be used within 7 days if stored in Optisol at 4 °C.
2. Microscope for tissue dissection.
3. Tissue dissection tools: forceps, scissors, and scalpels.
4. TrypLE express enzyme.
5. Human corneal tissue wash: DMEM/F12 medium supplemented with GASP (gentamicin, amphotericin B, penicillin, and streptomycin mixture).

6. Culture dishes/25 cm^2 and 75 cm^2 culture flasks.
7. Fibronectin (FNC) coating mix.
8. Cell Strainer-70 μm nylon mesh.
9. TMSC culture medium: multipurpose reduced-serum media (OptiMEM-1), 5% fetal bovine serum (FBS), 10 ng/mL epithelial growth factor, 100 μg/mL bovine pituitary extract, 20 μg/mL ascorbic acid, 200 μg/mL calcium chloride, 0.08% chondroitin sulfate, 100 IU/mL penicillin, 100 μg/mL streptomycin, and 50 μg/mL gentamicin.
10. Trypan Blue Solution, 0.4%.
11. An automated cell counter or a hemocytometer.
12. Sterile CO_2 incubator: Set at 37 °C, 5% CO_2, and 100% humidity.
13. Freezing medium: 70% OptiMEM-1, 20% FBS, and 10% DMSO (*see* **Note 3**).
14. Freezing vials.
15. Mr. Frosty Freezing Container and 100% isopropyl alcohol.
16. Water bath.
17. Liquid nitrogen tank.
18. Centrifuge.

2.2 Flow Cytometry Determination of TMSC Purity

1. 1×PBS
2. Fc Blocker.
3. 1% BSA (bovine serum albumin): Dissolve 1 g of BSA in 80 mL 1×PBS, wait for 10 min or stir for a short time, and add 1×PBS to a total of 100 mL. Filter through a 0.22 μm filter and store at 4 °C. Alternatively, prepare a stock of 10% BSA (5 g of BSA in 50 mL of 1×PBS) and dilute the stock solution at 1:10 in 1×PBS before use (*see* **Note 4**). Stock solution can be stored at 4 °C.
4. Live/Dead Fixable dye: Add 50 μL of DMSO into one vial (commercially available) and store at −20 °C. Use 1:1000 for staining with the cell concentration at 1×10^6 cells/mL.
5. Antibodies targeting CD73, CD90, CD105, and CD166, each conjugated with distinct fluorescence markers.
6. Flow cytometer or access to a flow cytometer.

2.3 Evaluation of TMSC Clonogenic Potential

1. TMSC culture medium, as described in Subheading 2.1, **item 9**.
2. Six-well culture plates.
3. 1% or 4% Paraformaldehyde (PFA).

4. Crystal violet stain solution (0.5% in 25% methanol): If commercially available, dilute 50 mL of 1% crystal violet in 25 mL of water and 25 mL of 100% of methanol. If powder is used, dissolve 500 mg of crystal violet in 25 mL of methanol and 75 mL of water.
5. Light microscope.
6. A plate reader (optional).

2.4 Evaluation of TMSC Multipotent Potential

1. TMSC culture medium, as described in Subheading 2.1, **item 9**.
2. 12-well plates.
3. Osteogenic differentiation medium: commercially available.
4. Alizarin Red S staining solution: 2% in ddH_2O.
5. Adipogenic differentiation medium: commercially available.
6. Oil Red O staining solution: 0.5% in isopropanol.
7. Neural differentiation medium: neurobasal medium, 1×B27 supplement, 1×N2 supplement, 20 ng/mL of epidermal growth factors, and 20 ng/mL of fibroblast growth factors.
8. Anti-neurofilament and anti-β-III tubulin antibodies.
9. Immumount antifade mounting solution.
10. Confocal microscope.

2.5 Trabecular Meshwork Cell Differentiation

1. Cultured and identified human primary TM cells.
2. Condition medium from TM cells: Culture medium collected in log phase growth condition (60–70% confluence) and clarified by centrifugation at 1000× *g* to remove any cell debris (*see* **Note 5**).
3. Dexamethasone (100 nM): Dissolve 25 mg dexamethasone in 1 mL of methanol or 2 mL of absolute ethanol, and then add culture medium DMEM/F12 to 6.37 mL to make it a 10 mM stock solution. Aliquot and store at −20 °C. Dilute one aliquot with DMEM/F12 to 100 μM (1:100 from 10 mM) and store at −20 °C as aliquots. 1:1000 dilute the 100 μM stock solution to reach final working concentration at 100 nM.
4. Anti-human MYOC antibody.
5. *S. aureus* bioparticles conjugated with pHrodo Red for phagocytosis.

2.6 Delivery of TMSC into the Murine Conventional Outflow Pathway

1. Surgical forceps.
2. 30-gauge needles
3. 33-gauge Hamilton needles
4. 10 μL or 25 μL Hamilton syringes

5. Anesthesia: ketamine/xylazine (*see* **Note 6**).
6. 0.5% Proparacaine eye drops
7. 0.3% Gentamicin eye drops
8. 2.5% Gonak hypromellose ophthalmic solutions
9. Surgical microscope.
10. Vybrant dye DiO (green), DiI (red), or DiD (far red) to label cells.
11. Mice: open-angle glaucoma mice and WT mice as controls.

3 Methods

3.1 Isolation and Culturing of TMSC from Tissue Explants

1. Thoroughly wash corneal rims or corneal tissues in human corneal tissue wash.
2. Submerge corneal tissues in DMEM/F12 with antibiotics GASP for 5 min. Repeat three times.
3. In the meantime, coat a 25 cm^2 flask with FNC coating (*see* **Note 7**).
4. Under a dissecting microscope, carefully dissect the TM tissue by cutting along its edges [18, 19]. Be sure to include the insert region, where the TMSCs are located (Fig. 1).
5. Place the dissected TM tissue onto the coated flask and add 1.5 mL of TMSC culture medium.
6. Place the flask into a tissue culture incubator set at 5% CO_2 and 37 °C.
7. Do not disturb for 7 days to facilitate tissue attachment and cell migration. Then, carefully add 3.5 mL fresh medium to the flask.
8. Perform partial medium changes every 3 days.
9. After 2–3 weeks, trypsinize the outgrowth cells for passage.

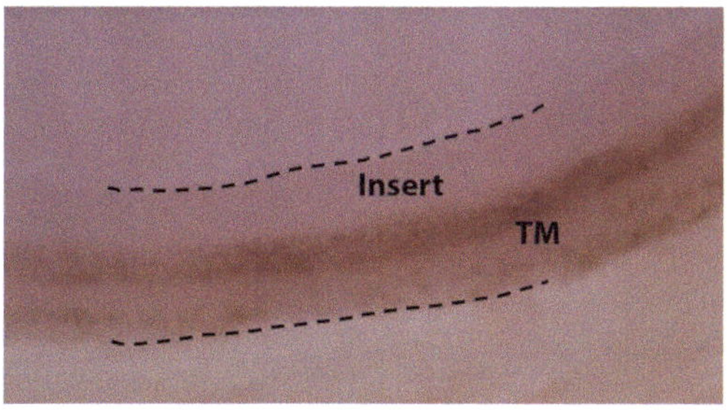

Fig. 1 Human trabecular meshwork brightfield view. The TM and insert regions are labeled. The dotted lines are the inner and outer edges for cutting and dissection for TM and TMSC culture

3.2 Isolation and Culturing of TMSC from Digested Single Cells

1. Follow **steps 1–4** in Subheading 3.1.
2. Using a pair of forceps, place the dissected TM tissue into a 15 mL conical tube.
3. Add 2 mL of TrypLE and loosely scroll the cap on, allowing air to enter the tube (*see* **Note 8**).
4. Place the tube into a tissue culture incubator set at 5% CO_2 and 37 °C for 30 min and gently agitate every 10 min.
5. To terminate the digestion, add 2 mL of DMEM/F12 with 2% FBS, pipetting up and down several times.
6. Pellet the cells by centrifugation at 400× *g* for 5 min. Discard supernatant.
7. Add 4 mL DMEM/F12–2% FBS and filter through a 70 μm Cell Strainer to remove any undigested tissue.
8. Centrifuge at 400× *g* for 5 min and discard supernatant.
9. Repeat **steps** 7 and **8**.
10. Determine cell viability and total cell density using Trypan Blue with an automated cell counter or a hemocytometer.
11. Seed the cells at $1–2 \times 10^3$ cells/cm^2 in TMSC culture medium onto FNC-coated dishes/flasks prepared in **step 1**.

3.3 Passaging of TMSC

Cells will be ready to passage when reaching ~80% confluence (Fig. 2) (*see* **Note 9**).

1. Aspirate culture medium and wash the cells twice with 1×PBS to completely remove FBS in the medium ready for digestion.

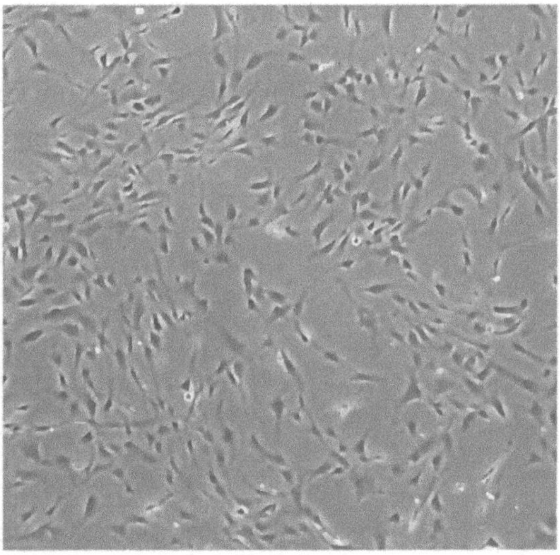

Fig. 2 Cultured human trabecular meshwork stem cells (TMSCs) that are ready to be passaged

2. Add a sufficient volume of TrypLE to cover the cells (1 mL in a 25 cm^2 flask or 3 mL in a 75 cm^2 flask), and incubate the flask in the incubator at 37 °C for approximately 5 min or until most of the cells appear rounded or detached from the flask surface.
3. Add the same volume of DMEM/F12–2% FBS as of TrypLE, and gently pipette up and down to completely detach the cells.
4. Pipette the cells into a 15 mL conical tube.
5. Determine cell viability and total cell density using Trypan Blue with an automated cell counter or hemocytometer.
6. Pellet the cells by centrifugation at 400× *g* for 5 min and wash one more time with DMEM/F12–2%FBS.
7. Add culture medium to seed the cells at 1–2 × $10^3/cm^2$.

3.4 Cryopreservation and Revival of TMSC

1. Follow Subheading 3.3, **steps 1–6**.
2. Resuspend the cells in freshly prepared freezing medium at 2 × 10^5–2 × 10^6 cells/mL, and aliquot into freezing vials at 1 mL/vial.
3. Place freezing vials into a Mr. Frosty Freezing Container filled with 100% isopropyl alcohol, allowing temperature to gradually reduced overnight. After 24 h, move cryovials into a liquid nitrogen tank for long-term storage (*see* **Note 10**).
4. To thaw TMSC, take one vial of the cells out of liquid nitrogen tank, and immediately put the vial into a prewarmed 37 °C water bath (*see* **Note 11**).
5. Wait for a minute for the cells to be thawed completely before taking the vial out of the water bath (*see* **Note 12**).
6. Gently, pipette the cells into a conical 15 mL tube and add 3 mL of DMEM/F12–2%FBS.
7. Centrifuge at 400× *g* for 5 min and discard supernatant.
8. Add 4 mL of DMEM/F12–2%FBS and gently suspend the cell pellet. Count cell number, and centrifuge again.
9. Resuspend the cells in the appropriate volume of TMSC culture medium and seed at a density of 5 × 10^3 cells/cm^2.
10. Replace the culture medium the following day.

3.5 Flow Cytometry Determination of TMSC Purity

TMSC share some characteristics as mesenchymal stem cells and express cell surface markers CD73, CD90, CD105, and CD166 which can be used to detect the stem cell purity by flow cytometry [2, 13, 14].

1. Trypsinize cultured TMSC when they reach 70–80% confluence as detailed in Subheading 3.3.
2. Wash cells with 1×PBS.
3. Resuspend the cells in DMEM/F12 at 1 × 10^6 cells/mL.

4. Add a Live/Dead Fixable dye at 1:1000 (choose the color distinguishable from antibody-conjugated colors).
5. Incubate 15 min on ice in dark.
6. Wash with 1×PBS and centrifuge at 500× *g* for 5 min.
7. Continue to next step or fix the cells in 1% PFA for 20 min and wash with 1×PBS once. Add 100 μL of 1×PBS-1% BSA and the fixed cells can be stored up to 7 days at 4 °C.
8. Resuspend the pellet cells in 75 μL of 1×PBS-1% BSA for 10 min on ice to block nonspecific sites.
9. Add antibodies or isotype controls: After blocking, no wash is needed. Directly divide each cell type into three groups (25 μL each) as no-stain control, isotype control, and staining (*see* **Note 13**). Dilute antibodies or isotype controls at 1:50 each in 1×PBS-1% BSA, and add 25 μL into each tube to make the final concentration of each antibody and isotype at 1:100. Add the same volume of 1×PBS-1% BSA into each no-stain control tube.
10. Incubate for 45 min on ice in dark.
11. Add 2 mL of 1×PBS-1%BSA and centrifuge at 500× *g* for 5 min. Discard the supernatant. Wash cells one more time.
12. Resuspend cells in 600 μL of 1×PBS and split into three tubes for triplicates. Alternatively, cells can be fixed with 1% PFA for 20 min on ice, washed in 2 mL of 1×PBS and stored in fresh 1×PBS at 4 °C in dark up to 1 week.
13. Run flow analysis in a flow cytometer.
14. Good TMSC should have more than 90% of the cells expressing these surface markers CD73, CD90, CD105, and CD166 (Fig. 3). Positive controls (other confirmed stem cell types or previously confirmed TMSC) and negative controls (nonstem cells such as TM cells and fibroblasts) should be included for every experiment. If TMSC purity is not good (less than 90%), the cells should be discarded or be passaged in a very low density (1000 cells/well of a 6-well plate = 100 cells/cm^2), and the colony-forming cells can be picked up as stem cells for further identification and experiments.

3.6 Evaluation of the TMSC Clonogenic Potential

1. Seed 1000 TMSC cells in a single well of a 6-well plate using TMSC culture medium.
2. At about 7 days, look for the presence of cell colonies under a microscope.
3. Fix the cells in 4% PFA for 15 min, followed by two of 5 min washes with 1×PBS.
4. Stain the colonies with 0.5% crystal violet staining solution for 30 min.

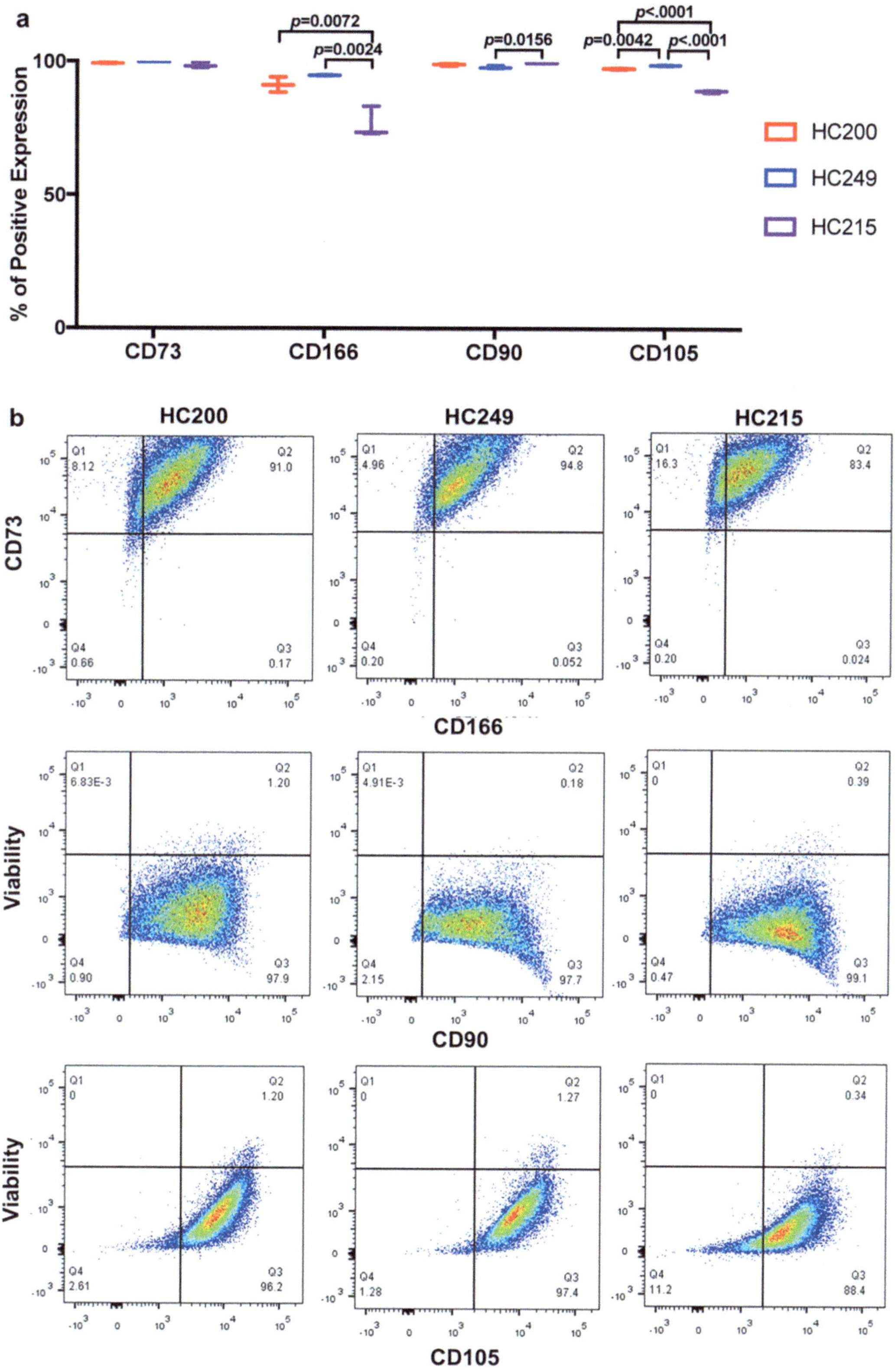

Fig. 3 Human trabecular meshwork stem cell identification. TMSC expression of cell surface markers CD73, CD166, CD90, and CD105 was assessed by flow cytometry. (**a**). Bars show the percentage of positive

5. Wash thoroughly with tap water (*see* **Note 14**).
6. Capture light microscopy images and count colonies containing more than 50 cells per colony (Fig. 4). The colony number indicates the quality of cultured stem cells, the more the better. Only stem cells can form colonies because of their self-renewal property.

[**Optional**] To assess the relative quantity of colonies, extract the crystal violet by incubating the stained colonies with 100% methanol (*see* **Note 15**) for 10 min. Measure the optical density at 570 nm using a plate reader.

3.7 Evaluation of TMSC Multipotent Potential

TMSCs are multipotent that they can be induced to differentiate into osteocytes, adipocytes, neural cells, and TM cells [2, 12, 14].

3.7.1 Osteogenic Differentiation

1. Seed TMSCs in TMSC culture medium at a density of 1×10^4 cells/well in 12-well plates. Allow cells to reach 70% confluence.
2. Switch culture medium to commercially available osteogenic differentiation culture medium. Replace the culture media every 3–4 days. Allow cells to differentiate for 21 days.
3. After the differentiation period, rinse the cells with 1×PBS, and fix them in 4% PFA at room temperature in a chemical hood for 15 min.
4. Stain cells with 2% Alizarin Red S for 2–3 min and rinse cells with distilled water.
5. Capture light microscopy images for quantitative analysis.
6. [Optional] For further quantification, Alizarin Red S can be extracted using cetylpyridinium chloride buffer, and the absorbance can be measured at 570 nm using a plate reader.

3.7.2 Adipogenic Differentiation

1. Follow **steps 1–4** in Subheading 3.7.1, using commercially available adipogenic differentiation medium in **step 2**.
2. Stain cells with Oil Red O to identify adipocytes that contain oil droplets.

Capture light microscopy images for quantitative analysis (i.e., calculate percentage of adipocytes containing oil droplets of the total cells per field).

Fig. 3 (continued) expression to CD73, CD166, CD90, and CD105 on TMSCs from different donors (HC200, HC249, HC215). Statistical analysis was done using two-way ANOVA followed by a Tukey posttest using SAS software. (**b**). Representative flow cytometry figures show the cell surface marker expression and viability, as assessed by Live/Dead staining. (Adapted from Yun et al. [13] under the Creative Commons Attribution 4.0 International (CCBY4.0) license)

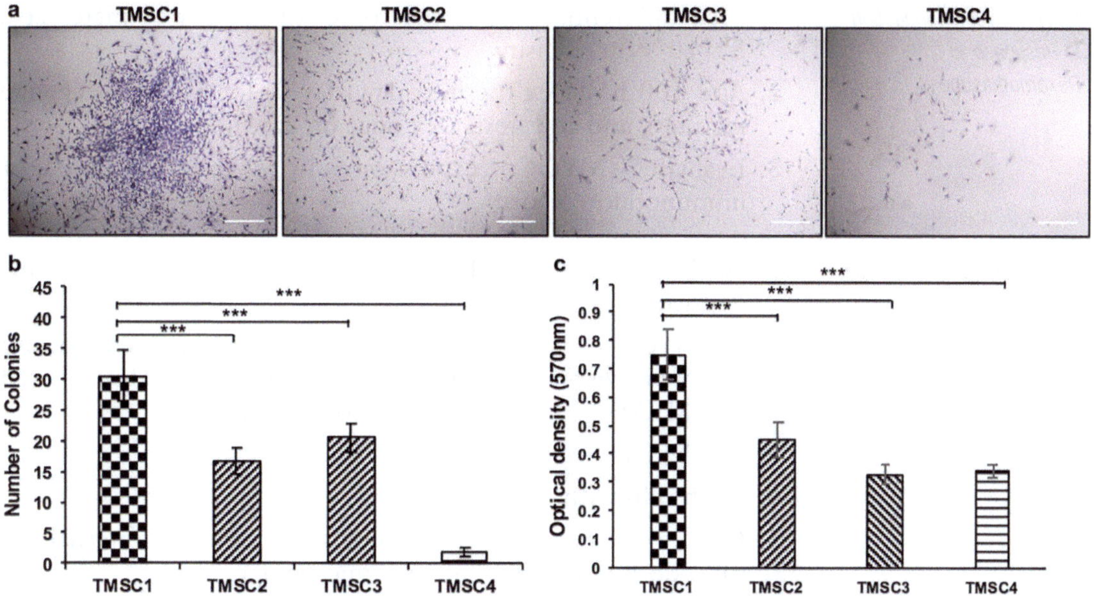

Fig. 4 Assessment of colony-forming efficiency. (**a**). Crystal violet staining for colonies formed by different TMSCs. (**b**). Comparison of colonies formed by different TMSCs. (**c**). Quantification of optical density from crystal violet-stained colonies in different TMSCs. Scale bars = 500 μm. ***$p < 0.0001$. (Adapted from Kumar et al. [14] with permission (license ID 1404147-1))

3.7.3 Neural Differentiation

1. Follow **steps 1–4** in Subheading 3.7.1, using neural differentiation medium in **step 2** and allowing cells to differentiate for 5 weeks.
2. Stain the cells with anti-neurofilament and anti-β-III Tubulin antibodies, using immunocytochemical techniques.

3.8 Differentiation of TMSC into TM Cells (See Note 16)

1. Plate TMSC into 6-well plates at a high density ($5 \times 10^3/cm^2$) in DMEM/F12–10% FBS for 10 days [2, 14]. Change medium every 3 days until day 10 (*see* **Note 17**). After 10 days, TMSC can differentiate into TM cells.

   Alternative: Although changing TMSC culture medium to DMEM/F12–10%FBS can induce TMSC to differentiate into TM cells, we use condition medium from primary TM cells to achieve a better induction rate as an alternative. We add 50% of condition medium into DMEM/F12–10%FBS culture medium for TM cell differentiation for 10 days. Change medium every 3 days.
2. Authenticate differentiated TM cells by evaluating myocilin induction in response to dexamethasone (Dex) treatment [19] (*see* Subheading 3.8.1) and phagocytic activity [20, 21] (*see* Subheading 3.8.2).

3.8.1 Myocilin Induction in Response to Dexamethasone

1. Seed differentiated TM cells onto 12- or 6-well plates at a $5 \times 10^3/cm^2$ density.
2. Add 100 nM Dex the next day (day 0) for 5–7 days, change medium, and add fresh Dex once on day 3.
3. Evaluate MYOC expression by Western blot or immunofluorescence.

3.8.2 Phagocytic Activity

1. Seed differentiated TM cells onto 6-well plates at $5 \times 10^3/cm^2$ density.
2. When cells reach 70% confluence, remove culture medium. and add *S. aureus* bioparticles conjugated with pHrodo Red diluted in DMEM/F12 at 1 mg/mL into the wells.
3. Incubate the cells for 4 h at 37 °C.
4. Wash cells with 1×PBS.
5. Cells can be fixed with 4% PFA or directly observe internalized pHrodo Red under a fluoresce microscope.

3.9 Delivery of TMSC into the Murine Conventional Outflow Pathway

3.9.1 Labeling of TMSC

1. Confirm stem cell purity of TMSC and their ability to differentiate into TM cells, as detailed in Subheadings 3.5 and 3.8.
2. Seed TMSC (passages 4–6) onto 75 cm^2 flasks and culture until reaching their log phase of growth at around 70–80% confluency.
3. Wash cells with 1×PBS, trypsinize, and evaluate cell number and viability as detailed in Subheading 3.3, **steps 1–5**.
4. Centrifuge cells at 400× *g* for 5 min.
5. Discard supernatant and wash with DMEM/F12–2% FBS.
6. Resuspend cells at a concentration of 1×10^6 cells/mL in DMEM/F12.
7. Add dye [vybrant dye DiO (green), DiI (red), or DiD (far red)] at a final 1:200 dilution to label the cell surface.
8. Incubate at 37 °C for 20 min.
9. Wash cells three times using DMEM/F12 to completely remove any unbounded dye.
10. Resuspend the cell pellet in OptiMEM-1 at a concentration of 5000 cells/μL (*see* **Note 18**).

3.10 Intracameral Injection of TMSC into the Mouse Eye

1. Anesthetize mice via intraperitoneal injection of ketamine and xylazine, as approved under your institutional animal care and use committee protocol (*see* **Note 19**).
2. Add a drop of 0.5% proparacaine onto the cornea surface for topical anesthesia.

3. Add a drop of antibiotic eye drops (such as 0.3% gentamicin eyedrops) onto the cornea surface for prevention of potential contamination.
4. Using a pair of forceps, protrude and hold the mouse eye for injection (*see* **Note 20**).
5. Use a 30 g needle to make a corneal tunnel that goes into the anterior chamber (*see* **Note 21**), and the aqueous humor will flow out of the eye.
6. Inject 1.5 μL air to fill up the anterior chamber using a 10 μL Hamilton microsyringe fitted with a 33 g blunt needle.
7. Gently inject 2 μL cells (10,000 cells) freshly filled in a 10 or 25 μL Hamilton microsyringe fitted with a 33 g beveled needle (*see* **Note 22**).
8. Hold the eye with the corneal tunnel on top so the injected air bubble can block the corneal tunnel to prevent cell leakage. This is a critical step to ensure the same cell number injection.
9. Add one drop of 2.5% Gonak onto the cornea surface.
10. Put the mouse on a warm pad to keep mouse warm and help recovery.

4 Notes

1. Human tissues should be handled in Biosafety Level 2 laboratories using a laminar flow hood and protective personal apparel. Serology should be obtained from each donor to exclude the possibility of contamination with HIV and hepatitis. A corneal rim after corneal transplant can only be used if the donated tissue has been obtained with informed consent and authorized for both clinical and research purposes.
2. Since TMSC cell numbers are reduced with age [9], similar to TM cell reduction with age [3,4], tissues from younger donors would have more chance to get TMSC.
3. The freezing medium should be made fresh each time when freezing cells. Since OptiMEM-1 is the basal medium of TMSC culture medium, it is better to use this in the freezing medium. DMEM or DMEM/F12 also works well.
4. BSA stock solution has to be stored at 4 °C to avoid potential contamination.
5. The condition medium can be kept at 4 °C if used within 1 week. Otherwise, the condition medium can be aliquoted and stored at −80 °C for later use.
6. For ketamine, DEA license is needed, and double-locked storage is necessary.

7. FNC coating solution contains fibronectin and collagen which can help the TM tissue attach to the culture dishes/flasks. After FNC coating, coated dishes/flasks can be used immediately and do not need to be dried out.
8. Assure that the tissue is completely submerged in TrypLE.
9. TMSC tend to differentiate when they reach 100% confluence. To better maintain their stemness, avoid complete confluency during culture.
10. If cells are used within a month, the cells in freezing vials can be stored at −80 °C without going into a liquid nitrogen tank.
11. Before taking a freezing vial out, prewarm the water bath to 37 °C, and warn other people not to put cold bottles into the water bath while thawing cells.
12. Do not take freezing vial out of 37 °C water bath and look at the cells within 1 min before cells completely thawed.
13. Antibody-conjugated colors should be easily distinguishable by the flow cytometer. If several cell strains are stained at the same time, a master mix of antibodies should be made and added with the same volume to avoid any possible pipetting errors with tiny volume of individual antibody for pipetting.
14. Both crystal violet and methanol are toxic and should be handled with caution. The stained solution can be collected and reused.
15. Using methanol to extract crystal violet should be performed in a chemical hood.
16. When doing cell-based therapies, the ability of stem cells differentiating into functional cells would be required. Whether TMSC can differentiate into functional TM cells should be evaluated to determine the TMSC quality.
17. We have reported that TMSC can differentiate into TM cells by changing medium from TMSC culture medium to DMEM/F12 containing 10% FBS and let them grow to 100% confluence. It means TMSC can differentiate into TM cells without adding TM condition medium, although the efficacy is lower than adding TM condition medium for induction.
18. We have injected 10,000 cells or 50,000 cells into mouse anterior chamber, and we did not see problems with such cell injection. Since 10,000 cells have effective effects in terms of TM cell replenishment and regeneration, we would recommend this cell number for injection.
19. An institutional animal care and use committee (IACUC)-approved protocol is required before any animal experiments.
20. When holding the eye with a pair of forceps, do not put much pressure over the eye and do not protrude the eye over.

21. Parallel the needle to the iris to avoid damaging the iris which could cause bleeding into the anterior chamber.
22. Fill 2 μL cells into a Hamilton microsyringe each time before injection. **Do not** fill cells full in the syringe, and inject 2 μL each time since cells would precipitate so the cell number would not be the same each injection.

References

1. Quigley HA, Broman AT (2006) The number of people with glaucoma worldwide in 2010 and 2020. Br J Ophthalmol 90(3):262–267. https://doi.org/10.1136/bjo.2005.081224
2. Du Y, Roh DS, Mann MM, Funderburgh ML, Funderburgh JL, Schuman JS (2012) Multipotent stem cells from trabecular meshwork become phagocytic TM cells. Invest Ophthalmol Vis Sci 53(3):1566–1575. https://doi.org/10.1167/iovs.11-9134
3. Alvarado J, Murphy C, Juster R (1984) Trabecular meshwork cellularity in primary open-angle glaucoma and nonglaucomatous normals. Ophthalmology 91(6):564–579. https://doi.org/10.1016/s0161-6420(84)34248-8
4. Alvarado J, Murphy C, Polansky J, Juster R (1981) Age-related changes in trabecular meshwork cellularity. Invest Ophthalmol Vis Sci 21(5):714–727
5. Gong HSD (2016) The histopathological changes in the trabecular outflow pathway and their possible effects on aqueous outflow in eyes with primary open-angle glaucoma. In: Knepper PA, Samples JR (eds) Glaucoma research and clinical advances 2016–2018. Kugler, Amsterdam, pp 17–40
6. Braunger BM, Ademoglu B, Koschade SE, Fuchshofer R, Gabelt BT, Kiland JA, Hennes-Beann EA, Brunner KG, Kaufman PL, Tamm ER (2014) Identification of adult stem cells in Schwalbe's line region of the primate eye. Invest Ophthalmol Vis Sci 55(11): 7499–7507. https://doi.org/10.1167/iovs.14-14872
7. Yun H, Zhou Y, Wills A, Du Y (2016) Stem cells in the trabecular meshwork for regulating intraocular pressure. J Ocul Pharmacol Ther 32(5):253–260. https://doi.org/10.1089/jop.2016.0005
8. Kelley MJ, Rose AY, Keller KE, Hessle H, Samples JR, Acott TS (2009) Stem cells in the trabecular meshwork: present and future promises. Exp Eye Res 88(4):747–751. https://doi.org/10.1016/j.exer.2008.10.024
9. Sundaresan Y, Veerappan M, Ramasamy KS, Chidambaranathan GP (2019) Identification, quantification and age-related changes of human trabecular meshwork stem cells. Eye Vis (Lond) 6:31. https://doi.org/10.1186/s40662-019-0156-z
10. Castro A, Du Y (2019) Trabecular meshwork regeneration—a potential treatment for glaucoma. Curr Ophthalmol Rep 7(2):80–88. https://doi.org/10.1007/s40135-019-00203-2
11. Kumar A, Gandhi K, Du Y (2021) Trabecular meshwork regeneration by stem cells for glaucoma treatment: rationale, feasibility, and mechanisms. In: Samples J, Knepper P (eds) Glaucoma research and clinical advances: 2020–2022. Kugler Publications, The Netherlands, pp 95–104
12. Coulon SJ, Schuman JS, Du Y, Bahrani Fard MR, Ethier CR, Stamer WD (2022) A novel glaucoma approach: stem cell regeneration of the trabecular meshwork. Prog Retin Eye Res 90:101063. https://doi.org/10.1016/j.preteyeres.2022.101063
13. Yun H, Wang Y, Zhou Y, Wang K, Sun M, Stolz DB, Xia X, Ethier CR, Du Y (2018) Human stem cells home to and repair laser-damaged trabecular meshwork in a mouse model. Commun Biol 1:216. https://doi.org/10.1038/s42003-018-0227-z
14. Kumar A, Xu Y, Du Y (2020) Stem cells from human trabecular meshwork hold the potential to develop into ocular and non-ocular lineages after long-term storage. Stem Cells Dev 29(1): 49–61. https://doi.org/10.1089/scd.2019.0169
15. Du Y, Yun H, Yang E, Schuman JS (2013) Stem cells from trabecular meshwork home to TM tissue in vivo. Invest Ophthalmol Vis Sci 54(2):1450–1459. https://doi.org/10.1167/iovs.12-11056
16. Xiong S, Kumar A, Tian S, Taher EE, Yang E, Kinchington PR, Xia X, Du Y (2021) Stem cell transplantation rescued a primary open-angle glaucoma mouse model. elife 10. https://doi.org/10.7554/eLife.63677

17. Xiong S, Xu Y, Wang Y, Kumar A, Peters DM, Du Y (2020) alpha5beta1 integrin promotes anchoring and integration of transplanted stem cells to the trabecular meshwork in the eye for regeneration. Stem Cells Dev 29(5): 290–300. https://doi.org/10.1089/scd.2019.0254
18. Stamer WD, Seftor RE, Snyder RW, Regan JW (1995) Cultured human trabecular meshwork cells express aquaporin-1 water channels. Curr Eye Res 14(12):1095–1100. https://doi.org/10.3109/02713689508995815
19. Keller KE, Bhattacharya SK, Borras T, Brunner TM, Chansangpetch S, Clark AF, Dismuke WM, Du Y, Elliott MH, Ethier CR, Faralli JA, Freddo TF, Fuchshofer R, Giovingo M, Gong H, Gonzalez P, Huang A, Johnstone MA, Kaufman PL, Kelley MJ, Knepper PA, Kopczynski CC, Kuchtey JG, Kuchtey RW, Kuehn MH, Lieberman RL, Lin SC, Liton P, Liu Y, Lutjen-Drecoll E, Mao W, Masis-Solano M, McDonnell F, McDowell CM, Overby DR, Pattabiraman PP, Raghunathan VK, Rao PV, Rhee DJ, Chowdhury UR, Russell P, Samples JR, Schwartz D, Stubbs EB, Tamm ER, Tan JC, Toris CB, Torrejon KY, Vranka JA, Wirtz MK, Yorio T, Zhang J, Zode GS, Fautsch MP, Peters DM, Acott TS, Stamer WD (2018) Consensus recommendations for trabecular meshwork cell isolation, characterization and culture. Exp Eye Res 171:164–173. https://doi.org/10.1016/j.exer.2018.03.001
20. Buller C, Johnson DH, Tschumper RC (1990) Human trabecular meshwork phagocytosis. Observations in an organ culture system. Invest Ophthalmol Vis Sci 31(10):2156–2163
21. Zhou Y, Xia X, Yang E, Wang Y, Marra KG, Ethier CR, Schuman JS, Du Y (2020) Adipose-derived stem cells integrate into trabecular meshwork with glaucoma treatment potential. FASEB J 34(5):7160–7177. https://doi.org/10.1096/fj.201902326R

Chapter 14

Aqueous Humor Angiography

Clemens A. Strohmaier, Fiona McDonnell, and Alex S. Huang

Abstract

Aqueous humor angiography, or aqueous angiography, is an anterior segment imaging technique capable of visualizing the conventional/trabecular aqueous humor outflow pathways. As a translational technique, it is applicable for in vivo imaging in living subjects and ex vivo imaging using whole-globe preparations or anterior segment perfusion setups. Excellent spatial and temporal resolution has enabled insights into the segmental distribution of aqueous humor outflow in physiological conditions as well as after trabecular bypass surgery. In this chapter, we thoroughly describe aqueous humor angiography in various experimental setups. The necessary materials for different settings and their application for in vivo and ex vivo experiments as well as notes on dye choice, dye sequences, and special considerations on performing aqueous humor angiography during surgery are presented.

Key words Aqueous humor outflow, Intraocular pressure, Angiography, Glaucoma

1 Introduction

Aqueous humor angiography, or aqueous angiography, is an anterior segment technique that images aqueous humor outflow (AHO), similar to how intravenous angiography for the posterior segment visualizes retinal and choroidal vessels. Its application has been focused on better understanding conventional/trabecular AHO and potentially improving glaucoma therapeutics that utilize this pathway.

For AHO research, aqueous angiography adds temporal and spatial dimensions to AHO understanding. Currently, the Goldmann equation expresses steady-state intraocular pressure (IOP) as the relationship between aqueous humor production and outflow facility with episcleral venous pressure (EVP) as an additive factor [1]. Thus, for the determination of steady-state IOP in this equation, trabecular outflow facility is reduced to a single number. This simplification, however, neglects the spatial as well as temporal aspects of trabecular outflow. Several clinical and experimental conditions highlight the necessity for a more detailed investigation

Tatjana Jakobs and Paloma B. Liton (eds.), *Glaucoma: Methods and Protocols*, Methods in Molecular Biology, vol. 2858, https://doi.org/10.1007/978-1-0716-4140-8_14,

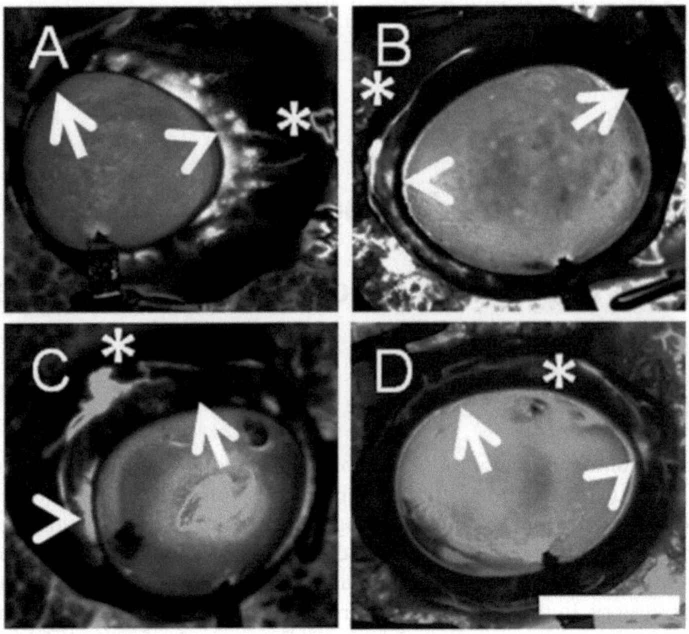

Fig. 1 Whole globe perfusion setup using postmortem pig eyes showing the segmental characteristics of AHO. Aqueous angiography distinguishes different AHO patterns: proximal high-flow regions (arrowheads), more distal high-flow regions (asterisks), and low-flow regions (arrows) [3]. (Figure acquired with author permission)

of AHO. First of all, trabecular outflow is segmental (*see* Fig. 1). This has been shown via spatial differences in AHO tracer-bead uptake during direct trabecular meshwork (TM) imaging [2] or via imaging of soluble tracers introduced into the eye from an external perspective [3]. Regions with greater (or faster) versus lower (or slower) AHO have been shown to differ in their extracellular matrix compositions and proteins as well as in TGFβ-related profibrotic pathways [4, 5]. Whether they differ in their local facility is currently unknown, even though such a difference is assumed.

Spatial information on AHO is also crucially important when TM interventions are studied, either in experimental settings (e.g., anterior segment perfusion setups) or in a clinical setting (e.g., surgical TM bypass) [6]. Acquiring AHO patterns may confirm successful TM bypass by differential AHO angiograms and could possibly guide the TM intervention to either high- or low-flow regions. The anatomy behind AHO is studied at an even deeper level when combining angiographic with structural imaging methods. Since the aqueous angiography technique as we regularly apply it and describe it in the present chapter is executed using a multimodal imaging device, optical coherence tomography (OCT) imaging of ocular anatomy within the depth of the tissue can also be acquired near-simultaneous to the angiographic outflow information.

Aqueous angiography was developed with translational purpose in mind and thus started with FDA-approved instrumentation and dyes (although off-label) for human applications. This approach provides the advantage that the same general method used for ex vivo eyes (e.g., whole eye perfusion setups and anterior segment perfusion setups) can be used for in vivo (e.g., living nonhuman primate and human subjects) AHO imaging. To the best of the authors' knowledge, aqueous angiography is currently the only outflow imaging technique with this translational potential.

In this chapter, we thoroughly describe relevant aspects for the use of aqueous angiography in ex vivo and in vivo eyes. In addition to the needed equipment and the acquisition of images, a detailed discussion of considerations for experimental design is given in the notes section.

2 Materials

2.1 Setup

AHO angiography can be performed using different setups. Up to now, we have used it for in vivo imaging in human subjects [7] and nonhuman primates [8]. Ex vivo imaging has been carried out in whole globe preparations for human [9], dog [10], cat [11], porcine [3], and bovine eyes [12]. Furthermore, anterior segment perfusion setups for porcine and human eyes have been recently performed. The basic components of the setup are the same across applications. This includes an imaging apparatus, imaging dyes, and a dye delivery system. Slight differences exist in how each component is arranged for each application. For example, pharmaceutical-grade agents as well as approved medical devices must be used for human subjects.

2.2 Imaging Apparatus

Typically, aqueous angiography is performed using the Heidelberg Spectralis (Heidelberg Engineering Gmbh, Heidelberg, Germany), a commercially available multimodal imaging device. It is available in the standard table-top configuration as well as in the Spectralis FLEX variant. In the FLEX, the camera is mounted on an adjustable arm suitable for imaging patients in a supine position (*see* Fig. 2) or ex vivo eyes on a table. Either variant is capable of all imaging modalities available on the Spectralis: fluorescein and indocyanine green (ICG) angiography using confocal laser scanning ophthalmoscopy, infrared confocal laser scanning ophthalmoscopy, and OCT. Through interchangeable lenses, the field of view, working distance, and image magnification can be adapted to the needs of the application. Built-in software and a PC supplied by the

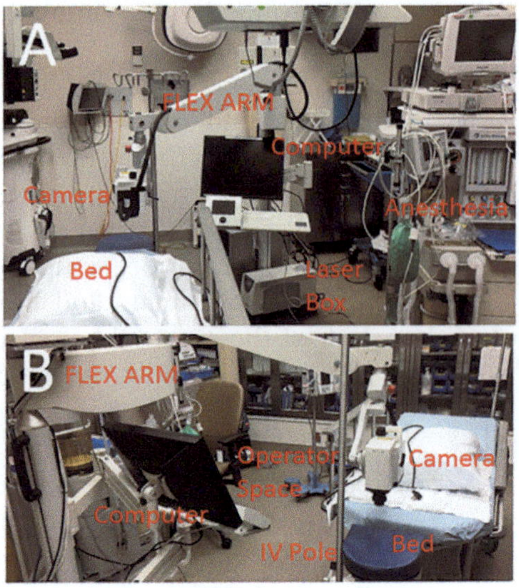

Fig. 2 Exemplary setup of the imaging system in the OR [15]. (Figure acquired with author's permission)

manufacturer handles the image acquisition, documentation, and data storage.

2.3 Imaging Dyes

The Spectralis device has inbuilt lasers and filters so that angiographically, it was originally used for intravenous delivery of fluorescein and ICG for retinal vasculature imaging as the FDA-approved human use. As such, intracameral dye delivery for AHO angiography is still off-label. The typical final dye concentrations are 2–2.5% for fluorescein and 0.4% for ICG. These are the same concentrations described for other anterior segment applications (e.g., staining the lens capsule in cataract surgery [13]) and have been found to provide good contrast in AHO angiography. Lower concentrations decrease contrast, but too high concentrations decrease it too, because of the well-known inner-filter effect of fluorescent dyes [12] (*see* **Note 1**).

The final fluorescein concentration can be easily diluted from a 10% or 25% commercially acquired stock solution using balanced salt solution. ICG, however, has limited solubility. Pharmaceutical-grade ICG comes as powder with a sterile solvent which can be used to achieve a 2% stock solution. Nonpharmaceutical grade ICG (for laboratory use) can be dissolved using sterile water to 2%. All ICG stocks must then be further dissolved to a 0.4% final solution using balanced salt solution. Fluorescein and ICG should be prepared and administered separately, as a combined solution alters obtained fluorescence intensity [12].

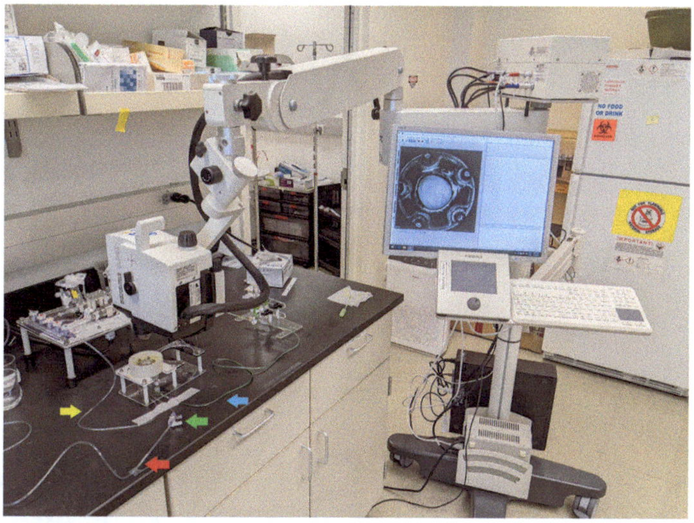

Fig. 3 Exemplary setup for aqueous angiography using an anterior segment perfusion system. The Spectralis FLEX is ideally suited for this kind of application. The iPerfusion system chamber uses two separate tubings for fluid delivery (red arrow) and drainage (blue arrow). Three-way stop-cocks are interposed in the tubing to allow for dye application with minimal dead volume (greed arrow). The third line (orange arrow) in the picture acts as a reference for hydrostatic pressure at the chamber height

2.4 Perfusion-Based Dye Delivery System (Using an Ex Vivo Perfusion Apparatus)

Depending on the application, an appropriate setup for perfusing the anterior chamber (AC) with the angiography dye is needed. The dye delivery system typically consists of one or two lines of tubing with three-way stop cocks and a syringe pump that provides constant flow prefusion. A pressure transducer can be added to measure IOP. In any case, the system used should allow for a quick volume exchange without increasing the anterior chamber pressure, so that the angiography imaging can be started at a defined timepoint by applying pressure to the system. We currently use the iPerfusion system [14] for anterior segment and whole globe perfusion setups (*see* Fig. 3) (*see* **Note 2**).

2.5 Gravity-Based Dye Delivery System (for Ex Vivo Eyes Mounted on a Styrofoam Head or In Vivo Imaging During Cataract Surgery in Patients)

If no Spectralis FLEX is available, a Styrofoam head can be used to hold whole globe preparations in the Spectralis tabletop configuration because the Styrofoam head chin can be seated in the Spectralis chinrest (*see* Fig. 4). In this case, dye delivery is accomplished using the same approach used during patient care. For patient care dye delivery, an IV pole is first acquired. The chandelier is removed from the pole to allow for more maneuverability. The perfusion apparatus is setup with a 10 cc syringe connected to a three-way stopcock (*see* Fig. 5). The side port of the three-way stopcock is connected to a 1 cc syringe, which is partially filled. Then the other end of the three-way stopcock is connected to 14–28 inches of

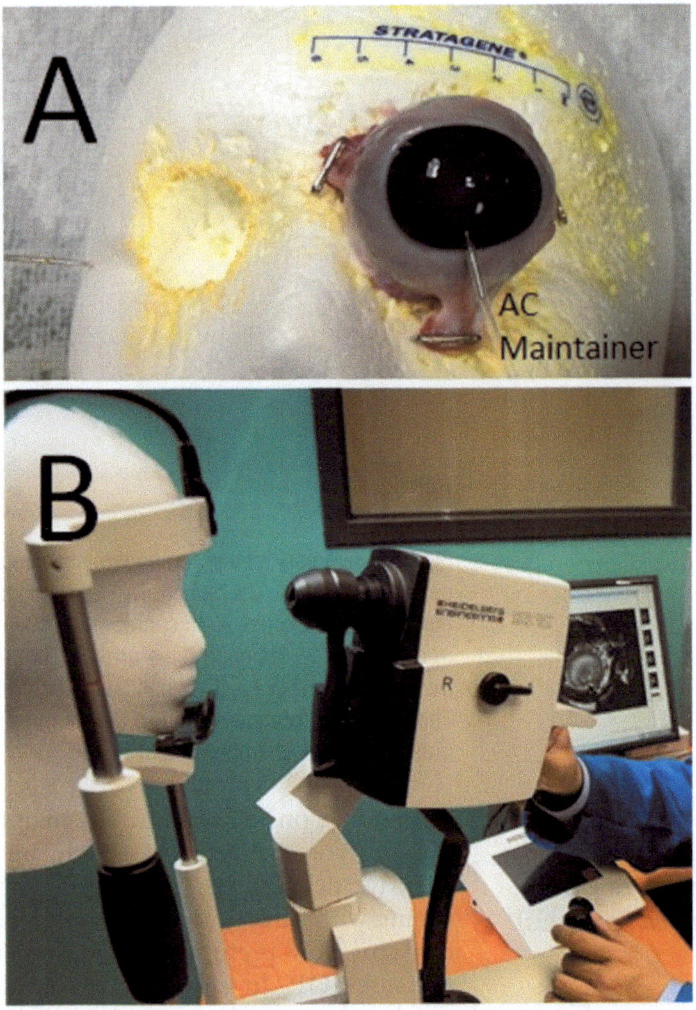

Fig. 4 Aqueous angiography in ex vivo whole globe preparations. This figure shows a bovine eye. (**a**) The eye is trimmed of excess tissue and the extraocular muscles are pinned to the Styrofoam head. An AC maintainer is used for anterior chamber fluid exchange. (**b**) The Styrofoam head can then be placed on the chin rest of the Spectralis device similar to what is done during patient care [12]. (Figure acquired with author's permission)

sterile tubing. Greater length allows for flexibility but increases the dead volume. The entire apparatus is primed with the dye of choice. The setup is then taped to the IV pole at a height above the eye for the desired gravity-driven pressure. For patient care and in vivo imaging, the entire dye delivery system is constructed in a sterile fashion and then taped to the IV pole that is sterile covered (e.g., multiple 3 M sterile drape 1000) (*see* **Note 3**).

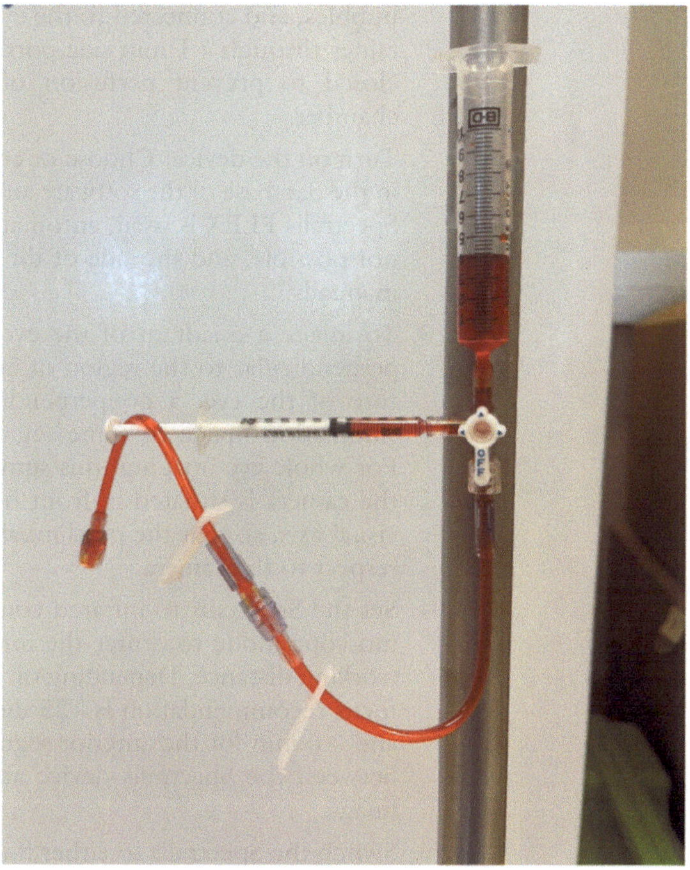

Fig. 5 Gravity based dye delivery system as used for in vivo imaging or ex vivo whole globes mounted on Styrofoam heads. For in vivo imaging, the IV pole is sterile-draped and all syringes and tubings are connected using sterile techniques

3 Methods

3.1 General Angiography Methods

First, decide on the region of interest (either whole eye or single quadrant imaging), and choose the appropriate Spectralis lens. Most commonly, the 55-degree lens will give a good overview of the entire eye. If either higher magnification or near-simultaneous OCT is desired, the blue Heidelberg anterior segment module lens should be used.

3.2 Angiography of Ex Vivo Eyes

1. Prepare the perfusion system. This will depend on the setup used (either with an eye placed in a table-top perfusion chamber [see Subheading 2.4] or mounted on the Styrofoam head [see Subheading 2.5]). Given that different experimental perfusions systems can be customized and lab-specific, the primary goal is to have the system readily filled with dye, free of air

bubbles, and connected to the eye (needle in AC or AC maintainer through a 1 mm side port wound). Keep the stopcocks closed to prevent perfusion of the dye into the anterior chamber.

2. Turn on the device. Choose or create the desired subject entry in the database of the software and start the examination. If the Spectralis FLEX is used, automatic eye detection (OD/OS) is not possible, and the side of the studied eye must be entered manually.
3. To image a quadrant of the eye, align the Spectralis camera perpendicular to the region of interest. Because of the curvature of the eye, a nonperpendicular alignment will yield a summation image of some regions with lesser spatial detail. For whole eye imaging, this summation cannot be avoided as the camera is situated in front of the eye, and pointed at the visual axis, so that the postlimbal area is naturally curved with respect to the camera.
4. Set the Spectralis to infrared confocal scanning laser ophthalmoscope mode to center the image and adjust the focus and working distance. Depending on the lens used (see above), the focus recommendation is ~25 diopters for the 55-degree lens and ~ 0 mm for the anterior segment lens. Adjust the distance between the Spectralis device and the eye to obtain a sharp image.
5. Switch the Spectralis to either fluorescein or ICG angiography mode. For fluorescein angiography, a starting sensitivity setting of ~60 works well for the given dye concentrations in our previous studies. For ICG, a higher sensitivity setting of ~80 is initially used. Image averaging (ART setting) can be used to increase image signal-to-noise ratio. Take an image of the eye without tracer using the respective settings. This step establishes the baseline background signal intensity for each experiment, tests for any fluorescent contaminants on the eye, and distinguishes the start of each experiment in the Spectralis software. Then proceed with the experiment.
6. Engage the perfusion system to flush dye into the anterior chamber. This step should be done at a low IOP, by either withdrawing volume prior to the dye injection or opening the abducent line if a two-line system is used.
7. Start the angiography timer on the Spectralis device to get accurate time stamps on all images. If this step is missed, all images are time-coded in the "information" tab. In this case, the preperfusion background image (*see* step F) can serve as the zero time.
8. Reset the IOP to the desired level by engaging the syringe pump for the perfusion-based dye-delivery system. In the

gravity-based dye delivery system, the eye will quickly reach the desired IOP based upon the reservoir height once the eye is filled.

9. Acquire images at all desired time points. If the Spectralis FLEX is used, operating the device with the supplied food pedal is recommended to avoid motion artifacts induced by operating the touch panel. Holding the food pedal switches the device into averaging mode. Short taps take pictures.

3.3 Angiography of In Vivo Eyes (During Cataract Surgery)

1. Perform routine preoperative preparation of the patient (anesthesia, sterile prep, drape, and speculum placement). The Spectralis FLEX is sterile covered (e.g., Oculus Surgical).
2. One-port approach (*see* Fig. 6, left panel): In this approach, one 1 mm side port wound is made temporal. The location is where the surgeon feels comfortable for cataract surgery second instrument access after aqueous angiography and during surgery. The advantage of this approach is that only one side port is made. The disadvantage is that, for a tracer exchange, the anterior chamber will need to be evacuated of aqueous humor before tracer delivery to ensure proper final tracer concentration.
3. Two-port approach (alternative) (*see* Fig. 6 [right panel] and Fig. 7): In this approach, two 1 mm side port wounds are made. One will continue to serve as the cataract surgery second instrument access point once transitioning to cataract surgery. The second port can be converted to the beveled keratome main wound for the phacoemulsification handpiece during cataract surgery. The advantage of this approach is that a tracer exchange can be performed without collapsing the anterior chamber. The disadvantage is the need for two ports where one is converted into a keratome wound for the

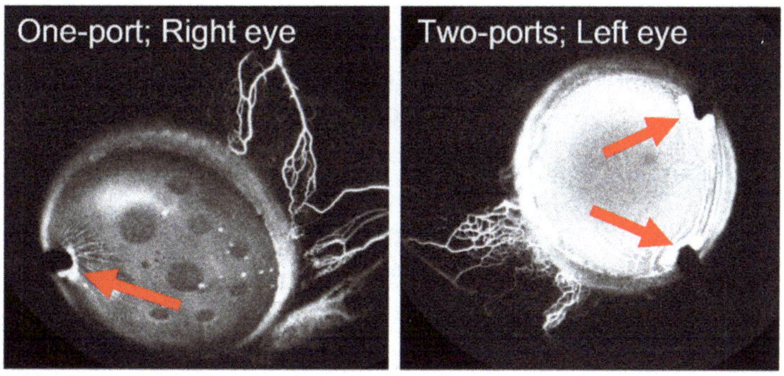

Fig. 6 Comparison of one-port versus two-port dye delivery system in human patients during cataract surgery. The anterior chamber maintainers (ACM, red arrows) appear as dark structures entering the eye during fluorescent imaging. Modified from [6, 7]. (Figure acquired with author's permission)

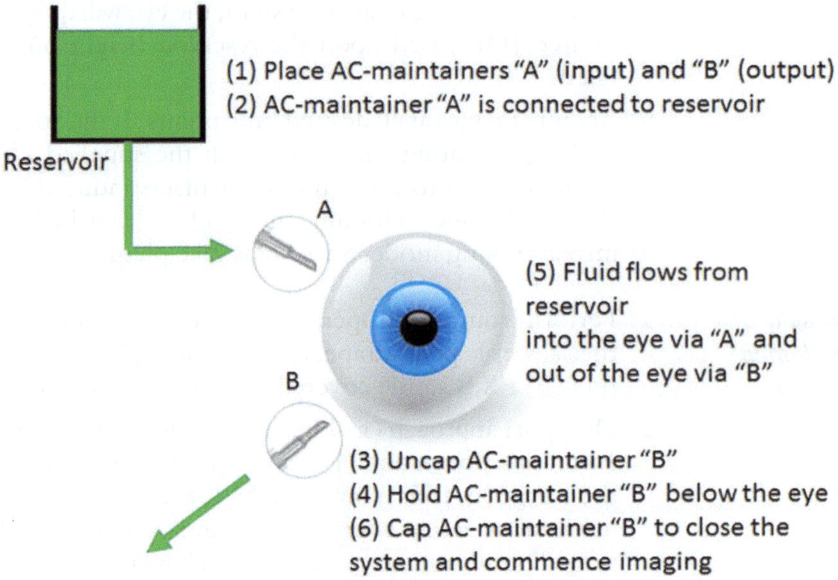

Fig. 7 Schematic drawing of a two-port dye delivery system and the steps needed for in vivo imaging. Steps B2-F in the text give further details on the use during cataract surgery [6]. (Figure acquired with author's permission)

phacoemulsification handpiece. Here, the surgeon needs to be cognizant of wound leakage during cataract surgery.

4. A sterile anterior chamber maintainer is primed with the intended perfusate for cataract surgery (e.g., balanced salt solution) using a 3 cc syringe that is only half-filled. With a twisting motion, the tip of the ACM is inserted through the 1 mm side port into the anterior chamber with a bevel-up final position. The eye is now a closed system, connected to the 3 cc syringe. The syringe can be used to add or remove fluid from the eye to maintain the chamber. This step is done once (one-port method) or twice (two-port method).
5. An assistant or the surgeon will bring the IV perfusion apparatus to the head of the bed that is primed with the tracer of choice (*see* Fig. 5).
6. One-port system: The surgeon will then push down on the heal of the ACM to point the ACM away from the iris in the anterior chamber. Withdrawal on the 3 cc syringe will evacuate the aqueous and collapse the anterior chamber. Too much withdrawal is to be avoided as air will enter the eye. Posterior direction of the ACM during withdrawal should be avoided as iris will plug the ACM. Then the 3 cc syringe is disconnected and one drop of perfusate added to the exposed female end of the ACM to make sure it is fully primed. At this point, the male end of the perfusion apparatus (*see* Fig. 5) will be joined to the

exposed and primed female end of the ACM. The perfusion apparatus is opened to flow toward the eye using the three-way stop cock (*see* Fig. 5). This is time-zero of the imaging (start the injection timer on the Spectralis).

7. Two-port system: Fig. 7 provides step-by-step guidance. The surgeon will remove both 3 cc syringes from both ACM. The perfusion apparatus (*see* Fig. 5) is joined to the first ACM, identical to the one-port system. The perfusion apparatus is opened to allow tracer flow toward the eye via its three-way stop cock (*see* Fig. 5). The second ACM is held below the level of the eye to elicit the aqueous/dye exchange (dye enters into the eye via the first ACM and then out of the eye via the second ACM). After six drops leave the second ACM, a 3 cc syringe is used to cap it. This step closes the system again and pressure builds. This is time-zero of the imaging.
8. If forward flow is not noted, there may be a clog in the system. This can occur during the exchange step in the one-port system with iris entering the ACM. This is much less likely to occur in the two-port system but still possible via the second ACM. In this case, the perfusion apparatus (on the IV pole, Fig. 5) will be opened to the partially filled side 1 cc syringe (via the three-way stop cock). Gentle pressure on this syringe will push fluid through the perfusion apparatus and relieve all clogs. Then the flow is returned to the tracer reservoir using the three-way stop cock. In the two-port system, the 3 cc syringe attached to the second ACM can also be used to relieve clogs.
9. Imaging proceeds using the Spectralis FLEX, identical to the above ex vivo experiments.
10. At the end of imaging, all ACM can be directly pulled from the eye. Irrigation of the anterior chamber using cataract surgery perfusate through a blunt cannula will wash the tracer out. Viscoelastic is added to the eye, and surgery is commenced.

4 Notes

1. Both dyes give very similar qualitative angiography patterns (*see* Fig. 8). The time course of the signal, however, can differ between the two dyes, and this can be species dependent [3, 9, 12]. In ex vivo eyes, fluorescein signal develops faster than ICG and also exhibits faster signal saturation. In in vivo eyes, the time course of aqueous angiographic signal is similar for fluorescein and ICG. Usually, the averaging function of the Spectralis software is not needed for fluorescein, whereas averaging can improve ICG image contrast.

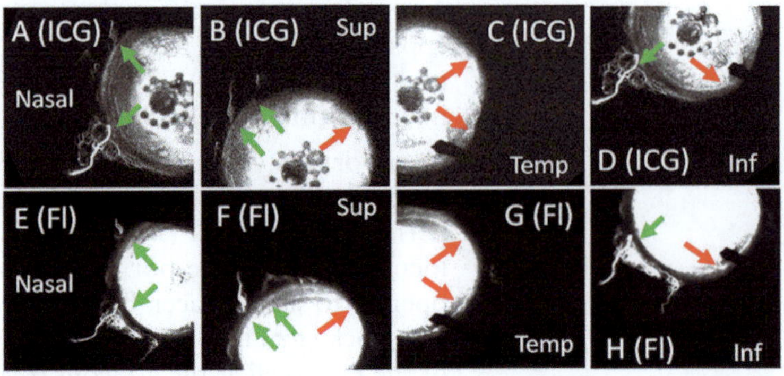

Fig. 8 Comparison of AHO outflow imaged using fluorescein and ICG in a live human subject. All images were acquired from a single subject using ICG (A-D) subsequently followed by fluorescein (E-H). (A-D) ICG aqueous angiography showed segmental regions with (green arrows) and without (red arrows) angiographic signal that were similar to the patterns obtained using fluorescein (E-H). ICG, indocyanine green. FI, fluorescein. Temp, temporal. Sup, superior. Inf, inferior. (Modified from Huang et al. [15]. Figure acquired with author's permission)

2. Anterior segment preparations typically include a perfusion chamber with tubing delivering and draining liquid. The eye is clamped to the perfusion chamber using a rigid ring and cushioning to protect the tissue (e.g., a rubber O-ring or foam) held in place by screws. The O-ring as well as the clamping ring and screws should be made of a material that can be treated with solvent and/or soaked in water for long periods of time. Fluorescein can be dissolved easily using water, but ICG stains strongly and requires more time to clean. Fluorescein, however, is particularly adhesive to materials commonly used in rapid prototyping (three-dimensional printing), and background fluorescence can be seen after several experiments. Structures casted from acrylic do not show this behavior. Unfortunately, they can be brittle and therefore brake easily when bent during clamping.
3. The space and layout of each operating room (OR) is unique. Given the equipment and staffing requirement, preoperative consideration of cramped ORs is critically important for in vivo imaging. ORs with ceiling mounted surgical microscopes will allow for more space to accommodate the FLEX and personnel. The FLEX module stand can be positioned on either side of the patient (*see* Fig. 1). Otherwise, surgical microscopes supported by a stand should be positioned on either the left or the right side of the gurney without subsequent movement. The FLEX module stand is then positioned on the other side of the patient with a small space for the photographer to stand and image either eye. Proper attention for arrangement of the

FLEX computer monitor and keyboard for easy access is important to consider prior to imaging. The IV pole (with the perfusion setup) needs space to be wheeled toward and away from the head as needed. Anterior segment OCT is more difficult in patients in the OR. Patients are draped with only the operative eye exposed. This eye is dilated in the case of cataract surgery and thus blurred. The patient is sedated by anesthesia. Overall, this makes it difficult for patient to follow instructions and to take and hold eccentric gazes necessary to expose postlimbal regions of interest for imaging. To improve imaging, two (instead of one) photographers can work together to control the FLEX camera and software for placing the OCT B-scan on the eye at the desired locations and acquiring the image. Also, decreasing the amount of image averaging or size of the scanned region of interest can help as this diminishes the time necessary for imaging.

Acknowledgments

Funding for this work came from the National Institutes of Health, Bethesda, MD (Grant Numbers R01EY030501 [ASH] and P30EY022589 [Core grant UCSD], an unrestricted grant from Research to Prevent Blindness (New York, NY) [UCSD], the Advanced Clinician Scientist Program/Johannes Kepler University (CAS), and the Adele Rabensteiner Foundation (CAS).

References

1. Goldmann H (1950) Abflussdruck, Minutenvolumen und Widerstand der Kammerwasser-strömung des Menschen. Doc Ophthalmol 5–6:278–356. https://doi.org/10.1007/BF00143664
2. Acott TS, Vranka JA, Keller KE, Raghunathan VK, Kelley MJ (2021) Normal and glaucomatous outflow regulation. Prog Retin Eye Res 82:100897. https://doi.org/10.1016/J.PRETEYERES.2020.100897
3. Saraswathy S, Tan JCH, Yu F, Francis BA, Hinton DR, Weinreb RN, Huang AS (2016) Aqueous angiography: real-time and physiologic aqueous humor outflow imaging. PLoS One 11:e0147176. https://doi.org/10.1371/JOURNAL.PONE.0147176
4. Saraswathy S, Bogarin T, Barron E, Francis BA, Tan JCH, Weinreb RN, Huang AS (2020) Segmental differences found in aqueous angiographic-determined high—and low-flow regions of human trabecular meshwork. Exp Eye Res 196:108064. https://doi.org/10.1016/J.EXER.2020.108064
5. Vranka JA, Staverosky JA, Reddy AP, Wilmarth PA, David LL, Acott TS, Russell P, Raghunathan VK (2018) Biomechanical rigidity and quantitative proteomics analysis of segmental regions of the trabecular meshwork at physiologic and elevated pressures. Invest Ophthalmol Vis Sci 59:246–259. https://doi.org/10.1167/IOVS.17-22759
6. Huang AS, Penteado RC, Papoyan V, Voskanyan L, Weinreb RN (2019) Aqueous angiographic outflow improvement after trabecular microbypass in glaucoma patients. Ophthalmol Glaucoma 2:11. https://doi.org/10.1016/J.OGLA.2018.11.010
7. Huang AS, Camp A, Xu BY, Penteado RC, Weinreb RN (2017) Aqueous angiography: aqueous humor outflow imaging in live human subjects. Ophthalmology 124:1249–1251. https://doi.org/10.1016/J.OPHTHA.2017.03.058

8. Huang AS, Li M, Yang D, Wang H, Wang N, Weinreb RN (2017) Aqueous angiography in living nonhuman primates shows segmental, pulsatile, and dynamic angiographic aqueous humor outflow. Ophthalmology 124:793–803. https://doi.org/10.1016/J.OPHTHA.2017.01.030
9. Huang AS, Saraswathy S, Dastiridou A, Begian A, Mohindroo C, Tan JCH, Francis BA, Hinton DR, Weinreb RN (2016) Aqueous angiography-mediated guidance of trabecular bypass improves angiographic outflow in human enucleated eyes. Invest Ophthalmol Vis Sci 57:4558–4565. https://doi.org/10.1167/IOVS.16-19644
10. Burn JB, Huang AS, Weber A, Komáromy AM, Pirie CG (2021) Aqueous angiography in pre-glaucomatous and glaucomatous ADAMTS10-mutant canine eyes: a pilot study. Vet Ophthalmol. https://doi.org/10.1111/VOP.12938
11. Snyder KC, Oikawa K, Williams J, Kiland JA, Gehrke S, Teixeira LBC, Huang AS, Mc Lellan GJ (2019) Imaging distal aqueous outflow pathways in a spontaneous model of congenital glaucoma. Transl Vis Sci Technol 8:22. https://doi.org/10.1167/TVST.8.5.22
12. Huang AS, Saraswathy S, Dastiridou A, Begian A, Legaspi H, Mohindroo C, Tan JCH, Francis BA, Caprioli J, Hinton DR, Weinreb RN (2016) Aqueous angiography with fluorescein and indocyanine green in bovine eyes. Transl Vis Sci Technol 5:5. https://doi.org/10.1167/TVST.5.6.5
13. Jacobs DS, Cox TA, Wagoner MD, Ariyasu RG, Karp CL (2006) Capsule staining as an adjunct to cataract surgery: a report from the American Academy of ophthalmology. Ophthalmology 113:707–713. https://doi.org/10.1016/J.OPHTHA.2006.01.024
14. Sherwood JM, Boazak EM, Feola AJ, Parker K, Ethier CR, Overby DR (2019) Measurement of ocular compliance using iPerfusion. Front Bioeng Biotechnol 7. https://doi.org/10.3389/FBIOE.2019.00276
15. Huang AS, Penteado RC, Saha SK, Do JL, Ngai P, Hu Z, Weinreb RN (2018) Fluorescein aqueous angiography in live Normal human eyes. J Glaucoma 27:957. https://doi.org/10.1097/IJG.0000000000001042

Chapter 15

Retinal Ganglion Cell Transplantation: Differentiation and Quantification Strategies

Jonathan R. Soucy, Volha V. Malechka, and Petr Baranov

Abstract

Glaucoma is a leading cause of irreversible blindness worldwide. Current treatments focus on reducing intraocular pressure but cannot restore lost visual function once it is lost due to retinal ganglion cell (RGC) degeneration and death. Recent advances suggest that transplantation of stem cell-derived RGCs could offer new therapeutic approaches for glaucoma and vision restoration. Here, we present a detailed protocol for differentiating human RGCs from embryonic stem cells using both three-dimensional retinal organoid and two-dimensional culture approaches. Following differentiation, we describe methods for isolating and purifying retinal ganglion cells from these cultures and their subsequent transplantation into the mouse retina, with careful monitoring and postoperative care to ensure successful integration. Finally, we describe a quantitative method for assessing transplantation outcomes involving confocal imaging of retinal flat-mounts and custom ImageJ and MATLAB scripts to map and analyze the spatial distribution of donor RGCs within the host retina. Altogether, this approach provides a robust framework for exploring RGC transplantation as a potential therapy for vision loss in glaucoma and other optic neuropathies.

Key words Retinal ganglion cells, Human embryonic stem cells, Organoid culture, Magnetic beads, Subretinal injection, Cell transplantation

1 Introduction

Approximately 3.5% of the world's population over 40 have glaucoma, the most common optic neuropathy [1], with an expected increase to 110 million affected by 2040 as the population ages [2]. Up to 10% of this cohort would have moderate-to-severe vision impairment, with the vision loss likely higher within a medically underserved population. Available glaucoma treatments reduce intraocular pressure (IOP) medically or surgically, but IOP reduction can only slow or halt disease progression. Currently, no therapies exist to restore lost visual function and target RGCs directly to improve their survival [3, 4]. Functional replacement of RGCs is needed to recover sight loss to glaucoma. The transplantation of primary and stem cell-derived RGCs [5–7],

Tatjana Jakobs and Paloma B. Liton (eds.), *Glaucoma: Methods and Protocols*, Methods in Molecular Biology, vol. 2858,
https://doi.org/10.1007/978-1-0716-4140-8_15,

differentiation of RGCs from human pluripotent stem cells [8, 9], and functional axon regeneration to the brain suggest that transplantation-mediated vision repair may be feasible [10]. The induced pluripotent stem cell-derived RGCs [11–13] survive following intravitreal transplantation (IVT) into healthy and damaged retinas [14]. These pioneering studies highlighted the need for the adjuvant therapy that can be used to boost cell survival [15] and structural and functional integration. The assessment of these combinatorial approaches requires rapid and robust quantification of the transplantation outcome. Here we summarize our strategy for RGC differentiation and transplantation that can be utilized beyond cell replacement studies and used to explore retinal neuron differentiation and maturation, as well as to study the host retina response and the role of the microenvironment on human retinal ganglion cell metabolism, neurite, and axon outgrowth. The cytoplasm transfer and cell fusion are other important phenomena that one has to check in cell transplantation studies—these have been extensively addressed in recent publication [16].

1.1 Human Retinal Ganglion Cell Differentiation with Three-Dimensional Protocol

Here, we describe a protocol for differentiating human retinal ganglion cells (RGCs) from embryonic stem cells (hESCs) in three-dimensional retinal organoid cultures. The hESCs were maintained in Matrigel-coated six-well plates with mTeSR1 media in a low-oxygen environment. At 70% confluency, hESCs were enzymatically passaged and split into a new Matrigel-coated six-well plate. Next, embryoid bodies are formed by aggregating 7500 hESCs/well with ultralow attachment U-bottom 96-well plates in a low-oxygen environment for 24 h. The plate is then transferred to a standard culture environment, and the culture media is gradually transitioned from mTeSR1 to BE6.2-NIM. Media is exchanged daily and supplemented with Y-27632, Matrigel, IWR-1-endo, and BMP4 to promote neural development and early retinal differentiation. On day 8, the organoids were collected and randomly chopped to excise the optic vesicles. The chopped aggregates were seeded in LT-RDM on tissue culture-treated plastic to encourage attachment and retinal epithelium formation. Culture media is exchanged every other day with a gradual transition to RDM by day 17 and supplemented with SAG to enhance retinal progenitor expansion. On day 17, the retinal tissue aggregates were carefully scrapped and lifted off the tissue culture plastic, so their neural epithelium remained attached. The detached retinal aggregates are then transferred to a poly(2-hydroxyethyl methacrylate)-coated flask and cultured in suspension with RDM supplemented with SAG. The culture media is exchanged every other day and gradually transitioned to LT-RDM by day 24. From days 26 and 32 onward, culture media is supplemented with taurine and all-transretinoic acid, respectively. LT-RDM is exchanged every other day until retinal maturation between days 42 and 50 (Fig. 1).

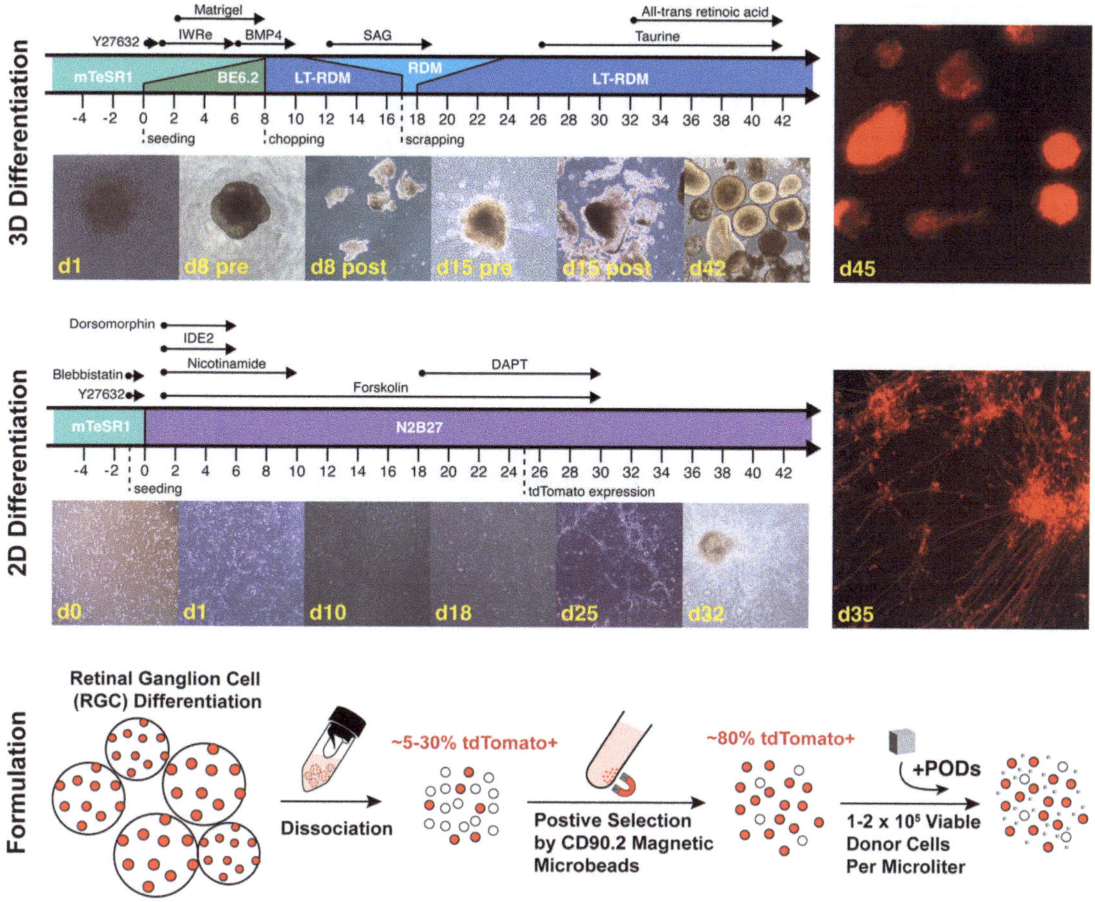

Fig. 1 Human retinal ganglion cell differentiation and formulation

The protocol describes a method for differentiating human retinal ganglion cells from embryonic stem cells in three-dimensional retinal organoid cultures. The process involves maintaining the stem cells in Matrigel-coated plates with mTeSR1 media in a low-oxygen environment, forming embryoid bodies with the cells, gradually transitioning the culture media to promote neural and retinal differentiation, excising the optic vesicles, seeding the aggregates on tissue culture-treated plastic to encourage attachment and retinal epithelium formation, and transferring the detached retinal aggregates to a poly(2-hydroxyethyl methacrylate)-coated flask for suspension culture with retinal differentiation medium supplemented with various factors until retinal maturation occurs between days 42 and 50.

2 Materials

- H9-BRN3B:tdTomatoThy1.2-hESCs
- Matrigel-coated (2%) six-well plates
- mTeSR1 media
- Accutase
- Ultralow attachment U-bottom 96-well plates
- DMEM/F12 (3500 mg/L dextrose)
- L-Glutamine
- Sodium pyruvate
- Antibiotic-antimycotic
- B27 without vitamin A
- NaCl
- Insulin
- L-Ascorbic acid
- Selenium
- Transferrin
- NaHCO3
- Y-27632
- IWR-1-endo
- BMP4
- Nonessential amino acids
- FBS
- Smoothened agonist (SAG)
- Poly(2-hydroxyethyl methacrylate)-coated flask
- Taurine
- All-transretinoic acid

2.1 Medium

BE6.2-NIM (B27 + E6 at 2× concentration—neural induction medium):

- 1× L-glutamine
- 1× sodium pyruvate
- 1× antibiotic-antimycotic
- 1× B27 without vitamin A
- 0.88 mg/mL NaCl
- 38.8 mg/L insulin
- 128 mg/L L-ascorbic acid

- 28 μg/L selenium
- 21.4 mg/L transferrin
- 38.8 mg/L NaHCO3 in DMEM/F12 (3500 mg/L dextrose)

RDM (Retinal Differentiation Media):

- LT-RDM without FBS

LT-RDM (Long-Term Retinal Differentiation Media):

- 50:50 1× DMEM/F12 (3500 mg/L dextrose):DMEM (4500 mg/mL dextrose)
- 1× L-glutamine
- 1× sodium pyruvate
- 1× antibiotic-antimycotic
- 1× B27
- 1× nonessential amino acids
- 10% FBS

2.2 Procedure

1. Culture H9-BRN3B:tdTomatoThy1.2-hESC colonies in Matrigel-coated (2%) six-well plates with mTeSR1 media in a low-oxygen environment (5% CO_2, 3.5% O2, >95% humidity, 37 °C).
2. Change media daily with room temperature mTeSR1 media.
3. At 70% confluency, after approximately 4–5 days of culture, enzymatically passage hESCs with accutase for 8 min at room temperature, and split at a ratio of 1:10 to 1:20 into a new Matrigel-coated six-well plate.
4. Dissociate colonies for four additional minutes (12 minutes total) to yield a single-cell suspension and form embryoid bodies by aggregating 7500 hESCs/well with ultralow attachment U-bottom 96-well plates in a low-oxygen environment for 24 h.
5. Transfer the plate to a standard culture environment after the first 24 h and gradually transition the culture media from 3:1 mTeSR1:BE6.2-NIM to >90% BE6.2-NIM by day 8.
6. Exchange media daily until day 6 and supplement it with 20 μM Y-27632 on day 0, 1% Matrigel on days 2–6, 3 μM IWR-1-endo on days 1–4, and 55 ng/mL BMP4 on day 6 to promote neural development and early retinal differentiation.
7. On day 8, collect organoids and randomly chop to excise the optic vesicles to allow for better propagation and maintain the size below the diffusion limit.

8. Seed the chopped aggregates in LT-RDM on tissue culture-treated plastic to encourage attachment and retinal epithelium formation.
9. Exchange culture media every other day with a gradual transition to 1:1 LT-RDM:RDM by day 17, and supplement it with 100 nM smoothened agonist (SAG) on days 12–16 to enhance retinal progenitor expansion.
10. On day 17, carefully scrape and lift the retinal tissue aggregates off the tissue culture plastic, so their neural epithelium remains attached.
11. Transfer the detached retinal aggregates to a poly (2-hydroxyethyl methacrylate)-coated flask and culture in suspension with RDM supplemented with 100 nM SAG.
12. The next day (day 18), replace the culture media with 1:3 LT-RDM:RDM (2.5% FBS) supplemented with 100 nM SAG.
13. From day 18 onward, exchange the culture media every other day and gradually transition to LT-RDM by day 24.
14. From days 26–32, supplement the culture media with 1 mM taurine and 250 nM all-transretinoic acid, respectively.
15. Exchange the LT-RDM every other day until retinal maturation between days 42 and 50.

Note: All the above steps should be performed using aseptic techniques to prevent contamination.

3 Human Retinal Ganglion Cell Differentiation with Two-Dimensional Protocol

Here, we describe a protocol for differentiating human retinal ganglion cells (RGCs) from embryonic stem cells (hESCs) using a two-dimensional approach. The first step is to prepare a 2% Matrigel (MG)-coated 6-well plate. Next, human embryonic stem cells (hESCs) are seeded onto the MG-coated plate at a density of 52.6 k cells/cm2 or approximately 500 k cells per well in a 6-well plate. The hESCs are cultured in mTeSR1 medium supplemented with 5 μM blebbistatin and 20 μM Y27632. The next day, the medium is replaced with N2B27 medium, a 1:1 mix of DMEM/F12 and Neurobasal medium supplemented with 1x GlutaMAX, 1× antibiotic-antimycotic, 1% N2 supplement, and 2% B27 supplement. From day 1 to day 5, the medium is replaced with N2B27 supplemented with 1 μM dorsomorphin (DSM), 2.5 μM IDE2, 10 mM nicotinamide (NIC), and 25 μM forskolin (FSK) daily. On day 6, the medium is changed to N2B27 supplemented with 10 mM NIC and 25 μM FSK and is replaced every other day until day 10. On day 10, the medium is changed to N2B27 supplemented with only 25 μM FSK and replaced every other day until day 16.

From day 18 to day 26, the medium is replaced every 2 days with N2B27 supplemented with 25 μM FSK and 10 μM DAPT to promote RGC differentiation. On day 30, the medium is changed to N2B27 without supplements and exchanged every other day until the RGCs are ready for transplantation between days 32 and 40.

3.1 Protocol for Making RGCs Using a Two-Dimensional Approach

This method describes a step-by-step protocol for making retinal ganglion cells (RGCs) using a two-dimensional approach. The protocol involves seeding human embryonic stem cells (hESCs) onto the plate and culturing them in a series of specific media with various supplements to promote RGC differentiation. The medium is replaced regularly with N2B27 supplemented with specific factors such as dorsomorphin, IDE2, nicotinamide, and forskolin. After 30 days, the RGCs are ready for transplantation.

3.2 Materials

- DMEM/F12
- Matrigel-coated (2%) six-well plates
- mTeSR1 medium
- Blebbistatin
- Y27632
- Neurobasal medium
- GlutaMAX
- Antibiotic-antimycotic
- N2 supplement
- B27 supplement
- Dorsomorphin (DSM)
- IDE2
- Nicotinamide (NIC)
- Forskolin (FSK)
- DAPT

3.3 Procedure

1. Prepare a 2% Matrigel (MG)-coated 6-well plate by mixing 8.3 mL of DMEM/F12 and 720 μL of 25% MG and adding 1.5 mL per well of a 6-well plate.
2. Incubate the plate at 37 °C and 5% CO2 for 1 h to allow the MG to coat the surface.
3. Seed human embryonic stem cells (hESCs) onto the MG-coated plate at a density of 52.6 k cells/cm2 or approximately 500 k cells per well in a 6-well plate.
4. Culture the hESCs in mTeSR1 medium supplemented with 5 μM blebbistatin and 20 μM Y27632.

5. Replace the medium the next day with N2B27 medium, a 1:1 mix of DMEM/F12, and Neurobasal medium supplemented with 1× GlutaMAX, 1× antibiotic-antimycotic, 1% N2 supplement, and 2% B27 supplement.
6. From day 1 to day 5, replace the medium daily with N2B27 supplemented with 1 μM dorsomorphin (DSM), 2.5 μM IDE2, 10 mM nicotinamide (NIC), and 25 μM forskolin (FSK).
7. On day 6, change the medium to N2B27 supplemented with 10 mM NIC and 25 μM FSK, and replace it every other day until day 10.
8. On day 10, change the medium to N2B27 supplemented with only 25 μM FSK and replace it every other day until day 16.
9. From day 18 to day 26, replace the medium every 2 days with N2B27 supplemented with 25 μM FSK and 10 μM DAPT to promote RGC differentiation.
10. On day 30, change the medium to N2B27 without any supplements, and replace it every other day until the RGCs are ready for transplantation between days 32 and 40.

Note: All the above steps should be performed using aseptic techniques to prevent contamination.

4 Retinal Ganglion Cell Purification

The protocol describes the dissociation and isolation of RGCs from mature human retinal organoids and two-dimensional cultures using enzymatic dissociation and magnetic bead sorting. For retinal organoids, the dissociation process involves using an enzymatic dissociation solution prepared by adding Enzyme P and A to Buffer X and Y, respectively. After collecting the organoids in a MACS M-tube, they are incubated for 5 min at 37 °C in the dissociation solution. The tube is placed in a MACS dissociator, and the brain_1 and brain_2 programs are run. For dissociating two-dimensional cultures, the process involves collecting stem cell-derived retinal neurons using accutase. After the dissociation, the cell suspension is washed and filtered through a 70 um cell strainer to remove debris.

For the isolation of RGCs, the cell suspension is transferred to a 2 mL Eppendorf tube and mixed with CD90.2 antibody, followed by incubation at 4 °C for 10 min. The cell suspension is then transferred to a 15 ml tube, washed with isolation buffer, and centrifuged to form a cell pellet. The resulting pellet was resuspended and combined with magnetic microbeads in an isolation buffer. After 10 min incubation, the magnetic microbeads were removed using a magnet, and the CD90.2-positive cells were released from the microbeads using a release buffer. The isolated RGCs can be counted and analyzed for their viability.

It is important to note that the protocol involves several critical steps, including carefully removing culture media and excess HBSS, resuspension of organoids in HBSS, accurate pipetting of the dissociation solution, and the filtration of the cell suspension to remove debris. The protocol provides detailed instructions for each step, including the volumes of each reagent and the required equipment, to ensure the successful dissociation and isolation of RGCs. Additionally, the viability of the isolated RGCs can vary based on the expected cell number, and the cutoff for viability is 10%, as measured by Trypan Blue.

4.1 Protocol for the Dissociation and Isolation of RGCs

This protocol describes the dissociation and isolation of retinal ganglion cells (RGCs) from mature human retinal organoids and two-dimensional cultures. The organoid dissociation step involves collecting the retinal organoids, rinsing them with HBSS, transferring them to a MACS M-tube, adding the dissociation solution, incubating the M-tube, and running the MACS dissociator. The two-dimensional culture dissociation involves enzymatic dissociation with accutase. The dissociated cells are then passed through a 70um cell strainer, counted, and sorted using magnetic microbeads against CD90.2.

4.2 Materials

- Embryoid body dissociation kit (Miltenyi Biotec, 130-096-348)
- Dynabeads™ FlowComp™ Mouse Pan T (CD90.2) Kit (Invitrogen, 11465D)
- HBSS w/o Ca2+, Mg2+
- 0.5 M EDTA
- HI-FBS
- 10% BSA
- Sterile filter with 0.22 μm syringe filter
- MACS M-tube
- MACS Gentle Dissociator
- DNAse I solution (1 mg/mL)
- 50 mL tube
- 15 mL tube
- 2 ml Eppendorf tube
- 70 μm cell strainer
- CD90.2 antibody
- Rolling shaker
- Magnetic rack
- Accutase

4.3 Procedure

Step 1: Solution Preparation

1. Prepare dissociation solution for MACS Gentle Dissociator.
   - Solution PX—Add 50uL of Enzyme P to 1900uL Buffer X, vortex briefly, and incubate at 37 °C for 30 min at bath or longer if needed.
   - Add 10 uL of Enzyme A to 20 uL of Buffer Y, do *not* vortex, and keep on ice (or at 4 °C) until use.
   - Dissociation solution: when the organoids are ready, and Enzyme P is activated (30 min), combine the total volumes of each solution (1950 uL + 30 uL = 1980 uL) and pipette mix.
2. Prepare the isolation buffer.
   - 50 mL HBSS w/o Ca2+, Mg2+.
   - 200 uL 0.5 M EDTA (2 mM final concentration).
   - 1 mL HI-FBS (2% final concentration).
   - 500 μL of 10% BSA (0.1% final concentration).
   - Sterile filter with 0.22 μm syringe filter.
   - Warm the isolation buffer at 37 °C before use.
   - Note: excess isolation buffer may be stored at 4 °C and is stable for 1 week.

Step 2.1: Organoid Dissociation

1. While solution PX is incubating, collect the retinal organoids from 5 to 15 96 well plates in a 50 mL tube, carefully removing any excess culture media as needed.
2. Let the organoids settle to the bottom of the tube, and carefully remove as much culture media as possible (~1 mL volume for semidry organoid sediment)
3. Rinse the organoids with ~15 mL of HBSS.
4. Transfer to a MACS M-tube.
5. Let the organoids settle (2 min) again before removing as much HBSS as possible.
6. Resuspend the organoids in another ~15 mL of HBSS.
7. Once all organoids have been transferred to the M-tube and the dissociation solution has been fully prepared, aspirate any remaining liquid—make it almost dry.
8. Add the total volume (~2 mL) of dissociation solution to the M-tube
9. Optional: add 2 μL of DNAse I solution (1 mg/mL).
10. Incubate the M-tube 37C for 5 min at the bath.

11. Invert the M-tube and place it into the MACS dissociator, making sure that all the organoids remain in solution (Note: this may require several inversion attempts).
12. Run the brain_1 program.
13. Remove the M-tube from the MACS dissociator and incubate at 37 °C for 5 min.
14. Carefully invert the M-tube again and place it into the MACS dissociator.
15. Run the brain_2 program.
16. Add 10 mL of the isolation buffer and triturate the solution 7–10 times with a 1000 microliter pipette tip to break up any remaining clumps.
17. Transfer the cell suspension (~12 mL) to a 15 mL tube.
18. Centrifuge for 200 g for 5 min.
19. Resuspend in 500 μL of isolation buffer.
20. Pass the suspension through a 70um cell strainer to remove debris.
21. Wash the strainer once with 500 μL of isolation buffer.
22. Count the cells.
    (a) Dilute at 1:10 or 1:20 based on the expected cell number to get approximately 1e6/mL for accurate cell count.
    (b) Cutoff for viability: 10% as measured by Trypan Blue.

Step 2.2: Two-Dimensional Culture Dissociation

1. Incubate two-dimensional RGC cultures for 8 min at room temperature in accutase (0.5 mL/well in a 6-well plate).
2. After enzymatic dissociation, dilute the accutase using isolation buffer (1.5–2 mL/well in a 6-well plate).
3. Collect the dissociated cells into a 15 mL tube and centrifuge at 200 g for 5 min.
4. Resuspend the cell pellet in 500 μL of isolation buffer.
5. Pass the suspension through a 70um cell strainer to remove debris.
6. Wash the strainer once with 500 μL of isolation buffer.

Step 3: Magnetic Bead Sorting (CD90.2)

1. Transfer 1 mL of the cell suspension to a 2 mL Eppendorf tube.
2. Add 50 uL of CD90.2 antibody (Thermo Fisher kit) and pipette mix.
3. Incubate cells with the antibody on a rolling shaker at 4 °C for 10 min.

4. Transfer the cell suspension into a fresh 15 mL tube.
5. Wash the Eppendorf tube with 2 mL of isolation buffer and add to the 15 mL tube with cell suspension.
6. Add 7 mL of isolation buffer to the 15 mL tube, and wash the cells by inverting five times.
7. Centrifuge at 200 g for 8 min.
8. While centrifuging, prepare the FlowComp Dynabeads.
   - Resuspend the Dynabeads in the vial by vortex for >30 s.
   - Place 2–3 flow tubes (1 flow tube per 10 M of cells) on the magnetic rack.
   - Add 2 mL isolation buffer to each flow tube on the magnetic rack.
   - Add 100 uL Dynabeads to each flow tube on the magnetic rack.
   - Turn the flow tube 180 degrees 2–3 times on the magnetic rack to wash the Dynabeads.
   - Wait 1 min for the Dynabeads to be pulled out of the solution by the magnet, and discard the supernatant by collecting it (vacuum line or pipette).
   - Turn the flow tube 180 degrees.
   - Add 1 mL isolation buffer to the washed Dynabeads and leave until further use.
9. Remove the supernatant from the 15 mL tube with the cell pellet and resuspend the cell pellet in 2–3 mL of isolation buffer (1 mL per flow tube).
10. Remove isolation buffer from washed Dynabeads (on the magnet).
11. Remove the flow tube with Dynabeads from the magnet.
12. Transfer 1 mL of cell suspension into the flow tube with Dynabeads and resuspend each flow tube.
13. Transfer the content of each flow tube to 2 mL Eppendorf tube and incubate for 15 min on a rolling shaker in the fridge.
14. Prepare 2–3 fresh flow tubes on the magnet with 1 mL isolation buffer. Add cell/bead suspension after incubation and leave for 2 min on the magnet.
15. While the tube is still in the magnet, carefully remove the supernatant containing the CD90.2-negative cells (for automatic counting at this point, dilute at least 1:20).
16. Remove the tube from the magnet, add 1 mL of isolation buffer to each tube, mix, and put on the magnet for 2 min, and then again remove the supernatant.
17. Remove the tube from the magnet.

18. Resuspend the bead-bound cells in 1 mL release buffer and transfer them to individual Eppendorf tubes. Incubate 10 min on room temperature orbital shaker (lay down).
19. Mix ten times with a 1000 μL pipette to efficiently release the cells—avoid foaming.
20. Transfer 2 mL of the cell suspension to new flow tubes and place on the magnet for 2 min.
21. Transfer the supernatant containing the bead-free $CD90.2^+$ cells to a new flow tube, and place it on the magnet for 1 min to remove residual beads.
22. Transfer and combine the supernatant containing the bead-free cells to a 15 mL tube; add 7 mL of isolation buffer, followed by centrifugation for 8 min at 200 g
23. Remove the supernatant and resuspend the cell pellet in 1000 uL N2B27 or other mediums suitable for transplantation.
24. Measure the volume using the micropipette.
25. Count cells.
26. Concentrate the cells for transplantation using Eppendorf tube centrifugation.

5 Cell Transplantation

The technique of intraocular delivery is an efficient route for gene or cell therapy and drug delivery to the posterior segment of the eye in both research and clinical applications [17]. The subretinal technique allows to deliver cells to the subretinal space, the area between the retinal pigment epithelium (RPE) and photoreceptors.

Here, we describe the technique of subretinal delivery of donor RGCs in a mouse eye (Fig. 2). The procedure starts with the step of anesthetizing a mouse with Ketamine-Xylazine cocktail by intraperitoneal injection. After a mouse is anesthetized and asleep, it is placed on its side with an eye for subretinal injection facing up. Following this step, a one drop of Tropicamide and one drop of Proparacaine are instilled before beginning the procedure. It is recommended to wait at least 5 min to let the drops start working for proper pupil dilation. Using a sterile technique, a drawing of 1 μL of cells into the blunt glass capillary needle of microinjector precedes the injection. An anterior chamber paracentesis of 1 mm deep is made with a 30-gauge sharp sterile needle immediately close to the limbus at the superior part of the mouse eye; the vessels and lens should not be hit by the needle to avoid hemorrhage from the ocular vessels and trauma to the lens. An extra liquid is usually

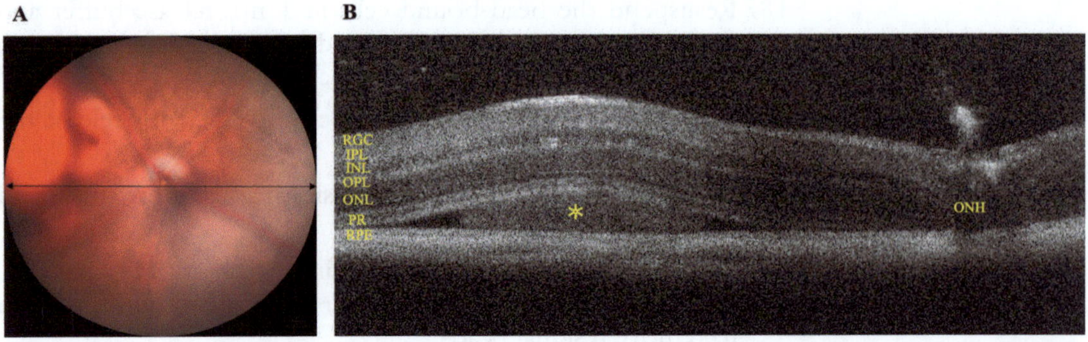

Fig. 2 Imaging of mouse retina after subretinal injection administered by transscleral route of delivery. (**a**) Representative image of the fundus following subretinal injection. (**b**) Representative horizontal SD-OCT scan showing the injection site (*). *INL* inner nuclear layer, *IPL* inner plexiform layer, *ONH* optic nerve head, *ONL* outer nuclear layer, *OPL* outer plexiform layer, *PR* photoreceptor layer, *RGC* retinal ganglion layer, and *RPE* retinal pigment epithelium

removed with a sterile cotton bud before starting the injection. The mouse eye should be fixed and held with the sterile ophthalmic surgical forceps in one hand. The positioning of the tip of a blunt glass capillary needle preloaded with drug or cells through the hole should be done with another hand. A glass capillary needle is inserted through the hole into 2 mm deep to reach the retina. Drug or cells are injected into the subretinal space slowly and carefully. After the injection is complete, a drop of antibiotic-antimycotic and a drop of GenTeal are applied to an injected eye to prevent infection and its dehydration. At the end of procedure, a mouse is placed into a clean cage on a heating pad with an injected eye facing up. It is recommended to wait until a mouse recovers from anesthesia and regains consciousness.

5.1 Materials

- Anesthetic cocktail of Ketamine-Xylazine
- Local anesthetic drops (e.g., Proparacaine)
- Tropicamide ophthalmic solution 1%
- GenTeal
- Antibiotic ointment (Neomycin and Polymyxin B sulfates and Bacitracin Zinc Ophthalmic ointment)
- Analgesic (e.g., Buprenorphine extended-release injectable suspension)
- Sterile cotton buds
- 30-gauge sharp sterile needle for paracentesis
- Sterile ophthalmic surgical forceps
- Microinjection system with blunt glass capillary needles with the inner tip about 100 μm
- Drug or cells for subretinal delivery (up to 20,000 cells per μL) stored on ice before injection

5.2 Procedure

1. Anesthetize a mouse with Ketamine-Xylazine cocktail. The dose of anesthesia is usually defined by animal facility core at the institution.
2. Place the mouse on its side with the eye for the injection facing up.
3. Instill a drop of 1% Tropicamide and Proparacaine before beginning the procedure and let the drops start working for at least 5 min.
4. Use a sterile technique to draw 0.5–1 μL of drug or cells (up to 20,000 cells per μL) into the glass capillary needle of microinjection system.
5. Make a 1 mm deep hole with a 30-gauge sterile needle immediately close to the limbus at the superior part of the eye trying to avoid hitting the vessels and lens.
6. Insert the tip of the glass capillary needle preloaded with drug or cells through the hole into 2 mm deep to reach the retina.
7. Slowly and carefully inject drug or cells into subretinal space.
8. Pull back the glass capillary needle.
9. Apply one drop of GenTeal and one drop of antibiotic-antimycotic ointment to an injected eye for avoiding its dehydration and infection prevention.
10. Inject intraperitoneally a dose of analgesic for pain relief of a mouse. The dose is usually defined by animal facility core at the institution.
11. Place a mouse into a clean cage with an injected eye facing up.

6 The Quantification of the Transplantation Outcome

Here, we describe a methodology for quantifying the position and number of donor retinal ganglion cells (RGCs) within the host neural retina. This was achieved using custom semiautomated ImageJ and MATLAB scripts. The first step was to image retinal flat-mounts using a confocal microscope with 20× magnification (UPlanSApo) and a Z-axis interval of 2 μm. Mosaic tiled images of the whole retinal flat-mount were taken at a resolution of 512 × 512 pixels per tile using the resonate scan on an Olympus IX83-FV3000 confocal microscope. Each tile from the retinal flat-mount was imported into ImageJ as an image sequence to identify donor RGCs within the host retina. The background was subtracted, and the three-dimensional object counter plugin was used to export the size and local position of donor RGCs in each tile to a ".csv" file. The MATLAB file containing the map data with the positions of each tile relative to each other was manually saved as a ".txt" file for every retina. These files were imported into MATLAB to calculate the global x, y, and z-positions of each identified donor

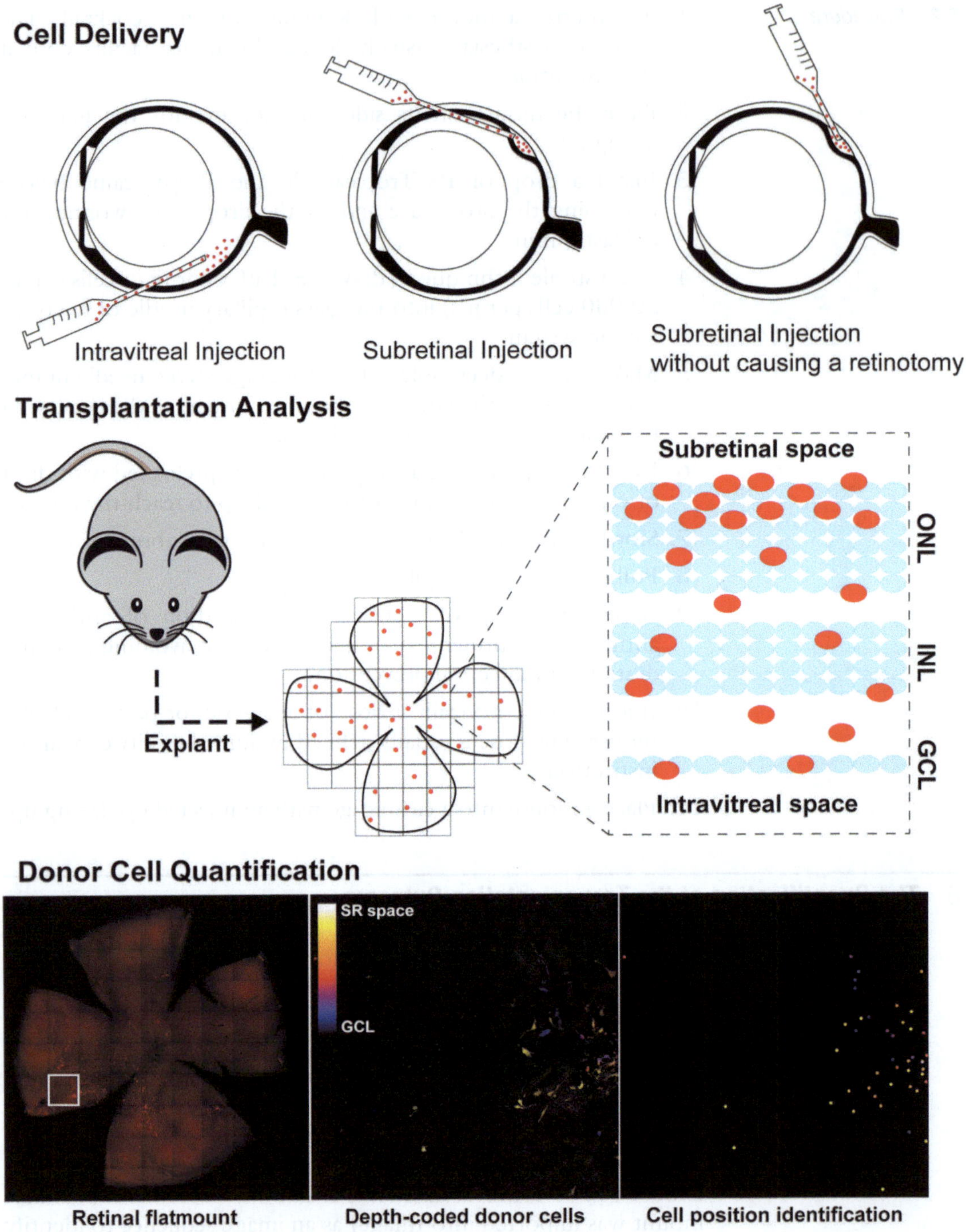

Fig. 3 Cell transplantation quantification

RGC and the total number of donor RGCs per retina. These coordinates were used to generate depth-coded color maps that could be manually overlayed on their corresponding retinal flatmount (Fig. 3). The number of cells within a cell cluster was calculated by dividing the volume of that cluster by 1.5× the average donor RGC volume. To calculate the percentage of donor RGC that migrated into the GCL (ganglion cell layer), the z-axis position of the GCL was manually inputted into the MATLAB script. The GCL's position was identified by averaging the z-plane containing RBMPS+ host cells in four randomly selected tiles from each retinal flat-mount. The z-position was normalized between 0 and 100 using min/max scaling to compare z-positions of donor RGCs across retinas. Finally, donor RGC coverage was calculated as the percentage of tiles per retina with one or more donor RGC. Overall, this methodology provides a quantitative approach to analyze the spatial distribution of transplanted RGCs in the host retina, which can be used to assess the effectiveness of RGC transplantation as a potential therapy for retinal degeneration.

6.1 Protocol for a Quantitative Approach to Assess RGC Transplantation

Here we describe a method to quantify the position and number of donor retinal ganglion cells (RGCs) within the host neural retina. This involves imaging retinal flat-mounts using a confocal microscope with 20× magnification and using custom semiautomated ImageJ and MATLAB scripts to identify donor RGCs within each tile of the retinal flat-mount. The global position of each identified donor RGC is then calculated, and depth-coded color maps are generated to visualize the spatial distribution of donor RGCs within the host retina. The number of cells within a cell cluster and the percentage of donor RGCs that migrate into the ganglion cell layer were also described using these data. This method provides a quantitative approach to assess the effectiveness of RGC transplantation as a potential therapy for retinal degeneration.

6.2 Procedure

1. Image retinal flat-mounts using a confocal microscope with 20× magnification (UPlanSApo) and a z-axis interval of 2 μm. Use tiled mosaic imaging to capture the entire retinal flat-mount at a 512 × 512 pixel resolution per tile.
2. Import each tile from the retinal flat-mount into ImageJ as an image sequence.
3. Subtract the background from each tile and use the three-dimensional object counter plugin to export the size and local position of donor RGCs in each tile to a ".csv" file.
4. Manually save the MATL file containing the map data with the positions of each tile relative to each other as a ".txt" file for every retina.
5. Import the ".txt" files into MATLAB to calculate the global x, y, and z-positions of each identified donor RGC and the total number of donor RGCs per retina.
6. Use the coordinates to generate depth-coded color maps that can be manually overlayed on their corresponding retinal flat-mount.

7. Calculate the number of cells within a cell cluster by dividing the volume of that cluster by 1.5× the average donor RGC volume.
8. Input the z-axis position of the GCL (ganglion cell layer) into the MATLAB script. Identify the GCL's position by averaging the z-plane containing RBMPS+ host cells in four randomly selected tiles from each retinal flat-mount.
9. Normalize the z-position of donor RGCs between 0 and 100 using min/max scaling to compare across retinas.
10. Calculate donor RGC coverage as the percentage of tiles per retina with one or more donor RGC.

References

1. Collaborators G et al (2019, 2020) Causes of blindness and vision impairment in 2020 and trends over 30 years, and prevalence of avoidable blindness in relation to VISION 2020: the right to sight: an analysis for the global burden of disease study. Lancet Global Heal. https://doi.org/10.1016/s2214-109x(20)30489-7
2. Tham Y-C et al (2014) Global prevalence of glaucoma and projections of glaucoma burden through 2040 a systematic review and meta-analysis. Ophthalmology 121:2081–2090
3. Almasieh M, Levin LA (2016) Neuroprotection in glaucoma: animal models and clinical trials. Annu Rev Vis Sci 3:1–30
4. Khatib TZ, Martin KR (2019) Neuroprotection in glaucoma: towards clinical trials and precision medicine. Curr Eye Res 45:327–338
5. Hertz J, Goldberg JL (2007) Retinal ganglion cell transplantation: survival and integration. Invest Ophthalmol Vis Sci 48:5092–5092
6. Hertz J et al (2014) Survival and integration of developing and progenitor-derived retinal ganglion cells following transplantation. Cell Transplant 23:855–872
7. Venugopalan P et al (2016) Transplanted neurons integrate into adult retinas and respond to light. Nat Commun 7:10472
8. Eiraku M et al (2011) Self-organizing optic-cup morphogenesis in three-dimensional culture. Nature 472:51–56
9. Eiraku M, Sasai Y (2012) Mouse embryonic stem cell culture for generation of three-dimensional retinal and cortical tissues. Nat Protoc 7:69–79
10. Benowitz LI, He Z, Goldberg JL (2017) Reaching the brain: advances in optic nerve regeneration. Exp Neurol 287:365–373
11. Perepelkina T, Kegeles E, Baranov P (2019) Optimizing the conditions and use of synthetic matrix for three-dimensional in vitro retinal differentiation from mouse pluripotent cells. Tissue Eng Part C Methods 25:433–445
12. Kegeles E, Perepelkina T, Baranov P (2020) Semi-automated approach for retinal tissue differentiation. Transl Vis Sci Technol 9:24–24
13. Kegeles E, Naumov A, Karpulevich EA, Volchkov P, Baranov P (2020) Convolutional neural networks can predict retinal differentiation in retinal organoids. Front Cell Neurosci 14:171
14. Oswald J, Kegeles E, Minelli T, Volchkov P, Baranov P (2021) Transplantation of miPSC/mESC-derived retinal ganglion cells into healthy and glaucomatous retinas. Mol Ther-Meth Clin D 21:180–198
15. Eriksen AZ et al (2018) Multifarious biologic loaded liposomes that stimulate the mammalian target of rapamycin signaling pathway show retina neuroprotection after retina damage. ACS Nano 12:7497. https://doi.org/10.1021/acsnano.8b00596
16. Johnson TV et al (2023) The importance of unambiguous cell origin determination in neuronal repopulation studies. Iscience 26:106361
17. Rowe-Rendleman CL et al (2014) Drug and gene delivery to the back of the eye: from bench to bedside. Invest Opthalmol Vis Sci 55:2714

Chapter 16

Retinal Ganglion Cell Subtypes and Their Vulnerability in Glaucoma

James E. Morgan, Ryan J. Bevan, and Gloria Cimaglia

Abstract

The detection of selective retinal ganglion cell damage in glaucoma has been a long sought-after goal, not just for the development of clinical tests for the early detection of glaucoma but for the elucidation of potential mechanisms underlying retinal ganglion cell loss. Early reports of the selective vulnerability of larger retinal ganglion cells (RGCs) in human studies did not translate simply to the loss of a particular class of RGC but more likely reflected shrinkage and degeneration across all RGC classes. Subsequent studies of nonhuman primate (NHP) models of glaucoma indicated some selectivity with great damage to the magnocellular vs parvocellular pathways. More recently, rodent models of experimental glaucoma have highlighted a selective vulnerability of OFF-centered RGCs—particularly those with transient responses. Selectivity for OFF pathway damage is also seen as a trend in a rat model of glaucoma. These data support the concept that some RGCs are more vulnerable to the effects of glaucoma damage. This chapter covers some of the methods to elucidate RGC damage and the relevance of model selection to mimic human glaucoma rather than just RGC death.

Key words ON and OFF retinal ganglion cells, Dendrites, Particle-mediated dye transfer (biolistics), Carbocyanine dyes, Scholl analysis

1 Introduction

The pathophysiology of glaucoma is characterized by the selective loss of retinal ganglion cells (RGCs) over other cells in the retina. In turn, this has driven considerable debate as to whether particular classes of retinal ganglion cells are vulnerable to the effects of glaucoma. The relevance of this point is twofold. Firstly, it can help in dissecting mechanisms that influence RGC vulnerability, and secondly, it can help in the development of tests for the early detection of RGC damage. This chapter does not attempt an exhaustive coverage of the literature. Rather, it will highlight the most salient evidence for selective damage and some of the potential pitfalls in interpreting changes in RGC structure as a function of RGC damage.

Tatjana Jakobs and Paloma B. Liton (eds.), *Glaucoma: Methods and Protocols*, Methods in Molecular Biology, vol. 2858,
https://doi.org/10.1007/978-1-0716-4140-8_16,

Glaucoma most commonly arises as a result of modest and chronic elevation of intraocular pressure (IOP) acting on the aged retina. Marked elevations in IOP will cause RGC death but also introduce the effects of ischemic damage as a confounding mechanism. While retinal ganglion cell death is the pathological endpoint, the canonical view is that RGCs undergo a slow process of degeneration in which their dendritic processes atrophy alongside axon damage [1–5]. Axotomy, acute, and extreme elevations in IOP may be informative in their own right and drive a similar pattern of degeneration [6], but extrapolation to IOP-related glaucoma should be made with caution, if at all. Selective retinal ganglion cell death should not be used as the validating factor for any particular mode of glaucoma.

1.1 Methods: Human and Primate Glaucoma Models

Human studies offered some early insights into the changes that might occur across visual pathways. The analysis of the change in axon size distributions suggests that a shift in the axon size distribution reflected a loss of larger axons [7]. In humans, this was matched by a shift in the size distribution away from larger cells [8] with a similar shift in the cell size distribution away from larger cells also seen in the nonhuman primate (NHP) model of glaucoma [9], regarded as the one that most closely resembles human glaucoma [10].

A reasonable interpretation of these changes was that larger RGCs and their axons were preferentially damaged. While this is a plausible conclusion, it relies in part on the assumption that retinal ganglion cells do not undergo any changes in structure or size as a result of glaucoma; a simple analysis of the change in RGC size as a function of the normal cell size distribution can generate the appearance of the selective loss of larger cells [11].

The importance of this possibility is that it questioned the presence (or not) of shrinkage and remodeling of retinal ganglion cells in glaucoma [12–14]. Rather than proceeding from a state of health and passing quickly to apoptosis [15], it suggested that RGCs underwent a prolonged period of degeneration. Subsequent work, based on intracellular labelling of RGCs supported with fluorescent dyes, supported the concept that larger parasol RGCs underwent a greater degree of degeneration than midget RGCS in the early stages of glaucoma [1]. Studies of the changes in cell density in the lateral geniculate nucleus found greater cell loss in the magnocellular layers (to which the parasol cells project) compared to the parvocellular layers [16] (the recipient zone for midget RGCs).

The analysis of the changes in RGC morphology in the NHP glaucoma model were undertaken using classical cell filling techniques using fluorescent dyes which have provided the basis for our knowledge of RGC morphology in humans and NHP [17, 18]. The quality of labelling in these studies is excellent and,

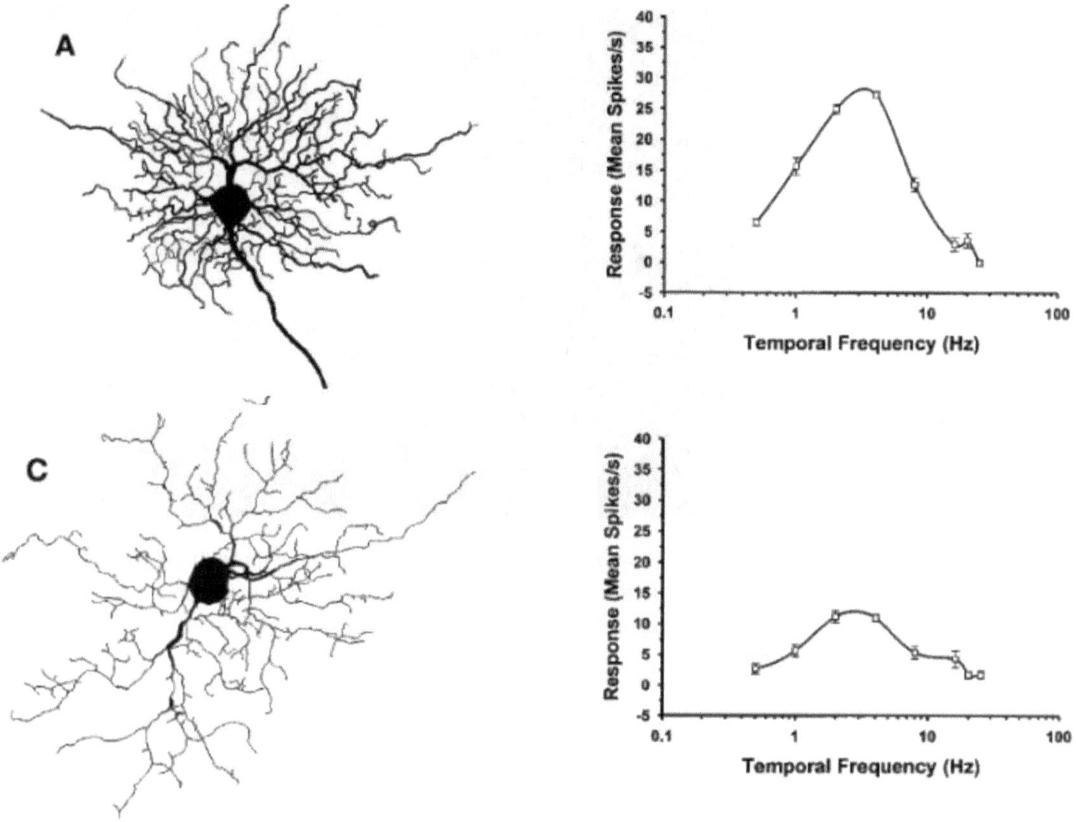

Fig. 1 Neurobiotin-filled parasol-type retinal ganglion cells in the NHP model of glaucoma. Top healthy cell. Bottom cell from a glaucomatous retina. The temporal frequency tuning curves were obtained from the same cells showing a marked reduction in dendritic integrity in the glaucoma cell and a corresponding reduction in temporal sensitivity (From Weber and Harman IOVS 2005)

importantly, the entire cell body and dendritic tree can be filled. Functional assessment can also be undertaken when RGCs can be stimulated using grating projects onto RGCs in explanted retinas [19] (Fig. 1) demonstrating the close relationship between RGC dendritic structure and function. RGCs with quite depleted dendritic processes are still able to generate a light response. However, labelling on a cell-by-cell basis is time-consuming, and retinal wholemount preparations comprise a population of axotomized retinal ganglion cells which limits the realistic availability of health cells for labelling; significant dendritic atrophy can occur in wholemount preparations within the first 24 h [20, 21]. In the analysis of changes in RGC dendritic structure regardless of technique, the time from death to getting the retinas should be as short as possible. RGCs can maintain largely intact dendritic structure even several hours after death allowing the analysis of RGC dendritic structure in fixed tissue (Fig. 2). The degree of beading within the dendritic tree increases with the delay in time from death to fix, but it is also influenced by the degree of fixation (*see* **Note 1**) [22].

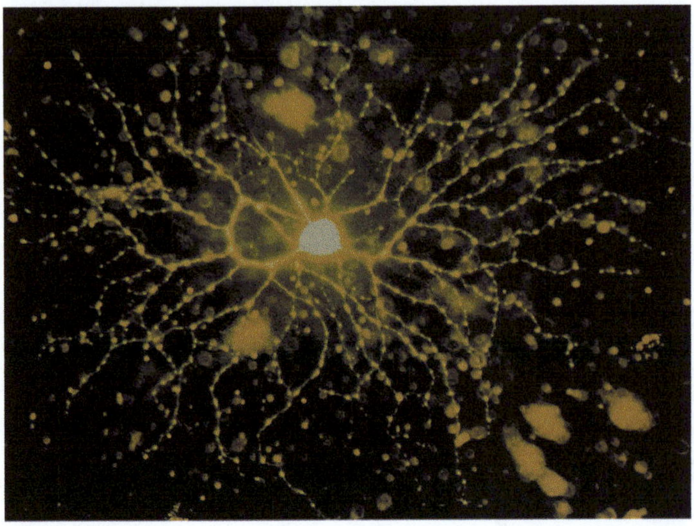

Fig. 2 Parasol retinal ganglion cell (human) labelled more than 20 h postmortem by intracellular filling with Lucifer Yellow. The degree of beading is likely to be an artifact of fixation but also reflects the prolonged death to preparation time (*see* **Note 1**)

Traditional intracellular labelling techniques carry the risk of bias in that healthier RGCs would preferentially be sampled since these are easier to fill resulting in an underestimate of dendritic degeneration. For the avoidance of bias, it is possible to bulk-fill RGCs in vivo. In NHPs this can best be done with direct implantation of tracers such as HRP into the optic nerve in vivo [21] (Fig. 3). It is notable that the degree of beading in the NHP model is considerably less than in the human retina, even following fixation by transcardiac perfusion with 1% paraformaldehyde, confirming the importance of time taken from sacrifice to processing as a factor in dendritic beading. Direct optic nerve labelling is effective in glaucoma models since the transit distance for the track to the optic nerve cell body is reduced, an important factor when retrograde transport is reduced. The method provides large numbers of labelled cells which can divided into parasol and midget cell classes based on the configuration of the primary and secondary dendrites which are relatively unaffected in glaucoma. In general, proximal dendrites are usually preserved so that these can be used to classify cells even when higher-order dendrites are undergoing degeneration [23]. The analysis of parasol and midget cell proportions following retrograde labelling did not confirm a propensity for selective loss. One of the limitations of retrograde labelling in the NHP model is that it does not provide reliable labelling of higher-order dendrites. It is not therefore possible to rule out the possibility of differential dendritic atrophy in parasol vs midget retinal ganglion cells.

The analysis of human tissue prior to fixation at the level of the connectome is possible but remains challenging. Human postmortem tissue can be labelled using HRP but the time from retrieval to injection should be minimal (typically under 2 h) [24]. When postmortem times are longer (24–48 h), tissues are best preserved in paraformaldehyde (1%) which renders them suitable for bulk labelling with DiI usually following the implantation of crystals within the optic nerve [25]. The location of crystal implantation is critical for RGC labelling. Insertion in the retrobulbar optic nerve does not provide suitable labelling of RGC possibly because of the restrictive effects of the myelin transition zone. When crystals are placed in the retinal nerve fiber layer, RGC axons, soma, and dendrites can be excellent though the retention of DiI within the retinal nerve fiber layer can be technically challenging. In the case of end-stage glaucoma, dendritic atrophy and cell soma shrinkage are widespread features, but they do not appear to be selectively greater in parasol cells [26] (Fig. 3). Carbocyanine dyes can also be implanted in the retinal nerve fiber layer/retinal ganglion cell soma of smaller rodent eyes using Diolistics [27], providing the fixation is light (c. 1% paraformaldehyde). This approach has not been attempted in human or NHP material. Given the greater thickness of the internal limiting membrane relative to that in rodents, higher injection pressures (in excess of 40 psi) would be required.

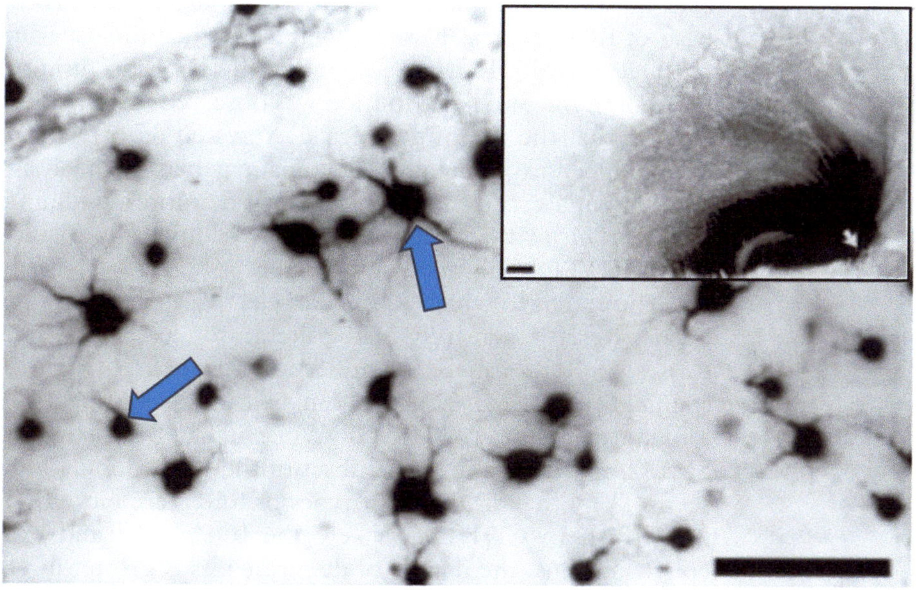

Fig. 3 Retinal ganglion cells labelled by the retrograde transport of Horse Radish Peroxidase (HRP) following direct implantation into the optic nerve (retrobulbar). The superior aspect of the retina is labelled. Scale bar 1 mm. Individual parasol and midget cells are shown. (From Morgan et al. [21])

The consistent observation in these models is that RGCs undergo shrinkage and remodeling at somal and dendritic levels. In the nonhuman primate, there is some evidence that parasol cells may be selectively damaged over midget cells in the early stage of disease, but this has not been a consistent finding. It is not clear whether this pattern of selective loss occurs in human glaucoma.

1.2 Rodent Models

Rodent models have the benefit that the level of IOP increase can be controlled and animal sacrifice and tissue processing timed for optimal RGC labelling. One of the clear benefits is the availability of mouse models in which RGCs are genetically labelled. Sparse RGC labelling using reporters such as YFP driven by Thy1 or using AAV is a model for RGC transfection. The former method has the advantage of sustained expression without the possible inflammatory effects of viral transfection. However, the commonly used Thy1 promoter is also downregulated in glaucoma [28] which can result in the undersampling of damaged cells. A good example of the issues that can arise with these models was provided by Williams et al. who studied dendritic changes in DBA2J mice crossed with Thy1-YFP transgenic mice [5]. In DBA2J -YFP mice, RGCs are sparsely labelled with expressed YFP which is ideal for RGC analysis since it excludes dendritic field overlap. Dendritic integrity was quantified using standard Sholl-based metrics. Surprisingly, YFP-positive cells did not demonstrate a left shift in the Sholl distribution previously reported for the mouse for cells labelled by intracellular filling [29] and subsequently on the basis of RGC synapse loss [30] (Fig. 4). When the experiment was repeated and the RGCs were labelled by Diolistics using DiI, the left shift in the Sholl distribution was observed. These observations caution that the use of genetically expressed reporters for chronically induced experimental glaucoma may bias the analysis of dendritic changes and underreport any dendrite loss in favor of healthier, more intact cells that were physiologically able to express sufficient YFP to fill the dendritic tree.

The extent to which RGCs are selectively damaged in mice has been covered extensively in the literature (see [31]). Since some classes of RGC can be identified on the basis of neurofilament staining (with SMI-32), this can provide a reasonable basis for looking at a subset of RGCs. While it has been suggested that SMI32 may label a distinct subset of the RGC population [32], it seems likely that at least four types of RGCs are picked up by this label [33]. In CD1 mice where the IOP is elevated by lasering episcleral veins, the degree of dendritic loss is greater in OFF-type RGCs with the effect particularly noticeable for the OFF transient RGCs when compared with ON-type cells (Fig. 5). These cells were labelled using biolistics ensuring that the labelling fluorescent protein (Td Tomato and PSD-95) is retained intracellularly which allows secondary immunofluorescent labelling with permeabilization. It is important to note that this is not possible with diolistic

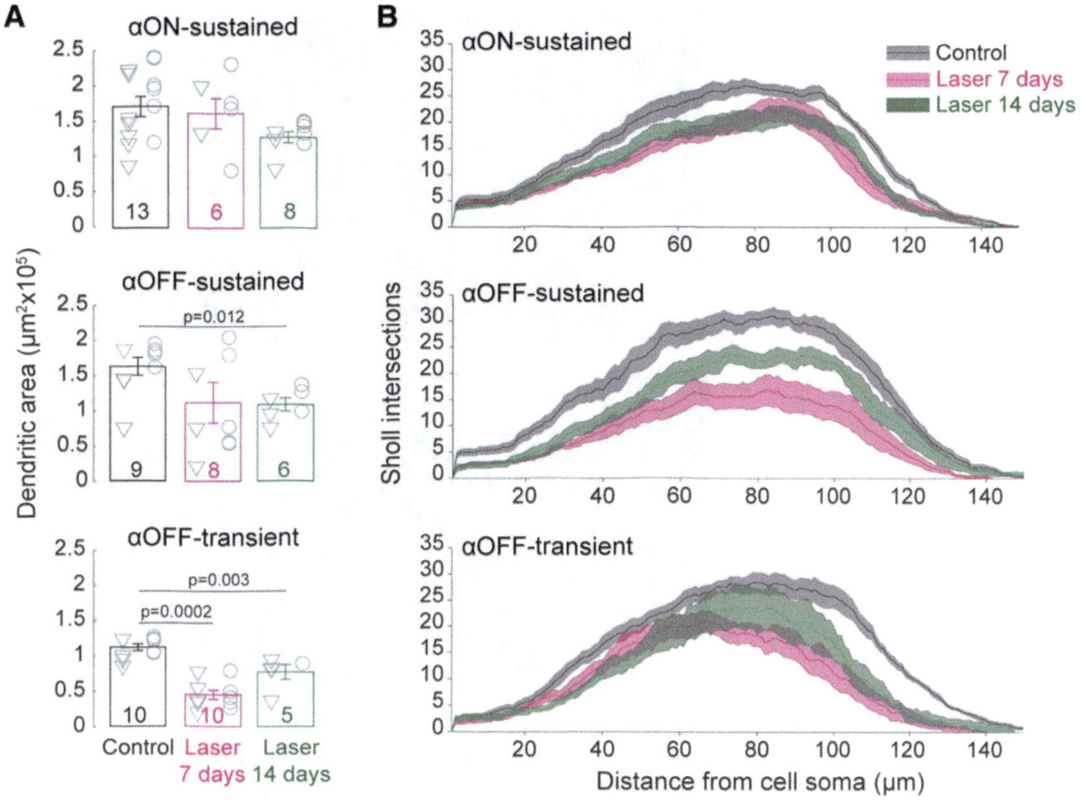

Fig. 4 Sholl plots summarizing dendritic integrity in alpha-type RGCs in mice with induced ocular hypertension. All ON- and OFF-type cells demonstrate reduced dendritic complexity, but this is greater for the OFF-type cells and in the OFF types for those with transient responses. The RGCs were labelled biolistically with a plasmi expressive dt Tomatro and then immunohistochemically for the neurofilament antibody SMI-32. (From Ou et al. [29])

labelling since the DiI is retained within the plasma membrane and is released on permeabilization thereby hindering the accurate quantification of dendritic structure, a problem that, in our hands, cannot be effectively overcome by the use of more persistent (chloromethylated) forms of carbocyanine dyes. Caution should be used when viewing IOP changes in the mouse since the IOP increases are short (typically 7–14 days) and the peak IOPs can be high (c 30 mmHg). A similar level of selective OFF-type RGC damage has also been reported for a microbead model of glaucoma based on the C57B6 strain (*see* **Note 2**) [34].

When studying glaucoma-related RGC damage, the selection of the model should be made with care. For example, rat glaucoma models present a better opportunity to observe changes in RGC structure following prolonged rather than acute increases in IOP. The relationship between IOP and axon loss is robust and modest, and sustained IOPs can be obtained following occlusion of the iridocorneal angles using magnetic microbeads [35, 36]. Furthermore, the rat eye is more resilient than in the mouse which can

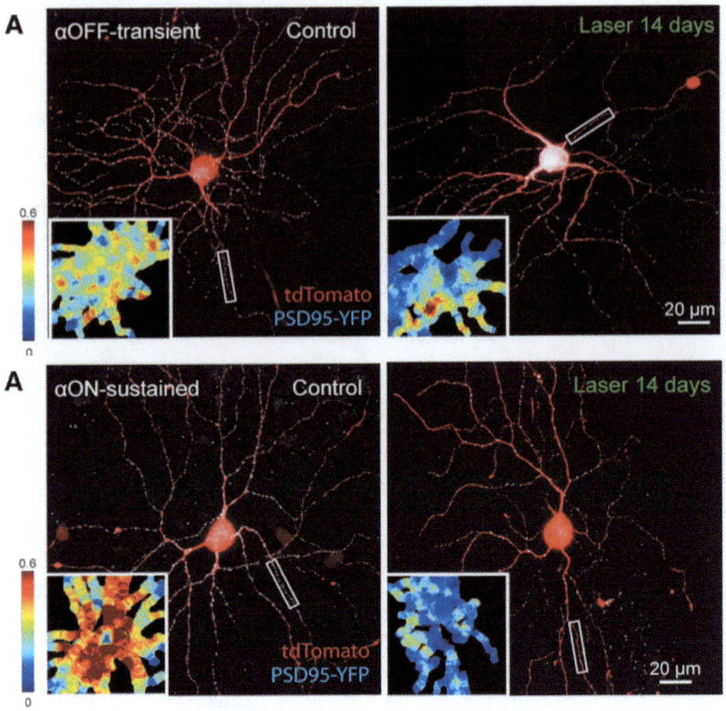

Fig. 5 Montage of alpha on sustained and alpha OFF transient retinal ganglion cells labelled biolistrically for TD Tomato and the synaptic marker PSD95. The loss of dendritic processes is minimal for the ON-type cells but significantly greater for the OFF-type cells. (From Ou et al. [29])

facilitate tissue handling in glaucomatous eyes. In our lab, we selected the Brown Norway rat for this reason and have sampled large numbers of RGCs regardless of type to obtain an overall estimate of dendritic changes across the RGC population, regardless of type. In the rat, we also see a trend for greater loss of OFF-type RGC dendrites, but this does not reach statistical significance (Fig. 6).

A comparison of the Sholl plots for the mouse (Fig. 5) and rat (Fig. 6) is of interest. Classical dendrite pruning with early neuronal degeneration commences with loss of higher-order dendrites—seen as a left shift in the Sholl distribution. By contrast, in the mouse, the reduction in the Sholl profile is more global including the involvement of primary and secondary dendrites [29, 34]. The implications of these differences are unclear but suggest that caution should be exercised in a simple comparison between models.

The reasons for selective damage to OFF-type cells remain unexplained. The activity levels of ON vs OFF RGCs will relate to the ambient luminance, and this may be a factor in determining vulnerability. For example, OFF center RGCs will fire at lower rates in dim illumination with ON center cells being more active with brighter illumination [37].

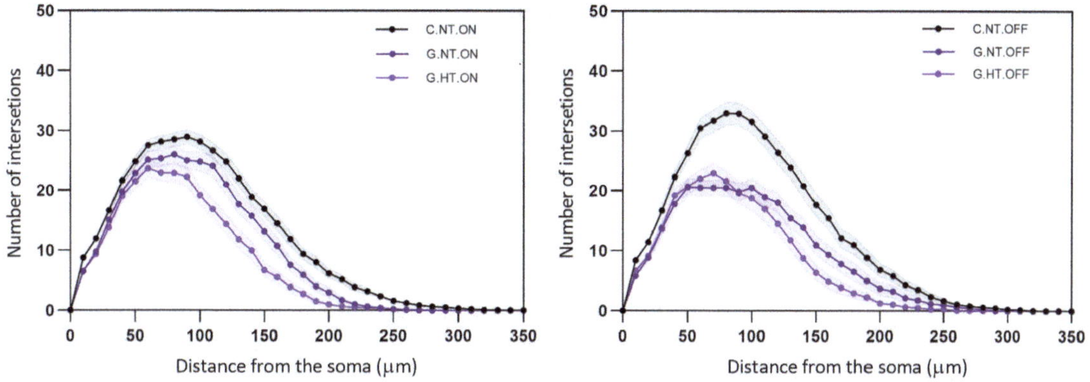

Fig. 6 Sholl plots summarizing dendritic complexity for ON- and OFF-type RGCs in a rat (magnetic microbead) models of glaucoma. There is a trend for the OFF-type cells to have a greater reduction compared to the ON-type cells, but this did not reach statistical significance. Shaded lines: SEMs C.NT: untreated control. G.NT: eye contralateral to the eye with the height IOP. G. HT: the eye with the increased IOP. Note that changes are also seen in the contralateral normotensive eye following the induction of unilateral glaucoma

It would be interesting to know if ON-OFF selectivity is a function of ambient (animal housing) luminance and certainly; the level of housing illumination should be reported in any study of ON-OFF selectivity. It is notable that in mouse models of compromised mitochondrial function such as OPA1 (autosomal dominant optic atrophy), greater damage was seen in dendrites terminating on the ON layer of the IPL [38]. Further work is required to determine if it reflects a fundamentally different mechanism of inducing RGC damage or simply the effect of housing illumination regimes.

2 Materials

2.1 Materials for RGC Labelling by Implantation of DiI Crystals into the Nerve Fiber Layer of Postmortem Human Eyes

Tweezers and scissors for dissection.

Paraformaldehyde 2–4% in phosphate buffer (pH 7.4).

DiI (1,1′-dioctadecyl-3,3,3′,3′-tetramethylindocarbocyanine perchlorate), crystalline.

Nitrocellulose paper.

2.2 Materials for Diolistic Labelling of RGCs

Tungsten bullets (Thermo Fischer Scientific). The particle size should be approximately 1 micron in diameter (*see* **Note 8** for safety in handling tungsten powder). Note that gold particles can also be used, but the injection pressure would need to be slightly increased to reflect the greater weight of gold.

DiI, DiO, or DiD: mixing three dyes will generate, potentially, nine spectral variants of labelled cells.

Dichloromethane (methylene chloride, *see* **Note 4**).

Large glass slide (75 mm × 50 mm), precleaned with 70% ethanol.

Clean razor blade.

1.5 mL Eppendorf tubes.

1 mL pipette tip.

Parafilm.

Tefzel tubing.

Gene gun system with tubing preparation stage (e.g., Helios gene gun). It is possible to fabricate a gene gun from parts at reduced cost.

N_2 and helium tanks.

3 Methods

3.1 RGC Labelling by Implantation of DiI Crystals into the Nerve Fiber Layer

1. Remove the anterior segment and the vitreous and fix the posterior eyecup in 2–4% paraformaldehyde in phosphate buffer. It is critical that fixatives such as glutaraldehyde are avoided since the tissue will show low-level autofluorescence.
2. Implant small DiI crystals into the nerve fiber layer of the retina. The crystals require direct and relatively deep implantation, ideally into the deeper parts of the retinal nerve layer close to the optic nerve head. A small patch of nitrocellulose filter paper (or similar) can be applied over the site of insertion to prevent crystal dislocation; this step is important since the DiI crystals can easily be dislodged.
3. Store the retinas in the same fixative in the dark. It is important that the samples are stored at room temperature (37 °C) and not refrigerated to facilitate dye diffusion within the plasma membrane. Diffusion times can vary from 4 to 24 weeks depending on the distance of the dye implant from the target neuron population. The sample can be inspected briefly during this period to check on dye transport.
4. Dissect the retina free of the eyecup and the pigment epithelium and cut the retina into four quadrants.
5. Whole-mount the retina pieces on Nitrocellulose filter paper.
6. Cover with antifade immersion medium and coverslip (*see* **Note 3**).

3.2 RGC Labelling Using Particle-Mediated Dye Transfer (Diolistics)

1. Take three or four Eppendorf tubes. One for the tungsten and one for each dye (DiI, DiD, and DiO).
2. Weigh 80 mg of Tungsten, 2 mg of DiI, 1 mg of DiD, and 4 mg of DiO.

3. Divide the tungsten in two or three equal parts on different glass slides according to a number of dyes that are going to be used.
4. Dissolve each dye in 400 μL of dichloromethane.
5. Once dissolved, add the mix drop by drop to the appropriate tungsten pile (max for drops at the time).
6. Wait until the solution dries out, scrap with the razor blade, and repeat until all the dye solution is used.
7. Mix the two/three coated tungsten piles together and grind finely with the razor blade.
8. Cut 30 cm of Tefzel tubing and cover one end with parafilm.
9. Insert the small part of a 1 mL pipette tip into the Tefzel tubing (it will be used to funnel the tungsten-coated particles).
10. Pour the coated tungsten particles into the larger part of the pipette tip.
11. Flick the pipette tip to transfer all the tungsten particles into the Tefzel tubing.
12. Cover the end part of the tube with parafilm and flick and spin the tube to evenly distribute the tungsten coated particles.

3.3 Retinal Preparation for Diolistic Labelling

1. Following euthanization, the eyes should be enucleated rapidly and the cornea marked with a handheld cautery to ensure correction orientation of the retina.
2. Subsequent processing depends on whether labelling is carried out on fresh or fixed tissue. Our parameters for rat eyes are that labelling is carried out on fresh tissue. For this, the eye is transferred to ice-cold HBSS, and the retinas are dissected out rapidly (ideally under 60 s) and placed ganglion cell side up, under HBSS for labelling.

   For mouse eye, retinas can be diolistically labelled fresh (using the same method as for the rat eye) or following fixation. For fixed tissue labelling, the optic nerve should be cut immediately flush with the globe and then the whole eye immersed in 1.5% formaldehyde. Eyes can then be stored for up to 6 months in 1.5% formaldehyde and used for diolistic labelling. The advantage of using fixed preparations is that eyes can be processed in batches and any delays from retinal preparation to labelling are not a confounding factor with regard to the quality of dendritic labelling. With fixed tissue, RGC structure is stabilized throughout the labelling process; however, labelling fixed tissue can be more challenging when trying to obtain high cell yield per retina (typically ten clearly identified RGCs per retina). The use of fixed retinal tissue for mouse models is now our preferred preparation method, for these reasons.

For unfixed tissue (rat), fire the gene gun with the distance from the nozzle to the retinal surface set to approximately 5 cm and a firing pressure set to 120–130 psi. For fixed tissue (mouse), the injection with the mouse retina distance can be reduced to 1.3–1.5 cm and lower pressures used (c 100–110 psi) (*see* **Note 6**). Ensure that the gun nozzle is orthogonal to the retinal surface since this will ensure even and sparse RGC labelling. A polyethylene terephthalate membrane filter (mesh size 3 μm, Fisher Scientific) should be placed between the nozzle of the gene gun and the tissue to avoid large clumps of tungsten to hit the retina (*see* **Note 7**).

3. For unfixed tissue, incubate the retinal segments, flat mounted for 30 minutes in Neurobasal-A media (Gibco; 37 ° C, 5% CO_2) to ensure dye diffusion and then fix for 1 h in 4% formaldehyde. Wash with 1 M PBS so that the retina can be counterstained with a nuclear marker (e.g., Hoechst, 1:1000 PBS), and then wash again in PBS. If fixed tissue is used, then keep the labelled retinas in the dark for 24 h at room temperature prior to fixation with 4% formaldehyde.
4. Mount with antifade-mounting medium (Flourosave, Millipore) and evaluate under fluorescent illumination immediately. DiI will diffuse over time, so the slides should be imaged as soon as possible. To minimize diffusion artefacts, imaging should be completed within 48 h.

3.4 Conclusions

The analysis of dendritic changes has revealed possible selective damage to parasol cells in the NHP models of glaucoma and selective damage to OFF cells in the mouse and possibly in the rat models of glaucoma. These studies illustrate the importance of using dendritic readouts as a sensitive indicator of retinal ganglion cell damage in glaucoma and related conditions. Although we do not have evidence of OFF-type RGC-selective damage in humans, there is evidence that recording responses to OFF stimuli may provide a useful method for the detection of functional damage [39] similar to ERG changes seen in mouse glaucoma [40]. The persistence of dendritic atrophy in the majority of RGCs from glaucomatous eyes suggests a neural substrate for the recovery of vision in glaucoma. The possibility that OFF pathways are selectively damaged suggests that targeted measurement of OFF responses may provide a novel and effective method for measuring this recovery.

4 Notes

1. Dendritic beading artefacts can be mitigated by the coadministration of sucrose (200 mM) and by the use of the lowest useful concentration of fixative (e.g., 1% formaldehyde). These artefacts will also be minimized with short dissection times.

2. A useful housekeeping note when using particle-mediated transfection of DNA (biolistics) and dye-based labelling (diolistics) in the same laboratory is that gold particles are used for biolistics since they are nontoxic. Gold particles can be used for diolistics too, but for reasons of economy, tungsten is still used for this application. Tungsten particles are not manifestly toxic for the 30–40 min required to label cells with carbocyanine dyes. The use of tungsten in fixed tissue does not pose any toxicity issues. However, any tungsten contamination in a gene gun used for biolistics will result in the death of labelled RGCs. The injection workstation should be cleaned of any particle debris—DiI/D staining is seen around the nozzle, and then it is important to check and replace the O-ring seals on the gun that clamp the cartridge in its carrier. These seals should be checked regularly since any damage reduce the pressure charge and diminish labelling. A sign of failure is that higher pressures may be required over time to achieve the same degree of labelling.
3. It is possible to photoconvert carbocyanine dyes with diaminobenzidine (DAB) for visualization under bright field illumination. For this, preincubate the retinas in the dark in DAB solution (1.5 mg/mL in 0.1 M Tris buffer pH 8.2). Immerse the tissue in fresh DAB solution with a change of solution every 10 min. Illuminate the tissue with fluorescent light through a 20× long working-distance objective. Fluorescent illumination is terminated when the desired labelling intensity under bright-field illumination is achieved [25]. DAB is toxic and should be handled with gloves in a chemical safety cabinet.
4. Dichloromethane is volatile. Handle under a fume hood.
5. The cartridges with tungsten/DiI can be stored in the dark in a light sealed container for up to 6 months at room temperature. Ideally, store in a desiccator under vacuum for optimal quality—but this is not essential [41].
6. The optimal pressure should be determined empirically. Some groups use a stand to support the gene gun so that the distance from the gun nozzle to the retinal surface can be calibrated. In general, higher pressures can be used at greater distances to provide more diffuse and sparser RGC labelling.
7. Labelling can be evaluated under fluorescent illumination immediately, and the same piece of retina can be shot 2–3 times with the gene gun until enough cells have incorporated the label.
8. Tungsten power (particles <2 microns) is flammable when combined with oxidants, and spontaneous combustion in air has been reported. It is important that sources of combustion are removed from the preparation area. It can also cause skin and respiratory irritation, so appropriate personal protective equipment should be used when preparing beads for labelling.

References

1. Weber AJ, Kaufman PL, Hubbard WC (1998) Morphology of single ganglion cells in the glaucomatous primate retina. Invest Ophthalmol Vis Sci 39:2304–2320
2. Santina LD, Inman DM, Lupien CB et al (2013) Differential progression of structural and functional alterations in distinct retinal ganglion cell types in a mouse model of glaucoma. J Neurosci 33:17444–17457
3. Morquette B, Morquette P, Agostinone J et al (2014) REDD2-mediated inhibition of mTOR promotes dendrite retraction induced by axonal injury. Cell Death Differ 22:612–625
4. Morgan JE (2012) Retina ganglion cell degeneration in glaucoma: an opportunity missed? A review. Clin Exp Ophthalmol 40:364–368
5. Williams PA, Howell GR, Barbay JM et al (2013) Retinal ganglion cell dendritic atrophy in DBA/2J glaucoma. PLoS One 8:e72282
6. Binley KE, Ng WS, Barde Y-A et al (2016) Brain-derived neurotrophic factor prevents dendritic retraction of adult mouse retinal ganglion cells. Eur J Neurosci 20:140–2039
7. Quigley HA, Dunkelberger GR, Green WR (1988) Chronic human glaucoma causing selectively greater loss of large optic nerve fibers. Ophthalmology 95:357–363
8. Quigley HA, Dunkelberger GR, Green WR (1989) Retinal ganglion cell atrophy correlated with automated perimetry in human eyes with glaucoma. Am J Ophthalmol 107:453–464
9. Glovinsky Y, Quigley HA, Dunkelberger GR (1991) Retinal ganglion cell loss is size dependent in experimental glaucoma. Invest Ophthalmol Vis Sci 32:484–491
10. Burgoyne CF (2015) The non-human primate experimental glaucoma model. Exp Eye Res 141:57–73
11. Morgan JE (1994) Selective cell death in glaucoma: does it really occur? Br J Ophthalmol 78: 875–880
12. Polo AD (2015) Dendrite pathology and neurodegeneration: focus on mTOR. Neural Regen Res 10:559–561
13. Liu M, Guo L, Salt TE et al (2014) Dendritic changes in rat visual pathway associated with experimental ocular hypertension. Curr Eye Res 39:953–963
14. Morgan JE (2002) Retinal ganglion cell shrinkage in glaucoma. J Glaucoma 11(4): 365–370
15. Kerrigan LA, Zack DJ, Quigley HA et al (1997) TUNEL-positive ganglion cells in human primary open-angle glaucoma. Arch Ophthalmol 115:1031–1035
16. Weber AJ, Chen H, Hubbard WC et al (2000) Experimental glaucoma and cell size, density, and number in the primate lateral geniculate nucleus. Invest Ophthalmol Vis Sci 41:1370–1379
17. Dacey D (1993) The mosaic of midget ganglion cells in the human retina. J Neurosci 12: 5334–5355
18. Dacey DM, Petersen MR (1992) Dendritic field size and morphology of midget and parasol ganglion cells of the human retina. Proc Natl Acad Sci USA 89:9666–9670
19. Weber AJ, Harman CD (2005) Structure–function relations of parasol cells in the Normal and glaucomatous primate retina. Invest Ophthalmol Vis Sci 46:3197–3207
20. Binley KE, Ng WS, Barde Y et al (2016) Brain-derived neurotrophic factor prevents dendritic retraction of adult mouse retinal ganglion cells. Eur J Neurosci 44:2028–2039
21. Morgan JE, Uchida H, Caprioli J (2000) Retinal ganglion cell death in experimental glaucoma. Br J Ophthalmol 84:303–310
22. Stradleigh TW, Greenberg KP, Partida GJ et al (2015) Moniliform deformation of retinal ganglion cells by formaldehyde-based fixatives. J Comp Neurol 523:545–564
23. Tribble JR, Samsel P, Cross SD et al (2014) A novel classification system for rat RGCs in retinal degeneration. Invest Ophthalmol Vis Sci 55:2389
24. Morgan JE, Jeffery G, Foss AJE (1998) Axon deviation in the human lamina cribrosa. Br J Ophthalmol 82:680–683
25. FitzGibbon T, Taylor SF (1996) Retinotopy of the human retinal nerve fibre layer and optic nerve head. J Comp Neurol 375:238–251
26. Pavlidis M, Stupp T, Naskar R et al (2003) Retinal ganglion cells resistant to advanced glaucoma: a postmortem study of human retinas with the carbocyanine dye DiI. Invest Ophthalmol Vis Sci 44:5196–5205
27. Coombs J, List DVD, Wang G-Y et al (2006) Morphological properties of mouse retinal ganglion cells. Neuroscience 140:123–136
28. Huang W, Fileta J, Guo Y et al (2006) Downregulation of Thy1 in retinal ganglion cells in experimental glaucoma. Curr Eye Res 31:265–271
29. Ou Y, Jo RE, Ullian EM et al (2016) Selective vulnerability of specific retinal ganglion cell

types and synapses after transient ocular hypertension. J Neurosci 36:9240–9252
30. Berry RH, Qu J, John SWM et al (2015) Synapse loss and dendrite remodeling in a mouse model of glaucoma. PLoS One 10:e0144341
31. Santina LD, Ou Y (2017) Who's lost first? Susceptibility of retinal ganglion cell types in experimental glaucoma. Exp Eye Res 158:43–50
32. Wang S, Masland R (2004) Retinal ganglion cell type, size, and spacing can be specified independent of homotypic dendritic contacts. Neuron 43:475
33. Coombs J, van der List D, Wang G-Y et al (2006) Morphological properties of mouse retinal ganglion cells. Neuroscience 140:123–136
34. El-Danaf RN, Huberman AD (2015) Characteristic patterns of dendritic remodeling in early-stage glaucoma: evidence from genetically identified retinal ganglion cell types. J Neurosci 35:2329–2343
35. Samsel PA, Kisiswa L, Erichsen JT et al (2011) A novel method for the induction of experimental glaucoma using magnetic microspheres. Invest Opthalmol Vis Sci 52:1671
36. Tribble JR, Otmani A, Kokkali E et al (2021) Retinal ganglion cell degeneration in a rat magnetic bead model of ocular hypertensive glaucoma. Transl Vis Sci Technol 10:21
37. Kageyama G, Wong-Riley M (1984) The histochemical localization of cytochrome oxidase in the retina and lateral geniculate nucleus of the ferret, cat, and monkey, with particular reference to retinal mosaics and ON/OFF-center visual channels. J Neurosci 4:2445–2459
38. Williams PA, Piechota M, von Ruhland C et al (2012) Opa1 is essential for retinal ganglion cell synaptic architecture and connectivity. Brain 135:493–505
39. Kong AW, Turner ML, Chan H et al (2021) Asymmetric functional impairment of ON and OFF retinal pathways in glaucoma. Ophthalmol Sci 1:100026
40. Kong AW, Santina LD, Ou Y (2020) Probing ON and OFF retinal pathways in glaucoma using electroretinography. Transl Vis Sci Technol 9:14
41. Bevan RJ, Cimaglia G, Morgan JE et al (2024) Improved DiOlistic labelling technique for neurons in situ: Detailed visualisation of dendritic spines and concurrent histochemical-detection in fixed tissue. Methods 229:82–93

Chapter 17

Full-Field Electroretinogram Responses in Rodent Models of Ganglion Cell Injury

Da Zhao, Pei Ying Lee, Vickie H. Y. Wong, Anh Hoang, Katie K. N. Tran, Anna K. Van Koeverden, Brianna C. Afiat, Christine T. O. Nguyen, and Bang V. Bui

Abstract

Preclinical studies of optic nerve injury models have led to significant insight into the mechanism underlying retinal ganglion cell neurodegeneration. During the process of ganglion cell injury, morphological changes can occur prior to gross structural changes and cell death. Similarly, following injury, functional changes can occur in the absence of substantive structural changes. These more subtle effects can often be detected using functional tools such as the electroretinogram. Moreover, the electroretinogram is a sensitive and complementary means to quantify treatment efficacy. Here, we describe in vivo electroretinography for assessing ganglion cell injury in rodent models.

Key words Small animal models, Rodents, In vivo retinal assessment, Electroretinogram, Retinal function

1 Introduction

There are a range of noninvasive behavioral [1] and electrophysiological assessment tools [2] that facilitate quantification of ganglion cell integrity in rodent models of optic nerve injury and ocular hypertension. The electroretinogram (ERG) continues to be one of the most widely employed preclinical approaches for functional assessment of the retina [3]. This is in part because the ERG waveform is well conserved across common laboratory species used to study glaucoma as well as in humans [4–6].

Several different types of stimuli can be used to elicit a signal containing information about ganglion cell health. The full-field (or Ganzfeld) ERG response elicited using short flashes of light is known to be dominated by ganglion cell-mediated spiking activity at very dim light levels that are close to the absolute detection threshold for rodents. Responses at these dim light levels are

Tatjana Jakobs and Paloma B. Liton (eds.), *Glaucoma: Methods and Protocols*, Methods in Molecular Biology, vol. 2858, https://doi.org/10.1007/978-1-0716-4140-8_17,

known as the scotopic threshold response (STR) [7, 8]. Information regarding ganglion cells can also be gleaned from the trough that follows the b-wave recorded under photopic conditions, known as the photopic negative response (PhNR) [9]. Finally, responses elicited using contrast reversing checkerboards (pattern ERG) are also highly sensitive to ganglion cell injury [10].

Some combination of the above approaches are specifically designed to provide information about the health of major cell classes in the retina. These cells sequentially communicate with each other, and these approaches provide a comprehensive means to determine the specificity of the injury or treatment for retinal ganglion cells. This manuscript describes a protocol for the recording and analysis of the full-field ERG to return quantitative measures of components reflecting photoreceptors, bipolar cells, and the inner retina, including ganglion cells.

2 Materials

2.1 Electroretinography

1. Electrode silver wire (99.9% Silver, 0.3 mm diameter round wire, A&E Metal Merchants).
2. Insulating tape (masking tape).
3. Chloriding battery (9 V battery, Energizer).
4. Normal saline (0.9%, GelFlex).
5. Platinum electrode leads (Grass Telefactor).
6. Electrode holders (micromanipulators, World Precision Instruments).
7. Ground electrode: F-E2-30 (needle electrode, Grass Telefactor).
8. Headlight for animal preparation (Energizer HD+ LED headlight, Energizer).
9. Mydriatic agent (0.5–1% tropicamide, Alcon).
10. Corneal anesthesia (0.5% proxymetacaine, Alcon).
11. General anesthesia (1.6 mL Ketamine [100 mg/mL, Troy Laboratory], 1.6 mL xylazine [20 mg/mL, Troy Laboratory], and 6.8 mL sodium chloride [0.9% w/v]).
12. 30-gauge needle (Terumo)
13. Lint-free tissue (Kimwipes, Kimberley-Clark).
14. Contact gel (carmellose sodium, Celluvisc 1.0%, Allergan).
15. Small scales (Digitech).
16. Light stimulus via Ganzfeld integrating bowl (Photometric Solutions International).

17. Bioamplifier (Grass P511, Grass Telefactor).
18. Data acquisition system (Powerlab data acquisition system, ADInstruments).
19. Data acquisition software (Scope or LabChart Software, ADInstruments).
20. Computer: personal computer (Windows based) for recording signals and offline analysis.
21. Temperature maintenance (circulating water bath, LAUDA-Brinkmann).
22. Faraday Cage (2 × 1.2 × 1.2 m, Photometric Solutions International).
23. Analysis Software (Excel, Microsoft).

3 Methods

3.1 Laboratory and Electrode Preparation

The scotopic threshold response is a sensitive indicator of early ganglion cell injury and loss [11]. This component is highly sensitive to background light and requires absolute dark adaptation and stable anesthesia due to its small signal size. The robustness of scotopic threshold response recording very much depends on the quality of light proofing (e.g., baffles on both sides of curtains, taping the edges of curtains to the walls, using multiple layers of curtains). Thus prior to experimentation, ensure that in and around the location of recording, all extraneous light sources (e.g., light from the edges of windows and under doors, computer equipment, indicator lights on wall switches, or other equipment) are minimized or preferably eliminated.

1. Dark-adapt animals in a well-ventilated space for longer than 4 h, preferably overnight.
2. Electrodes can be prepared beforehand or on the day. They should be chlorided immediately before use.
3. Use the same silver wire within an experiment as the purity of the metal can vary between batches.
4. Prepare four electrodes (two active, two reference) for recording from both eyes. Ensure that the leads of the same length are used to make active or reference pairs of electrodes. This eliminates the electrical resistance difference between the silver wires.
5. Prepare the active electrodes by firmly attaching (twisting) silver wire to platinum leads (with 2 cm of the plastic sleeve removed). Fold the silver so that the tip to contact the cornea is rounded. Use masking tape to insulate the connections

between the wire and lead leaving 1 mm of the rounded silver wire exposed.

6. The two reference electrodes are made the same way, but instead of a 1 mm rounded tip, create a ~ 4 mm diameter circle for mice or ~ 8 mm diameter circle for rats. This should be large enough to slide around the equator of the eye without compressing the eye. Insulate the connection between the silver and lead leaving the loop exposed.
7. Chloride the exposed silver tips or loops by immersing them into 0.9% saline, connecting the leads to a 9 V battery and completing the circuit. Chloride for 10 s, after which time, the silver wire should be coated with a fine layer of white chloride crystals. Lightly dust off any excess crystals to avoid them damaging the cornea.
8. Connect all electrodes to the preamplifier.
9. Use micromanipulators to hold the active electrodes to aid fine positioning.

3.2 Animal Preparation

1. Minimize exposure to light during anesthesia and electrode set up to maximize the size of the scotopic threshold response. To maintain dark adaptation, keep the room lights off and use a headlight to provide dim red illumination (e.g., <15 cd.m^{-2}, $\lambda max = 600$ nm) during anesthesia and electrode setup.
2. Weigh animals and anesthetize with a ketamine and xylazine cocktail delivered via an intraperitoneal injection using a 30G needle for mice and 27G for rats.
3. Dilate pupils using one drop of 0.5–1% tropicamide, and use a drop of 0.5% proxymetacaine for corneal anesthesia. Leave for 5 s and absorb any excess fluid from eyelid margins.
4. Check the depth of anesthesia and place the rodent on a warmed platform (37 °C) by using circulating heated water (Lauda). Avoid electrical heating pads as they contribute to electrical noise.
5. Insert the ground needle electrode into the tail (~2 mm subcutaneously) approximately halfway along the tail.
6. Gently place the reference electrode loop around each eye, using masking tape or a small velcro tab to secure in place (without squeezing the animal or changing its natural position) at the nape of the neck.
7. Use micromanipulators to place the tips of the active electrodes such that they gently touch the corneal apex. Place a small drop of contact gel onto the active electrode tip to improve electrical contact and maintain corneal hydration. Avoid excessively large drops of lubricant which can spread to contact both active and

reference electrodes, which will result in small signals. If needed, twist a piece of lint-free tissue into a fine tip and gently wipe along the margin of the lower lid to remove excess lubricating gel.

8. Move the stimulus so that the eyes are in the plane of the Ganzfeld sphere. Close the Faraday cage.
9. Check that the signals from both eyes are quiet.
10. Check that signals elicited using a moderate intensity light flash (e.g., −3.36 log cd.s/m^2) produce waveforms of an expected shape, amplitude, and intereye difference.
11. After the test flash, readapt for 5 min in total darkness to ensure full recovery from light used for setting up and any test flash.

3.3 Signal Acquisition

1. Suggested test intensities, signal averaging, and interstimulus intervals can be found in Table 1.
2. Stimuli are delivered starting with the dimmest light level (−5.53 log cd·s/m^2) and progressing to the brightest (2.07 log cd·s/m^2). Take care to ensure that adequate time is given between flashes so that signals do not decline due to light adaptation.
3. Signal averaging may be needed to remove random noise arising from animal breathing and other small involuntary movements, as well as environment related sources of noise. Average enough signals for a signal-to-noise ratio of >5. Increased signal averaging of 100–200 signals may be required at the very dimmest light levels [12] in the case of high noise.
4. Use an appropriate data acquisition system and software to record signals of a desired length. For example, an epoch of 500 ms is adequate for most short-flash ERG components. However, if the retinal pigment epithelium-derived c-wave is of interest, then an epoch of 2 s would be advised.
5. Choose the sampling rate by considering the Nyquist limit of the ERG signals 4 kHz is usually adequate.
6. Choose appropriate band-pass filter settings to ensure that all components of the ERG are not aliased. Band pass of 0.3–500 Hz will capture all components.
7. Include a prestimulus baseline (e.g., 10 ms of noise recording immediately before stimulus onset) to allow baseline correction in case of signal drift.
8. Cone responses can be acquired using a twin flash approach [13], whereby two bright flashes are presented with a short interstimulus interval (e.g., 500 ms). The first flash returns a mixed rod/cone response, whereas the second elicits only cone responses.

Table 1
Electroretinogram (ERG) light stimulus protocol. Different light levels elicit various components of the ERG including the ganglion cell scotopic threshold response (STR), the bipolar cell b-wave, the photoreceptor a-wave, and inner retinal oscillatory potentials (OPs). Repeating bright flashes with very short interstimulus intervals elicits a subsequent response that does not contain contributions from the rod pathway. Light adaptation isolates the cone pathway

Light level (log cd.s/m^2)	Number of repeats	Time between flashes (s)	ERG component elicited
Scotopic series			
−5.53	20	2	STR
−5.31	20	2	STR
−5.01	20	2	STR
−4.90	20	2	STR
−4.31	5	3	STR + b-wave
−3.36	5	3	Rod b-wave
−2.75	1	15	Rod b-wave, OPs
−1.61	1	30	Rod b-wave, OPs
−0.81	1	45	Mixed b-wave, OPs, a-wave
0.72	1	60	Mixed b-wave, OPs, a-wave
1.55	1	120	Mixed b-wave, OPs, a-wave
2.07	2	180 (500 ms for twin flash)	**1st flash:** Mixed b-wave, OPs, a-wave **Second flash:** Cone b-wave, OPs
Photopic series after 10 min of light adaptation			
0.77	10	1	Cone b-wave, OPs, a-wave
1.37	10	1	Mixed b-wave, OPs, a-wave
1.77	10	1	Mixed b-wave, OPs, a-wave
2.07	10	1	Mixed b-wave, OPs, a-wave
2.37	10	1	Mixed b-wave, OPs, a-wave
2.67	10	1	Mixed b-wave, OPs, a-wave

9. Cone responses can also be measured following light adaptation. Adapt to a bright background (e.g., 90 cd/m^2) for at least 10 min [14]. Use flashes ranging in intensity from 0 to 3 log cd.s/m^2. Signal averaging may be required; however, interstimulus intervals can be short (Table 1).

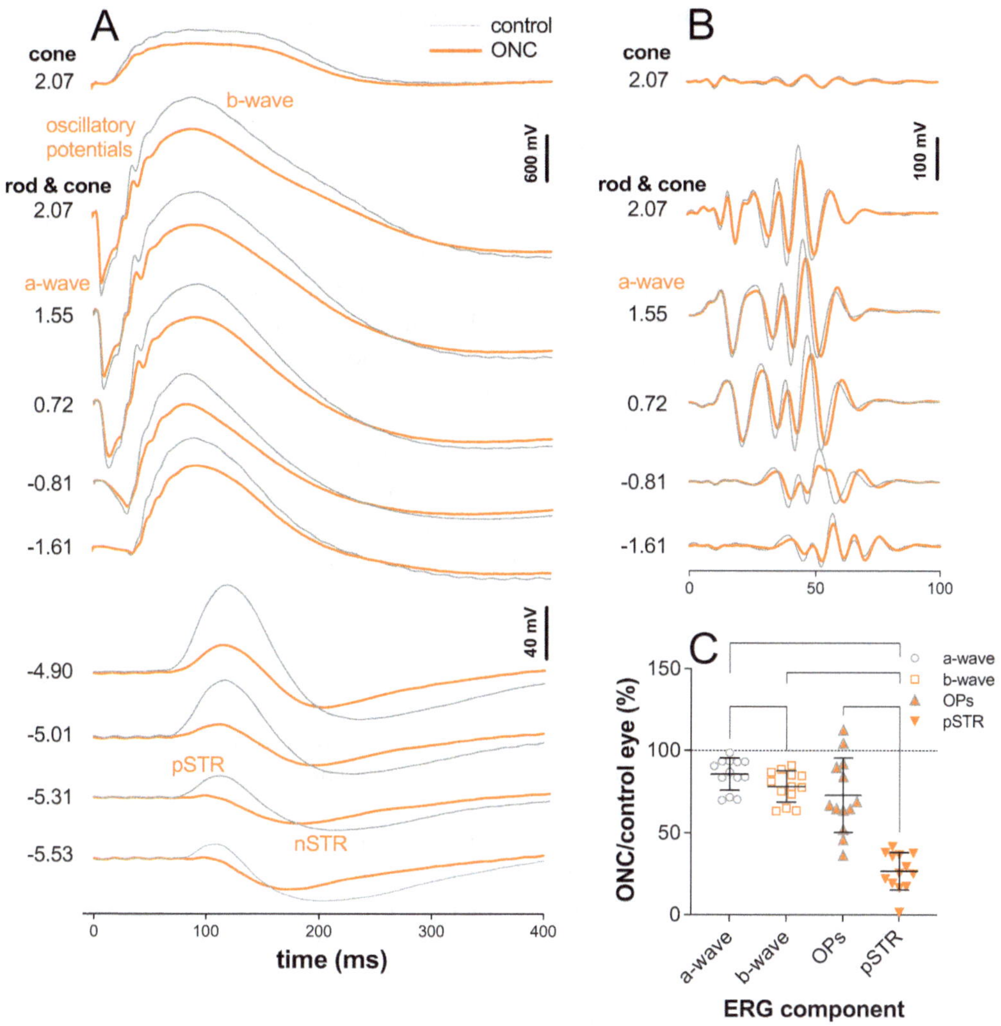

Fig. 1 Electroretinogram assessment of injury in a rat model of optic nerve crush. (**a**). Raw ERG waveforms from rats starting from the dimmest light level and progressing up to the brightest. At the top is the cone response elicited using a twin flash. (**b**). Responses are band-pass filtered (50–180 Hz) to isolate the inner retinal oscillatory potentials. (**c**). Optic nerve crush produced greater attenuation of the ganglion cell pSTR compared with outer retinal ERG components

10. At the end of the ERG protocol, measure pupil size to ensure that any reduction in signal size did not arise from poor mydriasis.

3.4 Signal Analysis

1. For an ERG waveform elicited by a bright flash of light, the very first electronegative component, known as the a-wave, comes from photoreceptors and can be described using a delayed Gaussian function (Fig. 1a). This equation models

the underlying P3 generated by photoreceptors [15] to return a maximal amplitude (RmP3, μV) indicating the number of photoreceptors (outer segment length or density of nonspecific cationic channels). The slope parameter (sensitivity, S, $m^2.cd^{-1}.s^{-3}$) provides a measure of the efficiency of phototransduction or the rate of amplification.

2. The second and largest component of the ERG waveform (the b-wave) is the voltage envelope comprising the corneal-negative photoreceptor P3 and positive P2, which is dominated by ON bipolar cells. Subtracting the P3 model from the raw ERG waveform returns a good approximation of the P2 along with the inner retinal oscillatory potentials (OPs) riding on the b-wave leading edge. Low-pass filtering (50 Hz) will remove the OPs (Fig. 1b) and high-frequency noise leaving the P2.
3. The amplitude of each P2 waveform can be plotted as a function of intensity and fit with a saturating hyperbolic function [16]. This model returns a maximum amplitude (Vmax, μV), which provides an index of bipolar cell integrity along with a light sensitivity parameter (1/K, log $cd.s/m^2$).
4. The dark-adapted ERG elicited with bright light levels (Table 1) contains contributions from both the rod and cone pathways. The long refractory time of the rods can be leveraged using repeated stimuli with short interstimulus intervals ($<$ 500 ms) to elicit subsequent responses that are cone dominated. Cone responses can be quantified by their peak amplitudes and implicit times (Fig. 1a). The cone response (second flash) can be subtracted from the mixed response (first flash) to return the rod response for a given stimulus intensity.
5. The OPs, which provide a measure of inner retinal inhibitory circuits involving amacrine cells [17], can be isolated using a band-pass filter (Fig. 1b, 50–180 Hz). OPs can be analyzed by taking the amplitude and implicit time of individual peaks or summarized as a root mean square amplitude across a selected epoch (e.g., between 25 and 75 ms). Alternatively, OPs can be examined in the frequency domain [18] or more comprehensively described using a time-frequency approach, such as wavelet analysis [19].
6. The positive scotopic threshold response (pSTR), which can only be measured at very dim light levels, is a good indicator of retinal ganglion cell function in rodents (Fig. 1a) [12, 20]. Quantify the pSTR by taking its peak amplitude and implicit time. As the STR is only apparent at very low light levels, it is important that STR analysis avoids intensities above -4.9 log $cd.s/m^2$, where components such as the scotopic

response and the b-wave make larger contributions to the rodent pSTR [7, 12].

3.5 Example ERG Responses in Optic Nerve Injury

1. *Optic nerve crush:* 14 days after optic nerve crush (optic nerve 2 mm behind the eye crushed for 5 s using microsurgical tweezers) in P18 Sprague Dawley rats, there were functional deficits throughout the retina (Fig. 1). The largest deficits were evident on the scotopic threshold response, the pSTR at the dimmest light levels. There were also more subtle deficits in the ERG a-wave, b-wave (Fig. 1a), and oscillatory potentials (Fig. 1b) evident toward brighter stimulus intensities. Comparatively across the group of animals, the a-wave was reduced by 18%, the b-wave by 25%, and the OPs by 29%, and the pSTR was most affected being attenuated by 75%. Using the full-field ERG in this way to elicit the spectrum of responses across the dynamic range of the rat retina helps to differentiate loss of input (i.e., loss of photoreceptor and bipolar cell function) to ganglion cells and direct deficits in ganglion cell-mediated responses. That is, this rules out the possibility that the reduction in the pSTR arises solely due to a smaller a-wave or b-wave.
2. *Recovery from acute IOP elevation:* The ERG is a highly sensitive indicator of both acute and chronic effects of intraocular pressure elevation. A subischemic injury that can be used to stress the retinal ganglion cell is an IOP elevation of 50 mmHg for 30 min [21, 22]. This can be achieved using a glass micropipette (50 μm tip) to connect the anterior chamber to a height adjustable water reservoir or a syringe pump. Figure 2 shows that the ganglion cell pSTR was more affected by acute IOP stress than the photoreceptor a-wave and/or bipolar cell b-wave. In young eyes, the pSTR takes 7 days to fully recover from a single episode of IOP stress (Fig. 2a). On the other hand, older eyes take 14 days to show full pSTR recovery (Fig. 2b). This protocol can be used to consider factors (e.g., aging) that may modulate ganglion cell adaption to IOP elevation.
3. *Chronic IOP elevation:* The ERG is very useful in quantifying both the degree of ganglion cell injury and progression of retinal dysfunction. Figure 3a shows ERG waveforms collected 8 weeks after chronic IOP elevation induced by placing a circumlimbal suture (10/0 nylon) around one eye of C57BL/6 J mice [20, 23]. There are small reductions across all ERG components after 8 weeks of chronic IOP elevation.

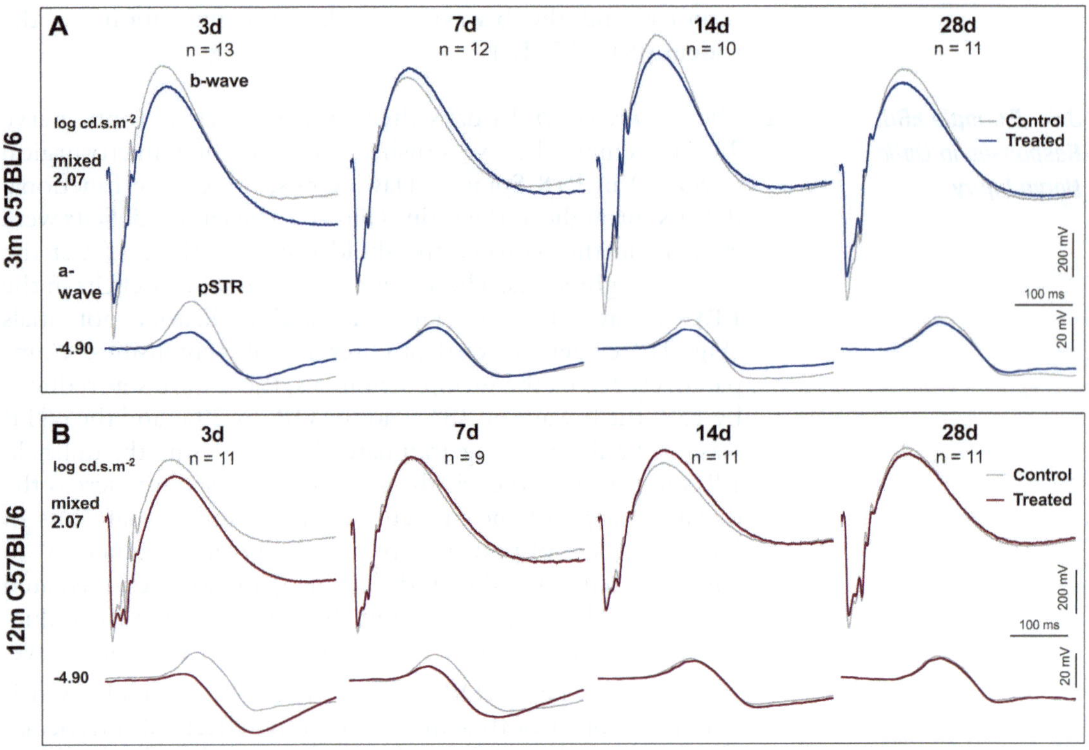

Fig. 2 Using the ERG to examine age-related differences in functional recovery from acute IOP elevation (50 mmHg for 30 min). (**a**). Group-averaged ERG waveforms in three-month-old mice (blue traces, treated eyes; gray traces, control eyes) at luminous energies representing predominantly ganglion cell responses (−4.90 log cd.s.m.$^{-2}$) and outer retinal function (2.07 log cd.s.m.$^{-2}$) at 3, 7, 14, and 28 days after IOP elevation. (**b**). Group-averaged ERG waveforms in 12-month-old mice (red traces, treated eyes; gray traces, control eyes). (Data from [21])

Figure 3b shows that in a cohort of mice subjected to IOP elevation for 16 weeks, the pSTR was more attenuated. In contrast, a-wave and b-wave attenuation was similar between weeks 8 and 16. The ERG can also be used to track recovery. Also shown in Fig. 3b are data from animals that had undergone 8 weeks of chronic IOP elevation, after which time the circumlimbal suture was removed to normalize IOP [23]. Four weeks later, assessment of the ERG showed that the ERG response in treated eyes had recovered to levels similar to contralateral control eyes (Fig. 3b).

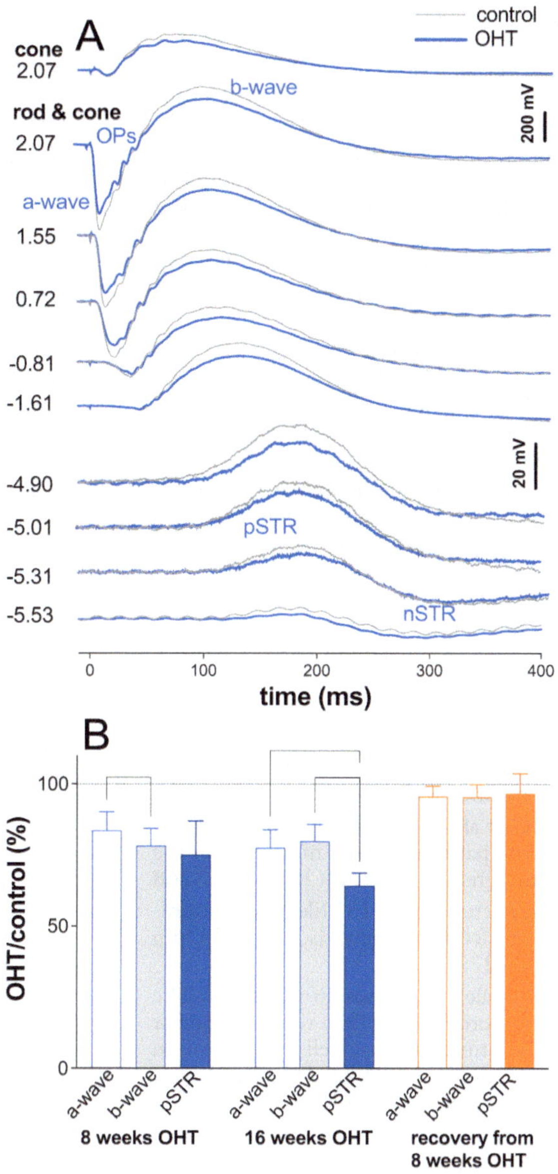

Fig. 3 Using the ERG to quantify progression in the circumlimbal suture model of chronic IOP elevation. (**a**). Group-averaged ERG waveforms in young adult mice (blue traces, treated eyes; gray traces, control eyes) at luminous energies representing predominantly ganglion cell responses (below -4.90 log cd.s.m.$^{-2}$) and outer retinal function (above -1.61 log cd.s.m.$^{-2}$) collected 8 weeks following placement of a circumlimbal suture to induce chronic ocular hypertension. A twin flash response at 2.07 log cd.s.m.$^{-2}$ is also included. (**b**). Group-averaged ($\pm$ SEM) a-wave, b-wave, and pSTR amplitude in OHT eyes expressed relative to contralateral control eyes. All ERG components are reduced after 8 weeks of ocular hypertension OHT ($n = 13$). There is a greater pSTR deficit after 16 weeks of ocular hypertension. Following 8 weeks of OHT, IOP was normalized via suture removal. All ERG components are fully recovered after 4 weeks. (Data replotted from [20, 23])

References

1. Grillo SL, Koulen P (2015) Psychophysical testing in rodent models of glaucomatous optic neuropathy. Exp Eye Res 141:154–163
2. Leinonen H, Tanila H (2018) Vision in laboratory rodents-tools to measure it and implications for behavioral research. Behav Brain Res 352:172–182
3. Pinto LH, Enroth-Cugell C (2000) Tests of the mouse visual system. Mamm Genome 11(7):531–536
4. Frishman L (2006) Origins of the electroretinogram. In: Heckenlively JR, Arden GB (eds) Principles and practice of clinical electrophysiology of vision. The MIT Press, Cambridge, pp 139–184
5. Granit R (1933) Components of the retinal action potential in mammals and their relations to the discharge in the optic nerve. J Physiol 77:207–238
6. Weymouth AE, Vingrys AJ (2008) Rodent electroretinography: methods for extraction and interpretation of rod and cone responses. Prog Retin Eye Res 27(1):1–44
7. Saszik SM, Robson JG, Frishman LJ (2002) The scotopic threshold response of the dark-adapted electroretinogram of the mouse. J Physiol 543(Pt 3):899–916
8. Robson JG et al (2004) In vivo studies of signaling in rod pathways of the mouse using the electroretinogram. Vis Res 44(28):3253–3268
9. Wilsey LJ, Fortune B (2015) Electroretinography in glaucoma diagnosis. Curr Opin Ophthalmol 27:118
10. Porciatti V, Saleh M, Nagaraju M (2007) The pattern electroretinogram as a tool to monitor progressive retinal ganglion cell dysfunction in the DBA/2J mouse model of glaucoma. Invest Ophthalmol Vis Sci 48(2):745–751
11. Kohzaki K et al (2013) Electroretinography in streptozotocin diabetic rats following acute intraocular pressure elevation. Graefes Arch Clin Exp Ophthalmol 251(2):529–535
12. Bui BV, Fortune B (2004) Ganglion cell contributions to the rat full-field electroretinogram. J Physiol 555(Pt 1):153–173
13. Nixon PJ et al (2001) The contribution of cone responses to rat electroretinograms. Clin Experiment Ophthalmol 29(3):193–196
14. Bui BV, Fortune B (2006) Origin of electroretinogram amplitude growth during light adaptation in pigmented rats. Vis Neurosci 23(2): 155–167
15. Lamb TD, Pugh ENJ (1992) A quantitative account of the activation steps involved in phototransduction in amphibian photoreceptors. J Physiol 449:719–758
16. Naka KI, Rushton WA (1966) S-potentials from colour units in the retina of fish (Cyprinidae). J Physiol 185(3):536–555
17. Wachtmeister L (1998) Oscillatory potentials in the retina: what do they reveal. Prog Retin Eye Res 17(4):485–521
18. Bui BV, Armitage JA, Vingrys AJ (2002) Extraction and modelling of oscillatory potentials. Doc Ophthalmol 104(1):17–36
19. Forte JD, Bui BV, Vingrys AJ (2008) Wavelet analysis reveals dynamics of rat oscillatory potentials. J Neurosci Methods 169(1): 191–200
20. Zhao D et al (2017) Characterization of the circumlimbal suture model of chronic IOP elevation in mice and assessment of changes in gene expression of stretch sensitive channels. Front Neurosci 11:41
21. Lee PY et al (2022) The effect of aging on retinal function and retinal ganglion cell morphology following intraocular pressure elevation. Front Aging Neurosci 14:859265
22. Crowston JG et al (2015) An acute intraocular pressure challenge to assess retinal ganglion cell injury and recovery in the mouse. Exp Eye Res 141:3–8
23. Zhao D et al (2019) Reversibility of retinal ganglion cell dysfunction from chronic IOP elevation. Invest Ophthalmol Vis Sci 60(12): 3878–3886

Chapter 18

Testing Visual Function by Assessment of the Optomotor Reflex in Glaucoma

Karen Chang, Julie Chen, Aishwarya Rajagopalan, Dong Feng Chen, and Kin-Sang Cho

Abstract

Optomotor response/reflex (OMR) is a fast and efficient first-in-line visual screening method, especially for rodents. It has the potential to evaluate both the scotopic and photopic visions of nonrestrained animals through tracking head movement, providing a quantitative estimate of visual functions. In restrained animals, optokinetic response (OKR), compensatory eye movements for visual shifts in the surroundings, is utilized. Both OMR and OKR capitalize on an individual's innate reflex to stabilize images for the purpose of capturing clear vision. The two reflexes have similar reliability when evaluating stimulus luminance, contrast, spatial frequency, and velocity. They have emerged as powerful tools to evaluate the efficacy of pharmacological treatments and phenotypes of subjects undergoing study. With OMR and OKR accurately assessing visual acuity (VA) as well as contrast sensitivity (CS), the gold standards for measuring clinical vision, they provide reliable and easily accessible results that further eye and brain research. These methods of sight evaluation have been used in multiple animal models, particularly mice and zebrafish. Through OMR assays, these animal models have been utilized to investigate retinal degenerative diseases, helping researchers differentiate between worsening stages. Alongside tests such as optical coherence tomography (OCT), OMR provides confirmation of visual status, where increased OMR function often correlates with improved visual status. OMR has continued to be used outside of glaucoma in various retinal diseases, such as retinitis pigmentosa (RP), diabetic retinopathy, and age-related macular degeneration.

In this chapter, we will introduce the concept and application of visual stimulus-induced head or eye reflex movement in different animal species and experimental models of eye diseases, such as glaucoma and other neurodegenerative disorders, and in patients with glaucoma.

Key words Retinal ganglion cells, Visual acuity, Contrast sensitivity, Rodent glaucoma models, Behavioral tests

1 Introduction

1.1 OMR in Insects, Fish, and Rodents

The optomotor response (OMR) is a reflexive behavior in which an animal's head moves in the direction of the detection of visual motion for the purpose of orienting itself with respect to the visual environment. This occurs especially during locomotion, such as

Tatjana Jakobs and Paloma B. Liton (eds.), *Glaucoma: Methods and Protocols*, Methods in Molecular Biology, vol. 2858, https://doi.org/10.1007/978-1-0716-4140-8_18,

swimming, flying, or walking. The optokinetic response (OKR), on the other hand, is the eye movements that follow objects in motion when the head remains stationary [1, 2]. These innate reflexes are widespread across the animal kingdom and essential for survival. This animal behavior has been studied extensively across many species.

In flying insects, such as flies and honeybees, OMR is often used to understand the functional properties of neural circuits for a specific behavior and examine the sensorimotor transformations underlying that behavior [3, 4]. OMR has been the most influential experiment for studying the motion vision of insects. When a drosophila is tethered in the center of a rotating striped drum, the insect will have the tendency to turn clockwise or counterclockwise reflexing the direction of the moving strips [3]. In free-flight conditions, the flying behavior of drosophila is also dramatically influenced in response to a rotating patterned drum. In a stationary visual environment, saccade-like flight behavior with rapid changes of flying direction is found. In contrast, the flying path changes toward a concentric circular pattern followed with the direction of the rotating drum [5]. This reaction helps insects maintain a straight course by compensating undesired deviations, for example, when the wind blows the insect to the left, causing the image in the eyes to move toward the right, the insect will generate a compensatory yaw to the right to stabilize and guide its flight through the environment. In the insect's visual system, the movement-detecting system underlying the OMR depends on the temporal frequency of optical simulation induced by the width of stripes, not by the angular velocity (rotational speed, in degree(s)) of the stripes [6]. Typically, narrow stripes produce weaker tracking responses than wider stripes [7].

Both OKR and OMR responses have also long been studied in both adult and larvae zebrafish [8–10]. The OKR response develops between 73 and 80 h postfertilization and persists throughout adulthood [11]. Zebrafish larvae embedded in methylcellulose will track gratings on a drum rotating clockwise or counterclockwise around the fish. The eye movements consist of smooth tracking of the gratings across the visual field (pursuit movement) followed by fast saccade movements to reset the eyes back to the initial position when they first saw the object [10]. When zebrafish are presented with a whole-field moving stimulus with black and white grating patterns, they turn and swim in the direction of motion perceived either when swimming freely or restrained by embedding their head in agar [12].

Rodents, particularly mice, are the most used mammalian research animals. Current methods for assessing the visual function of mice can be classified into two models: the discriminative learning model and the natural visual reflex model. The discriminative learning model usually requires training of the animal either with reward or penalty for the animal to react to the visual stimuli. The natural visual reflex model, on the other hand, based on the instinctive reflex responses that do not require training can be easily acquired [13]. The neuronal circuits that elicit OMR in mice remain unclear. Although most RGCs project axons to the superior colliculus, Douglas et al. suggested that instead of the cortex, RGC-projecting axons that connect to the accessory optic system play a critical role in OMR [14, 15]. Further studies are needed to understand the visual circuitry controlling the OMR and the similarity comparing to human. As preclinical studies are highly dependent on mouse models, assays assessing visual functions based on natural visual reflexes including OKR and OMR are well accepted and established [13, 16–18]. They are essential for phenotypic studies in disease models or animals with developmental defects or for treatment development of eye and even brain disorders. Most OMR assays do not require animal restraint and allow the animals to move freely on the testing platform. Thus, subtle head movements of mice can be easily missed during visual assessment. To enhance efficiency and accuracy, automated OMR devices are available. In recent years, semiautomated OMR devices have been developed and rapidly gained popularity for visual assessments [13, 18]. Visual functions, such as visual acuity (VA) and contrast sensitivity (CS), are surrogate measures of clinical assessment of vision. VA can be referred to the clarity of vision, with higher scores indicating animals' ability to detect thinner stripes. CS measures the ability to distinguish contrast, with higher scores signifying animals' improved ability to differentiate, less contrast stripes. In normal C57BL/6 J mice, the reported VA values range from 0.4 to 0.6 cycles per degree (cpd), and CS values range from 6 to 25 [18].

Algorithms and systems of standardization are being created to refine the consistency of these measurements [13]. Several methods of analysis utilize video tracking programs to determine the position of the subject's head in real time and manipulate a stimulus relative to this location [13]. Stimuli presented to the animals are often a repetitive pattern, such as rotating stripes [18]. In restrained animals, for OKR, this method is integrated with commercial eye trackers that measure the angular eye velocity [13]. Over the years, researchers have been working to fine-tune and improve the automation and precision of these measurements. Nevertheless, the fundamental issue with the current semiautomated OMR devices on the market is that they were only designed to detect positive OMR responses (tracking behaviors). When the visual stimuli are getting more difficult for the mice—either with thinner strips (higher spatial frequencies) or with less contrasted strips—the OMR responses will become less obvious and ambiguous [13]. When the stimulus approaches the visual threshold, weak OMR responses may be mixed with many other voluntary head or body movements that lead to false-positive results. Therefore, a negative OMR indicator, such as the head pausing behavior of staring, can be applied to accurately pinpoint the visual thresholds in mice with fast and reliable results. In retinal degenerative disease mouse models, CS was shown to be more sensitive than VA readings, especially at the early stage of retinal degeneration [19]. This result is in line with a clinical finding in human patients [20], although CS measurement is not routinely performed in humans. Further investigation of the sensitivity of CS and VA in retinal degeneration in both animals and humans is needed to thoroughly understand the implication of OMR scores in preclinical and even clinical studies.

1.2 Application of OMR in Glaucoma

Glaucoma is a retinal degenerative disease characterized by progressive degeneration of RGCs, their axons, and the higher visual centers. RGC axons in rodents mainly project to the lateral geniculate nucleus (LGN and superior colliculus [21]. Most experimental glaucoma models are performed in rodents, especially mice and rats [22], and some studies were reported in rabbits [23, 24] and nonhuman primates [25].

Visual impairment in glaucoma is attributed to the degeneration of RGCs and subsequent target neurons along the visual pathways. To investigate the visual changes in experimental glaucoma, rodents are the most popular choice as they have a well-studied anatomy and physiology in the visual system and are affordable [26]. To evaluate the changes in spatial vision in rodents, OMR and OKR assays are visual behavioral assays to track the head and eye movement, respectively. In both assays, the animals are trying to fix the moving object on the retina. OKR necessitates fixing the head position and requires imaging technologies to track a slight change of position in eye movement. For OMR, a mouse can freely move on a small platform during the OMR assay, and no prior training is required [18]. Both OKR and OMR have similar psychometric curves, although OKR showed a higher gain in eye movement than that is observed with the head movement in OMR [13].

Different laboratories detected a similar mouse visual acuity among the young to aging C57BL/6 mice and Long-Evans rats; however, the contrast sensitivity may decrease with age [27]. Currently, mouse OMR can be recorded manually by experienced observers or semiautomatically using a commercially available machine. Detection of negative OMR is particularly important to identify whether a mouse is blind or just not focusing on the task. It was reported that decreased locomotor activity and increased anxiety-like behavior are found in aging mice that may lead to a more subtle head movement in aged mice [28].

In glaucoma, in addition to assessing the survival and electrical activity of RGCs, documenting the changes in OMR is a major readout to evaluate the spatial vision in mice. However, the background strain should be taken into account as it can affect the OMR. The DBA/2 J strain of mice is a well-known genetic model of glaucoma [29]. However, the OMR behavior of DBA/2 J mice is controversial. Studies showed reduced visual acuity [30] and contrast sensitivity in DBA/2 J mice by OMR assessment [15]. Surprisingly, the level of IOP does not correlate to the reduced visual performance in this study [30]. On the contrary, Barabas et al. reported an optomotor reflex deficit in young DBA/2 J mice before the onset of IOP elevation and RGC degeneration [31]. Such discrepancies in OMR assessment in DBA/2 J mice may limit their application for glaucoma drug screening using this mouse strain.

Many reports documented the impact of OMR in various experimental glaucoma models. Intracameral injection of hydrogel in mice led to a progressive reduction of VA [32] and CS [33]. Similarly, Feng et al. reported a reduction of VA in microbead-injected model [34]. In a study by van der Heijden et al., in scotopic rather than photopic condition, CS is directly impacted by IOP levels as examined in both microbead- and sodium hyaluronate-injected models [35]. Additionally, Feng et al. showed that laser photocoagulation-induced sustained ocular hypertension in mice led to both VA and CS reductions [36]. Reduction of VA was detected in Norway brown rats with experimentally induced glaucoma by hypertonic saline injection [37, 38]. Collectively, OMR assay is a convenient approach for detecting spatial visual changes in glaucoma.

Interestingly, the application of OMR has been extended beyond glaucoma. It has been used to detect spatial vision changes in other neurodegenerative diseases. Mouse models of retinitis pigmentosa such as Rd10 mice showed a reduction of VA [39, 40]. Rhodopsin-deficient mice showed reduced VA and CS over time, but the reduction did not go to a similar profile. CS is a more sensitive indicator of spatial vision [19]. Beyond retinal degenerative disease models, reduction of spatial vision was reported in the brain neurodegenerative diseases such as Alzheimer's disease model (5xFAD mice) at a young age [41].

2 Materials

1. An arena made from computer monitors to display rotating stripes (Fig. 1, also *see* **Note 1**).
2. Computer and software to generate the stimuli (*see* **Note 2**).
3. Small platform in the center of the arena (*see* **Note 3**).
4. Video camera to record the behavior of the mouse (*see* **Note 4**).
5. Disposable pads.
6. Alcohol or disinfectant wipes.

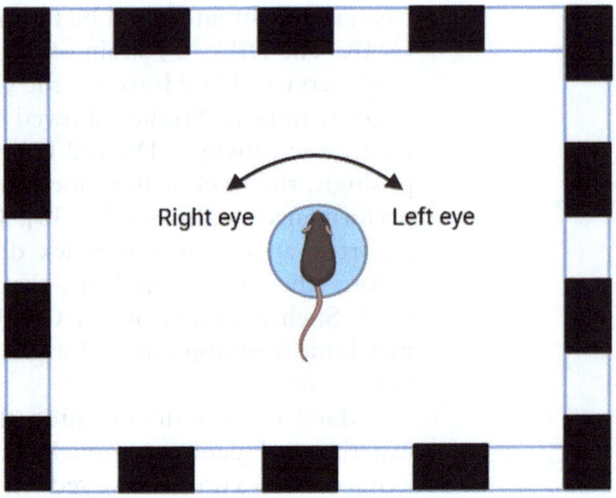

Fig. 1 Schematic Diagram of Mouse Optomotor Response (OMR) Setup. A mouse was placed on a small stage (blue) which is placed in the mid-level of the monitor height and at the center surrounded by 4 monitors with dynamic black and white stripes. Stripes can be set to move clockwise and anti-clockwise to stimulate the left and right eye, respectively. By manipulating the width or the contrast of stripes, researchers can investigate the threshold of visual acuity and contrast sensitivity, respectively. The bi-directional arrow represents the direction of moving stripes. (Created with BioRender.com)

3 Methods

3.1 Measurement of Visual Acuity (VA)

1. Place a clean disposable pad at the bottom of the arena.
2. Turn on the computer and start the software.
3. Place the mouse on the center platform. No pretreatment of the animal is needed.
4. Usually, the mouse will explore the new environment or even try to climb off the platform. Wait until the mouse has calmed down (about 2 min).
5. Perform a training step for both eyes with the easiest stimulus: black and white stripes at 100% contrast and 0.186 cycle/degree. Clockwise and counterclockwise movements of black and white stripes stimulate the left and right eyes, respectively. Observe the corresponding head tracking response (*see* **Note 5**).
6. After passing the training step, start testing the threshold of visual acuity on one or both eyes.
7. To determine the thresholds of visual acuity, one should start from low to high cycles/degree with 100% contrast sensitivity. The threshold of visual acuity is the highest cycles/degree that a mouse shows a positive OMR (*see* **Note 6**).
8. Wipe the platform with disinfectant between animals.

3.2 Measurement of Contrast Sensitivity (CS)

Perform **steps 1–5** as described for VA. However, to determine the threshold of contrast sensitivity, first, the optimal spatial frequency that produces the best threshold of contrast sensitivity should be identified. Thomas et al. showed that the best parameters of the speed of the grating and the width of the grating are different in mice and rats and also the optimal grating speed changes during the disease progression of retinal degeneration [42]. Based on the optimal spatial frequency, the contrast of the strips is progressively reduced. The threshold of contrast sensitivity is defined as the positive OMR of the mouse in responding to the lowest contrast of stripes one can detect [16]. The threshold is presented as Michelson contrast based on the screen's luminance (maximum − minimum)/(maximum + minimum), and CS is calculated from the reciprocal value of the threshold.

4 Notes

1. We use 17 inch flatscreen monitors. The dimensions of the arena in our setup are 14.5 * 14.5 inches.
2. Software for stimulus generation can be found at: https://bitbucket.org/luolab/omr-stimuli
3. A suitable platform can be custom-made (e.g., from acrylic). The dimensions should be: 6.3 cm in diameter.
4. It is preferable to record the experiment for documentation and to allow an unbiased observer to assess the tracking behavior. If this is not feasible, the arena can be covered by a black cardboard top with a small viewing window over the platform with the animal. An observer ignorant of the genotype or IOP history of the animal can visually assess tracking behavior through the viewing window. Care must be taken that the observer cannot see the stimulus monitors to avoid bias.
5. Tracking behavior refers to a head movement that is matched to the stimulus speed. It can be fairly subtle, and some experience is required to identify it with certainty. Please refer to movies m1 and m2 for examples of tracking behavior.
6. To calculate cycles/degree from the width of the stimulus pattern on the monitor use: Number of black and white stripes on a flatscreen monitor divided by 90°.

References

1. Allen RS et al (2018) TrkB signalling pathway mediates the protective effects of exercise in the diabetic rat retina. Eur J Neurosci 47(10): 1254–1265
2. Kretschmer F et al (2017) Comparison of optomotor and optokinetic reflexes in mice. J Neurophysiol 118(1):300–316
3. Borst A, Haag J, Reiff DF (2010) Fly motion vision. Annu Rev Neurosci 33:49–70
4. Lehrer M (1994) Spatial vision in the honeybee: the use of different cues in different tasks. Vis Res 34(18):2363–2385
5. Mronz M, Lehmann FO (2008) The free-flight response of Drosophila to motion of the visual

environment. J Exp Biol 211(Pt 13): 2026–2045

6. Srinivasan MV (2011) Honeybees as a model for the study of visually guided flight, navigation, and biologically inspired robotics. Physiol Rev 91(2):413–460
7. Duistermars BJ et al (2007) The spatial, temporal and contrast properties of expansion and rotation flight optomotor responses in Drosophila. J Exp Biol 210(Pt 18):3218–3227
8. Najafian M, Alerasool N, Moshtaghian J (2014) The effect of motion aftereffect on optomotor response in larva and adult zebrafish. Neurosci Lett 559:179–183
9. Matsuda K, Kubo F (2021) Circuit Organization Underlying Optic Flow Processing in Zebrafish. Front Neural Circuits 15:709048
10. Easter SS Jr, Nicola GN (1997) The development of eye movements in the zebrafish (Danio rerio). Dev Psychobiol 31(4):267–276
11. Portugues R, Engert F (2009) The neural basis of visual behaviors in the larval zebrafish. Curr Opin Neurobiol 19(6):644–647
12. Bollmann JH (2019) The Zebrafish Visual System: From Circuits to Behavior. Annu Rev Vis Sci 5:269–293
13. Kretschmer F et al (2015) A system to measure the Optokinetic and Optomotor response in mice. J Neurosci Methods 256:91–105
14. Douglas RM et al (2005) Independent visual threshold measurements in the two eyes of freely moving rats and mice using a virtual-reality optokinetic system. Vis Neurosci 22(5): 677–684
15. Burroughs SL, Kaja S, Koulen P (2011) Quantification of deficits in spatial visual function of mouse models for glaucoma. Invest Ophthalmol Vis Sci 52(6):3654–3659
16. Prusky GT et al (2004) Rapid quantification of adult and developing mouse spatial vision using a virtual optomotor system. Invest Ophthalmol Vis Sci 45(12):4611–4616
17. Benkner B et al (2013) Characterizing visual performance in mice: an objective and automated system based on the optokinetic reflex. Behav Neurosci 127(5):788–796
18. Shi C et al (2018) Optimization of optomotor response-based visual function assessment in mice. Sci Rep 8(1):9708
19. Xiao J et al (2019) Visual contrast sensitivity correlates to the retinal degeneration in rhodopsin knockout mice. Invest Ophthalmol Vis Sci 60(13):4196–4204
20. Jindra LF, Zemon V (1989) Contrast sensitivity testing: a more complete assessment of vision. J Cataract Refract Surg 15(2):141–148
21. Zhang S et al (2009) Detection of early neuron degeneration and accompanying glial responses in the visual pathway in a rat model of acute intraocular hypertension. Brain Res 1303:131–143
22. Pang IH, Clark AF (2020) Inducible rodent models of glaucoma. Prog Retin Eye Res 75: 100799
23. Johnson B et al (1999) Developing laser-induced glaucoma in rabbits. Aust N Z J Ophthalmol 27(3–4):180–183
24. Zhao J et al (2016) Optic neuropathy and increased retinal glial fibrillary acidic protein due to microbead-induced ocular hypertension in the rabbit. Int J Ophthalmol 9(12): 1732–1739
25. Weber AJ et al (2000) Experimental glaucoma and cell size, density, and number in the primate lateral geniculate nucleus. Invest Ophthalmol Vis Sci 41(6):1370–1379
26. Huberman AD, Niell CM (2011) What can mice tell us about how vision works? Trends Neurosci 34(9):464–473
27. Grillo SL, Koulen P (2015) Psychophysical testing in rodent models of glaucomatous optic neuropathy. Exp Eye Res 141:154–163
28. Shoji H, Miyakawa T (2019) Age-related behavioral changes from young to old age in male mice of a C57BL/6J strain maintained under a genetic stability program. Neuropsychopharmacol Rep 39(2):100–118
29. Libby RT et al (2005) Inherited glaucoma in DBA/2J mice: pertinent disease features for studying the neurodegeneration. Vis Neurosci 22(5):637–648
30. Rangarajan KV et al (2011) Detection of visual deficits in aging DBA/2J mice by two behavioral assays. Curr Eye Res 36(5):481–491
31. Barabas P et al (2011) Missing optomotor head-turning reflex in the DBA/2J mouse. Invest Ophthalmol Vis Sci 52(9):6766–6773
32. Chen K et al (2019) Stimuli-responsive polymer-doxorubicin conjugate: antitumor mechanism and potential as nano-prodrug. Acta Biomater 84:339–355
33. Zhu J et al (2021) Oral scutellarin treatment ameliorates retinal thinning and visual deficits in experimental glaucoma. Front Med (Lausanne) 8:681169
34. Feng L et al (2016) Long-term protection of retinal ganglion cells and visual function by brain-derived neurotrophic factor in mice with ocular hypertension. Invest Ophthalmol Vis Sci 57(8):3793–3802
35. van der Heijden ME et al (2016) Effects of chronic and acute intraocular pressure

elevation on scotopic and photopic contrast sensitivity in mice. Invest Ophthalmol Vis Sci 57(7):3077–3087

36. Feng L et al (2013) Sustained ocular hypertension induces dendritic degeneration of mouse retinal ganglion cells that depends on cell type and location. Invest Ophthalmol Vis Sci 54(2): 1106–1117
37. Stankowska DL et al (2015) Neuroprotective effects of transcription factor Brn3b in an ocular hypertension rat model of glaucoma. Invest Ophthalmol Vis Sci 56(2):893–907
38. Feola AJ et al (2019) Menopause exacerbates visual dysfunction in experimental glaucoma. Exp Eye Res 186:107706
39. Zhang J et al (2022) Mesenchymal stem cell-derived extracellular vesicles protect retina in a mouse model of retinitis pigmentosa by anti-inflammation through miR-146a-Nr4a3 axis. Stem Cell Res Ther 13(1):394
40. Martinez-Gil N et al (2022) Purinergic receptors P2X7 and P2X4 as markers of disease progression in the rd10 mouse model of inherited retinal dystrophy. Int J Mol Sci 23(23):14758
41. Zhang M et al (2021) Brain and retinal abnormalities in the 5xFAD mouse model of Alzheimer's disease at early stages. Front Neurosci 15:681831
42. Thomas BB et al (2010) Modulatory influence of stimulus parameters on optokinetic head-tracking response. Neurosci Lett 479(2): 92–96

Chapter 19

Controlled Elevation of Intraocular Pressure (CEI) Glaucoma Model in Rats

Diana C. Lozano, Elaine C. Johnson, William O. Cepurna, and John C. Morrison

Abstract

Experimental elevation of intraocular pressure (IOP), a major glaucoma risk factor, has been a mainstay of research into mechanisms of glaucomatous optic nerve damage for decades. Methods that produce sustained IOP elevation can mimic the chronic nature of glaucoma and produce optic nerve damage. However, the pressure course for individual animals can be variable, unpredictably high at times, and difficult to monitor with current tonometry methods. All of this can complicate correlations of pressure history with axonal injury. An alternative is to control the extent and duration of IOP elevation over a period of several hour—long enough to produce axonal injury and gene expression changes within the optic nerve head that may indicate cellular mechanisms of glaucomatous optic nerve damage. The prolonged general anesthesia that this requires does have the potential to reduce systemic blood pressure, which may contribute to axonal injury in the face of elevated IOP. This chapter will describe our Controlled Elevation of IOP (CEI) model in laboratory rats. We will include methods for applying this to several animals at a time, as well as how to maintain blood pressure, oxygenation, and body temperature to ensure that the resulting injury and tissue events reflect the effects of elevated IOP on optic nerve tissues and not simply reduced ocular perfusion and ischemia.

Key words Intraocular pressure, Glaucoma, Brown Norway rats, Aqueous humor, Tonometry, Balanced salt solution, Isoflurane anesthesia, Optic nerve

1 Introduction

Many experimental approaches have been developed in mice and rats to produce elevated intraocular pressure (IOP), a major glaucoma risk factor [1]. These have included laser treatments, particulate injections, and sclerosing methods to obstruct aqueous humor

Supplementary Information The online version contains supplementary material available at https://doi.org/10.1007/978-1-0716-4140-8_19.

Tatjana Jakobs and Paloma B. Liton (eds.), *Glaucoma: Methods and Protocols*, Methods in Molecular Biology, vol. 2858, https://doi.org/10.1007/978-1-0716-4140-8_19,

outflow [2–4]. Mean IOP elevations can be sustained for days and weeks, appropriate for modeling a chronic disease such as glaucoma. However, the pressure course for individual animals is often variable, and severe IOP spikes, which may be missed by intermittent, periodic tonometry, do occur [5]. Other factors that hamper detailed understanding of the true IOP include the use of anesthesia during tonometry, which can lower IOP [6], and measurement of IOP only during the day, which would miss significant pressure spikes that generally occur at night [7, 8].

Because undetected fluctuations in IOP can compromise our ability to correlate pressure with optic nerve injury, as well as to assess the neuroprotective effects of new treatments and manipulations, we have developed an additional strategy-controlled elevation of IOP (CEI) [9, 10]. This consists of cannulating the anterior chamber with tubing connected to an elevated reservoir to control the extent and duration of IOP elevation. This basic approach has long been used with pressures that exceed ocular perfusion pressure for a relatively short period of time (generally over 100 mmHg for 60–90 min) to produce ocular ischemia [11, 12]. While investigators have used lower pressures in mice for relatively short intervals [13–15], our approach uses longer exposure times of up to 8 h—long enough to produce gene expression changes resulting from pressure-induced stress and strain within the ONH, an important concept in understanding the mechanism of glaucomatous damage [16].

This model replicates many tissue responses and the pattern of axonal injury seen in more chronic models [9, 17, 18]. Because CEI allows the investigator to manipulate the level and duration of IOP elevation, correlations of these responses with IOP are more reproducible. In addition, by knowing exactly when the IOP was returned to normal, we have determined that IOP elevation produces a cascade of cellular events within the optic nerve head [9]. This may provide clues on how these changes might contribute to axonal injury and help determine factors that may contribute to ongoing vision loss, even after IOP has been apparently "controlled."

It is important to understand that prolonged exposure to general anesthetics can significantly lower systemic blood pressure [19]. Although pressures used to produce mild optic nerve damage in this model are higher than in human glaucoma, we have determined that these do not affect ocular perfusion, as long as systemic blood pressure is maintained [19–22]. This article will describe methods we have developed for producing this model, including techniques necessary to support ocular perfusion in the face of prolonged anesthesia.

2 Materials and Equipment

2.1 Materials

1. 31-gauge needle (outer diameter of 0.010″) attached to a 1 mm syringe or other handle. This should be plugged so aqueous will not escape through the needle.
2. Colibri forceps for grasping the limbal conjunctiva to stabilize the eye while making the needle track and inserting the cannula.
3. Curved forceps with a 0.010″ hole drilled through the interface of the tips for holding and guiding the cannula (Fig. 1).
4. Cannula (Fig. 2) made of polyurethane tubing (0.010″ OD/ 0.005″ ID; Instech Laboratories Inc., Plymouth Meeting, PA, Part # BTPU-010) connected with UV-activated resin (BONDIC® c/o Freight Boy 4450 Witmer Industrial Est Ste. 4 Niagara Falls NY 14305–1391 USA) to larger diameter tygon tubing (Component Supply Company, Fort Meade, FL, Part # TND80–040) and a blunt 18-gauge cannula (*see* **Note 1**). The tip of the cannula should be trimmed to create a beveled end for insertion. Gas sterilize or flush with 70% ethanol followed by 1 mL of balanced salt solution.
5. Tubing pinch clamp.
6. Proparacaine (Akorn, Inc., Lake Forest, IL).
7. Warmed saline in a 12 mL syringe connected to an intravenous catheter for subcutaneous injection (Insyte Autoguard Winged 22 GA x 1.00 inch) (BECTON DICKINSON INFUSION THERAPY SYSTEMS INC. One Becton Drive Franklin Lakes NJ 07417 US).

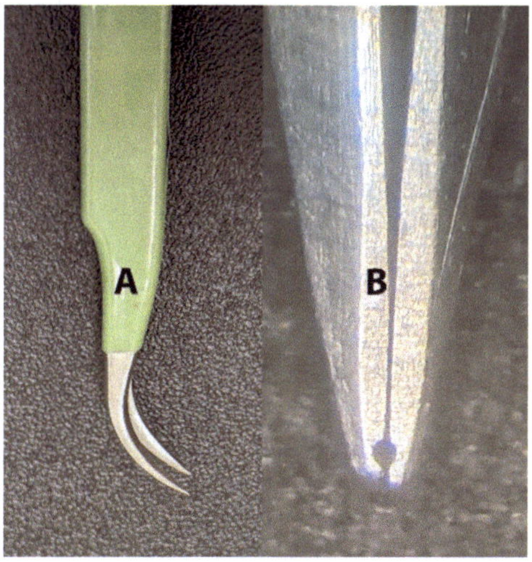

Fig. 1 (**a**) Curved forceps for cannula insertion. (**b**) High magnification view demonstrating 0.010″ hole in the tip

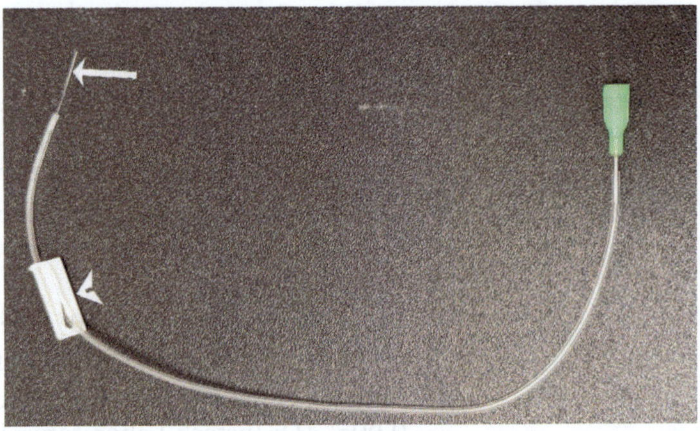

Fig. 2 Polyurethane cannula (arrow) with attached larger tubing connected to an 18-gauge blunt needle with green luer lock hub. Arrowhead indicates pinch clamp

8. Balanced salt solution-plus (BSS PLUS) (Alcon Laboratories, Inc., NDC 0065–0800-94, parts 1 and 2).
9. BSS reservoir on height-adjustable stand.
10. Isoflurane (NDC66794–017-25) (*see* **Note 2**).
11. Timers.
12. Weck-Cel® Cellulose Eye Spears (Beaver Visitec Intl Ltd. 500 Totten Pond Road, fifth floor 10 City Point, Waltham, MA 02451, USA).

2.2 Equipment/Instruments

1. Isoflurane delivery system (Table Top, Non-Rebreathing Anesthesia Machine) with active waste gas removal (Supera Anesthesia Innovations 1220 NW Noble Drive, Estacada Oregon 97,023), four O_2 flow meters, and nebulizers for humidification of the inspired gases (MicroMist nebulizer (catalogue #1880, Hudson Respiratory Care Inc., Temecula, California) (*see* **Note 3**).
2. Operating or dissecting microscope. When doing multiple animals, the microscope should be on a rolling base or suspended on a track that will allow the operator to move easily from one eye to the next for both cannula insertion and troubleshooting.
3. CODA Noninvasive Blood pressure System (Kent Scientific Corporation, Torrington, CT) with tail cuff and sensor.
4. Mouse Ox Plus Oximeter (STARR Life Sciences Corporation, Oakmont, PA) 4 channel physiology monitoring system with paw sensors for continuous monitoring of heart rate, respiration rate, and systemic oxygenation.

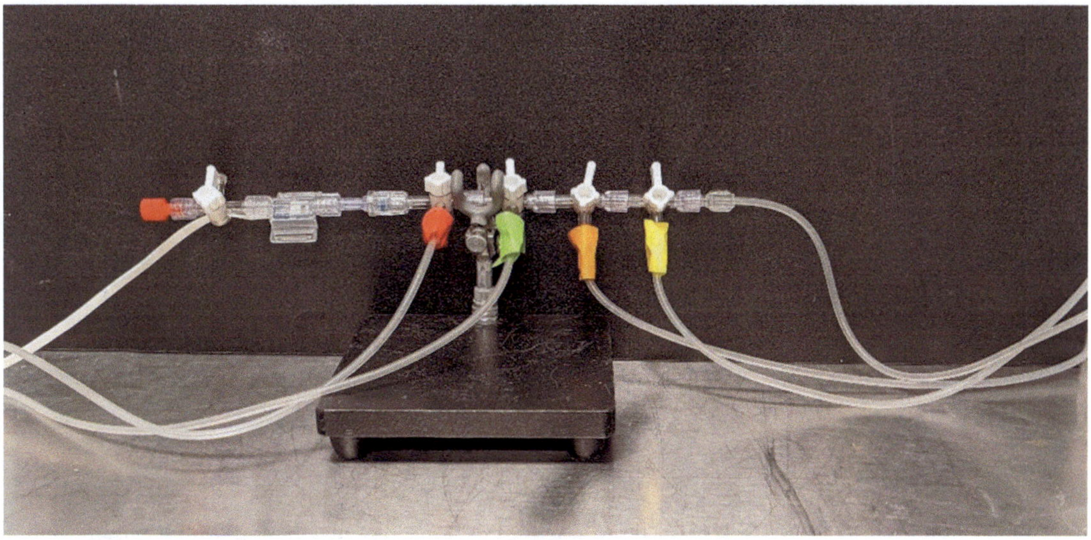

Fig. 3 Manifold from BSS reservoir leading to four animals and an "inline" pressure transducer. Note the use of colored tape. This helps distinguish each animal, which greatly simplifies checking to be sure that all connections are accurate, as well as trouble shooting and clearing air bubbles or other obstruction during an experiment

5. Pressure transducer (Transpac® IV Disposable Pressure Transducer ICU Medical, Inc. 951 Calle Amanecer San Clemente, CA 92673) with a Data acquisition system, DAQ, in line with elevated BSS+ reservoir.
6. Four-way manifold for distributing BSS+ to all animals equally (Fig. 3).
7. Custom-made stand for animals designed to stabilize the head, provide a platform for positioning and stabilizing the cannula, and allow delivery of isoflurane as well as active removal of waste gas and CO_2 (Fig. 4a, b).
8. Tonolab tonometer (Colonial Medical Supply, Franconia, NH, USA).
9. Water warming blanket (Heat Therapy Pad 14″× 20) (Adroit Medical Systems, 1146 Carding Machine Rd., Loudon, Tennessee 37774).
10. Rectal thermometer/probe (RET-2 Rat Rectal Temperature Probe) (World Precision Instruments 175 Sarasota Center Blvd. Sarasota, FL 34240), Six Channel Handheld Temperature Data Logger (Omega Engineering Inc. 800 Connecticut Ave. Suite 5 N01, Norwalk, CT 06854, USA).

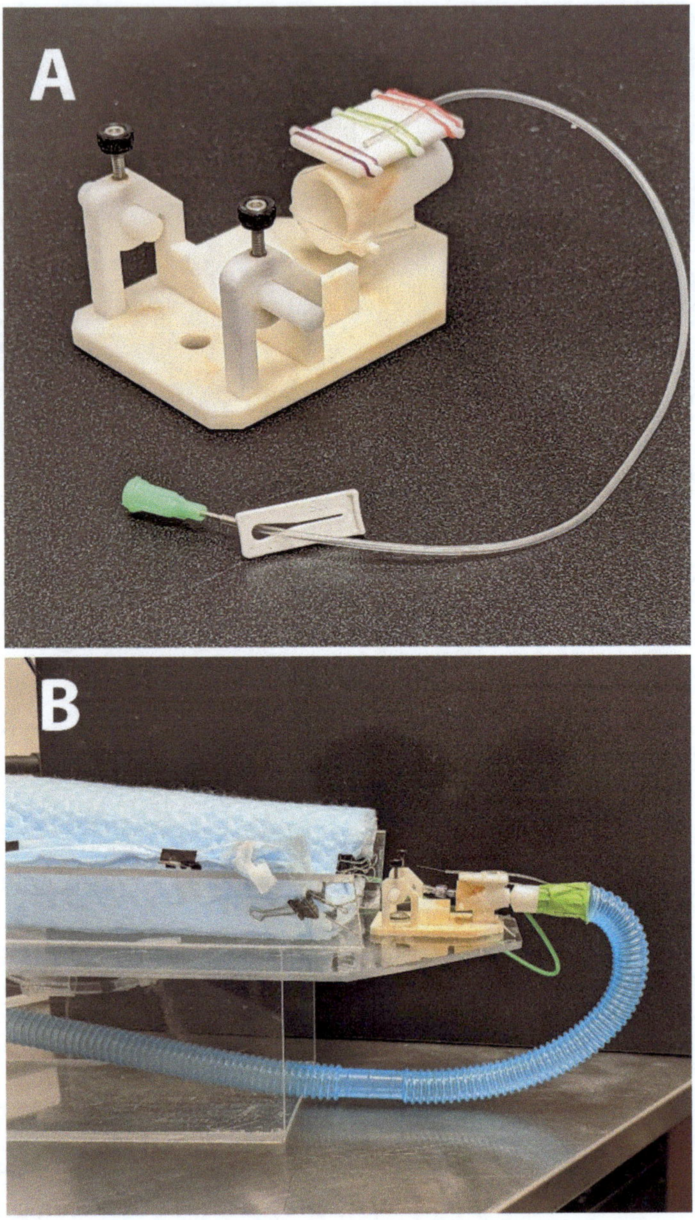

Fig. 4 (**a**) Custom head holder, demonstrating ear bars to fixate head, nose cone for isoflurane delivery, and waste gas removal and platform with rubber bands holding cannula and attached tubing in place. (**b**) Head holder in place on custom stand. Note blue water blanket, green tubing for gas delivery, and large blue tube leading to active waste gas removal. A three-dimensional print file for this is availalbe upon request

3 Methods

3.1 Animal Preparation

1. Initiate anesthesia with 5% isoflurane with 100% O_2 carrier gas. After no more than 20 min, reduce the flow to 3% and adjust as needed to maintain anesthesia.
2. Shave a small patch of fur on the back and insert a 22G IV catheter into the subdermal space. This is connected to a 12 cc syringe containing 0.9% normal saline that will be used for periodic saline hydration. Lay this on the heating blanket to keep it at the proper temperature (Fig. 5a).

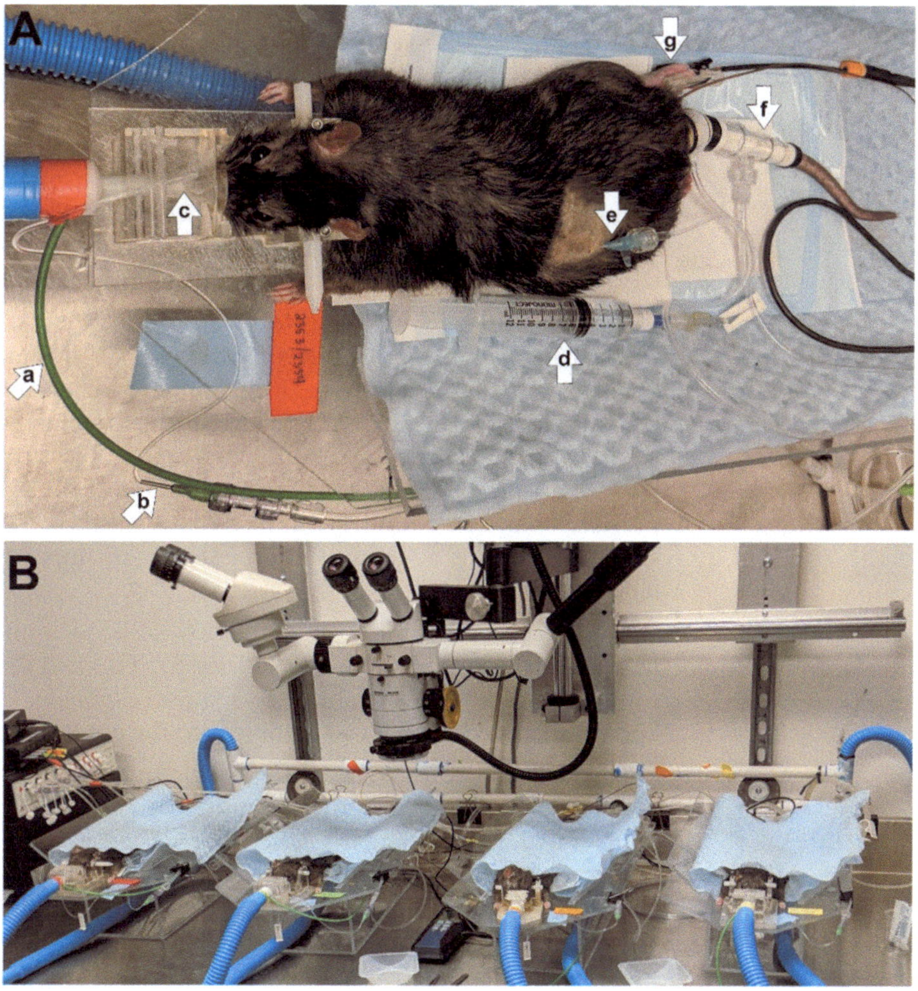

Fig. 5 (**A**) Animal in head holder, showing, counterclockwise: (**a**) green isoflurane tubing to nose cone; (**b**, **c**) BSS tubing to eye, (**d**, **e**) syringe with warm saline for periodic subcutaneous injection; (**f**) tail cuff for CODA blood pressure monitoring: and (**g**) foot sensor for MouseOx Plus. (**B**) Four animals undergoing simultaneous CEI. Note microscope on a wall-mounted track to allow movement from one animal to the next. Note also tape on nose cones that correspond to color coding on BSS manifold shown in Fig. 3

3. Transfer the animal to the animal stand, lying on a warm water blanket (set to 39 °C) which can be pulled over the animal as needed. Insert rectal probe thermometer, place the tail cuffs for CODA blood pressure monitoring, and place MouseOx paw sensor to record oxygen saturation and heart rate (Fig. 5a).
4. Repeat **steps 2** and **3** for all remaining animals. Lower isoflurane level to 2.25% once all animals are in their individual stands (Fig. 5b).
5. Ensure rectal temperature is between 37.5 °C and 38.5 °C throughout the experiment.

3.2 Eye Cannulation and CEI Experiment

1. Set the height of the reservoir to deliver a pressure of 20 mm Hg.
2. Each animal stand has its own platform to help hold the cannula in place. This platform should have at least three elastic bands (rubber or silicone) stretched over it. This allows the surgeon to position the tubing, so the tip is properly oriented toward the anterior chamber, with it extending just beyond the point at which the cannula will enter the cornea. Fixation with the two elastic bands closest to the animal allows the operator to make accurate, small corrections in positioning and will keep the cannula from pivoting out of position (Fig. 4a).
3. Place a drop of proparacaine on the eye and advance 31G needle, with the bevel down, into the anterior chamber at a shallow angle to produce a self-sealing corneal wound (*see* **Note 4**). This angle of entry can be further refined by bending the shaft of the needle, as necessary to accommodate the operator's preferred hand position. When the needle is withdrawn, only a small amount of aqueous should escape (*see* supplementary video).
4. Release the pinch clamp to start the flow of BSS+ immediately prior to insertion of cannula (*see* **Note 5**). This will flush fluid into the tip (which can otherwise acquire a small air column) and avoid introducing an air bubble into the anterior chamber.
5. Using curved forceps with a 0.010″ hole to grasp the cannula, insert the tip, bevel up, into the anterior chamber, avoiding contact with the lens and iris. Check for leakage at the insertion site with absorbent Weck spear. The cannula should have a slight curve leading to the eye to reduce the chance of accidental retraction.
6. Once all eyes are cannulated, adjust the height of the BSS+ reservoir to achieve the desired IOP, determined using the inline transducer connected to the manifold. Check all IOPs by Tonolab to verify that this corresponds to that set by the reservoir (*see* **Note 6**).

7. Once the reservoir IOP is attained and pressure verified, animals are monitored over a several hour period, as dictated by the experimental protocol.
8. Throughout IOP exposure, several variables, in addition to readouts from the CODA and MouseOx, must be actively monitored. These include IOP, animal temperature, systemic hydration, and corneal hydration. We have found that a set routine is most helpful for this, in which IOP is checked by Tonolab in each eye every half hour. Alternating ocular instillation of normal saline or proparacaine and subcutaneous injection of 0.5 ml normal saline via the intracatheter should be staggered by 15 min. Because multiple animals are monitored at the same time, we have found it very helpful to use an excel spreadsheet. This lists times of day, beginning with the onset of the experiment, and associated reminders to perform saline instillation, proparacaine instillation, and saline injection. Space is also provided to record Tonolab readings for each animal, with calculation of mean and SD over the entire experiment. Figure 6 shows a spreadsheet used for a modified CEI paradigm, called Pulse-Train CEI (PT-CEI), in which IOP is lowered to 20 mmHg for 5 min every hour. This demonstrates not only the flexibility of the CEI model but the organizational value of this spreadsheet.

3.3 Ending CEI Experiment

1. At the conclusion of an experiment, IOP is reduced to 20 mmHg for 5 min, and the cannula is then removed, allowing the corneal wound to self-seal. Due to the prolonged anesthesia, time should be planned to observe the animals, sometimes for 30 min or more, to allow them to recover sufficiently before returning them to the animal care facility.
2. Remove all physiological sensors and the IV catheter.
3. Connect a vacuum to the manifold and evacuate all remaining BSS+ from the tubing. Flush with sterile water.
4. Within the limits of general anesthesia, this approach allows the investigator to manipulate a range of experimental parameters, such as the level of IOP and duration, as well as the pattern of IOP elevation, as might be used to assess IOP fluctuation. This also includes the duration of time following pressure exposure, which we use to correlate timing and relationship of cellular events with axonal injury.
5. All physiologic parameters are recorded and are available for later analysis. This will allow correlation of blood pressure and systemic oxygenation with axonal injury or other responses. We typically perform euthanasia for injury analysis of myelinated optic nerve cross sections 10–14 days after IOP exposure, although evidence of axonal injury can appear as early as 7 days.

PT-CEI 60-8-2D	Pulse Train Controlled Elevation of Intraocular Pressure 60 mmHg-8 Hour-2 day survival									
PT-CEI date 1/29/2018			OD mmHg	OS mmHg	OD mmHg	OS mmHg	OD mmHg	OS mmHg	OD mmHg	OS mmHg
Start time and induction % of Isoflurane 7:40 AM, 5% 8:00 3%			2331	2332	2333	2334	2335	2336	2337	2338
	8:35 AM	TonoLab IOP SQ saline proparacaine	58	7	62	7	58	13	60	8
	8:35 AM	Saline on Eye								
	8:50 AM	TonoLab IOP SQ saline proparacaine	59	7	57	9	54	9	58	8
Lower Isoflurane to 2.25%	9:05 AM	Saline on Eye								
	9:20 AM	TonoLab IOP SQ saline proparacaine	60	7	59	12	64	9	64	8
	9:30 AM	IOP check (5 mins down to 20 mmHg)	22		19		21		19	
1	9:35 AM	Saline on Eye								
Hours 2-7 not shown										
7	3:35 PM	Saline on Eye								
	3:50 PM	TonoLab IOP SQ saline proparacaine	60	7	56	12	60	16	61	15
	4:05 PM	Saline on Eye								
	4:20 PM	TonoLab IOP SQ saline proparacaine	65	13	60	15	54	17	58	12
	4:30 PM	IOP check (5 mins down to 20 mmHg)	22		16		16		17	
8	4:35 PM	Saline on Eye								
extra 40 minutes (8 x 5 mins)	4:50 PM	TonoLab IOP SQ saline proparacaine	57	12	56	16	57	16	58	13
	5:05 PM	Saline on Eye								
	5:15 PM	Final IOP	58	10	63	16	60	14	58	15
		60 mean	60	8	59	12	58	11	58	10
		STDEV	3	2	3	3	4	3	3	3
		20 Mean	21		19		17		15	
		STDEV	3		2		2		3	

Fig. 6 Portions of a record of modified CEI performed simultaneously on four animals. In this paradigm, called Pulse-Train CEI (PT-CEI), IOP in the cannulated eye (OD) is returned to 20 mmHg (normal awake IOP) for 5 min every hour. Animal eye identification numbers are arrayed across the top. Time of day is indicated in the left-hand columns, with reminders for when to do Tonolab measurements, subcutaneous saline injections, and topical drop applications. A detailed record such as this is necessary when performing a complex, yet repetitive, experiment with these many animals. Two independent timers are very helpful for remaining on schedule

4 Notes

1. This plastic cannula has now replaced our originally described needle to reduce the chance of erosion and damage to the cornea and lens. The cannula is connected to the larger tubing with the aid of a piece of silicone tubing, to which UV-activated resin glue will not adhere (Fig. 7). To make this, one end of the cannula is sealed off by melting it with a battery-powered cautery. One end of the silicone tubing (which has an inner diameter equal to the larger polyurethane tubing) is filled with resin for a distance of 5 mm. The sealed end of the cannula is then held in the center of the resin and the resin activated by UV light to cure. The cannula with a surrounding resin plug is then slid out of the silicone tubing and the cured resin, and contained cannula is then cut in cross section with a razor blade. This produces a plug (attached to cannula that is now open) that will just fit into the larger tubing. A small bead of resin is placed around the plug, which is then inserted into the tubing, creating a thin, resin-filled interface that is then cured with UV light. Resin can be added to the junction of the cannula and tubing for added strength.
2. For prolonged anesthesia, inhalational isoflurane is preferable to injectable cocktail preparations such as ketamine and xylazine. This is because the level of anesthesia can be accurately titrated with minimal fluctuation. With injectable anesthetics, it is difficult to know when to use "booster" injections and at what dose. This makes it difficult to avoid too deep an anesthesia at some times, while at the same time avoiding letting the animal wake up.

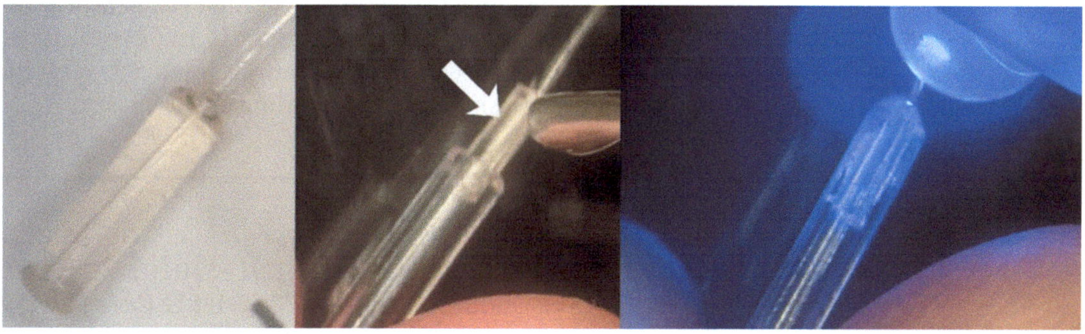

Fig. 7 Assembly of polyurethane cannula, demonstrating (left) plug with contained cannula, (middle) insertion of plug (arrow) into larger tubing; and (right) polymerization of glue with UV light

3. It is essential to actively, via a Waste Gas Interface Valve, remove waste anesthesia gas and exhaled CO_2 which can otherwise lead to significant reduction in systemic blood pressure, increasing the chance of optic nerve head and retinal ischemia. Passive connection of waste gas to a F/air Canister is not sufficient [19].
4. Orienting the needle bevel down will encourage a shallower entry into the cornea. A more traditional bevel-up orientation may result in the needle entering the eye more rapidly. This increases the chance of damaging the lens and iris and creating a less beveled wound that may not self-seal and be more likely to leak once the cannula is removed.
5. It is critical to eliminate air bubbles from all tubing leading to the eye. Regular two- and three-way stopcocks are adequate for connections leading from the reservoir to the manifold and to larger gauge tubing. However, when tubing is reduced to the diameter of the cannula, these types of connections are clumsy and can introduce air bubbles when opened and closed. Pinch-clamps on the tubing that leads to the final cannula are less likely to do this. Even with these, a small column of air can get drawn up into the cannula tip when the tubing is pinched off. If this occurs, releasing the clamp will generally restart flow. However, if the air persists, a sharp tap with a fingernail on the larger tube, which sends a mini shock wave down the tube, is required to restart the flow. This should always be done before looking for a greater systemic flaw.
6. The IOP set by the reservoir will accurately deliver the intended pressure to the eye. Tonolab readings primarily serve to indicate possible problems. Persistently low readings are a good indication that there is either a plugged tube, possibly by debris or potentially the iris, or an air bubble in the line that has produced an air lock. Careful examination with the operating microscope generally reveals the problem. If necessary, the cannula can be temporarily removed, cleared, and reinserted. Occasionally, a new cannula is necessary.

Acknowledgments/Support

NIH/NEI: R01EY010145-17S1 (DCL), R01EY-010145 (JCM), R01EY-016866 (ECJ), and P30 EY010572 (OHSU Core Grant), and an unrestricted grant from Research to Prevent Blindness (New York, NY).

References

1. Pang IH, Clark AF (2007) Rodent models for glaucoma retinopathy and optic neuropathy. J Glaucoma 16(5):483–505
2. Sappington RM et al (2009) The microbead occlusion model: a paradigm for induced ocular hypertension in rats and mice. Invest Ophthalmol Vis Sci 51(1):207–216
3. Morrison JC et al (1997) A rat model of chronic pressure-induced optic nerve damage. Exp Eye Res 64(1):85–96
4. Levkovitch-Verbin H et al (2002) Translimbal laser photocoagulation to the trabecular meshwork as a model of glaucoma in rats. Invest Ophthalmol Vis Sci 43(2):402–410
5. Samsel PA et al (2011) A novel method for the induction of experimental glaucoma using magnetic microspheres. Invest Ophthalmol Vis Sci 52(3):1671–1675
6. Jia L et al (2000) Effect of general anesthetics on IOP in rats with experimental aqueous outflow obstruction. Invest Ophthalmol Vis Sci 41(11):3415–3419
7. Jia L et al (2000) Patterns of intraocular pressure elevation after aqueous humor outflow obstruction in rats. Invest Ophthalmol Vis Sci 41(6):1380–1385
8. Kwong JM et al (2013) The dark phase intraocular pressure elevation and retinal ganglion cell degeneration in a rat model of experimental glaucoma. Exp Eye Res 112:21–28
9. Morrison JC et al (2016) A period of controlled elevation of IOP (CEI) produces the specific gene expression responses and focal injury pattern of experimental rat glaucoma. Invest Ophthalmol Vis Sci 57(15):6700–6711
10. Tehrani S et al (2016) Astrocyte structural and molecular response to elevated intraocular pressure occurs rapidly and precedes axonal tubulin rearrangement within the optic nerve head in a rat model. PLoS One 11(11):e0167364
11. Smith GG, Baird CD (1952) Survival time of retinal cells when deprived of their blood supply by increased intraocular pressure. Am J Ophthalmol 35(5):133–136
12. Buchi ER, Suivaizdis I, Fu J (1991) Pressure-induced retinal ischemia in rats: an experimental model for quantitative study. Ophthalmologica 203(3):138–147
13. Sun D, Moore S, Jakobs TC (2017) Optic nerve astrocyte reactivity protects function in experimental glaucoma and other nerve injuries. J Exp Med 214(5):1411–1430
14. Crowston JG et al (2015) An acute intraocular pressure challenge to assess retinal ganglion cell injury and recovery in the mouse. Exp Eye Res 141:3–8
15. Sun H et al (2011) Protective effect of a JNK inhibitor against retinal ganglion cell loss induced by acute moderate ocular hypertension. Mol Vis 17:864–875
16. Burgoyne CF (2010) A biomechanical paradigm for axonal insult within the optic nerve head in aging and glaucoma. Exp Eye Res 93(2):120–132
17. Johnson EC et al (2007) Global changes in optic nerve head gene expression after exposure to elevated intraocular pressure in a rat glaucoma model. Invest Ophthalmol Vis Sci 48(7):3161–3177
18. Johnson EC et al (2011) Cell proliferation and interleukin-6-type cytokine signaling are implicated by gene expression responses in early optic nerve head injury in rat glaucoma. Invest Ophthalmol Vis Sci 52(1):504–518
19. Zhi Z et al (2015) Evaluation of the effect of elevated intraocular pressure and reduced ocular perfusion pressure on retinal capillary bed filling and total retinal blood flow in rats by OMAG/OCT. Microvasc Res 101:86–95
20. Zhi Z et al (2012) Impact of intraocular pressure on changes of blood flow in the retina, choroid, and optic nerve head in rats investigated by optical microangiography. Biomed Opt Express 3(9):2220–2233
21. Jiang X et al (2018) The effect of age on the response of retinal capillary filling to changes in intraocular pressure measured by optical coherence tomography angiography. Microvasc Res 115:12–19
22. Pi S et al (2019) Monitoring retinal responses to acute intraocular pressure elevation in rats with visible light optical coherence tomography. Neurophotonics 6(4):041104

Chapter 20

A Comprehensive Protocol for Microbead-Induced Ocular Hypertension in Mice

M. Reza Bahrani Fard, Nina Sara Fraticelli-Guzmán, Jessica Chan, A. Thomas Read, Andrew Feola, W. Daniel Stamer, Simon W. M. John, C. Ross Ethier, and Rebecca M. Sappington

Abstract

Glaucoma is a common optic neuropathy characterized by degeneration of retinal ganglion cells (RGCs). Elevated intraocular pressure (IOP), that is, ocular hypertension, is the primary modifiable risk factor for glaucoma and the primary characteristic of most preclinical glaucoma models. Extensive genotype and phenotype diversity at relatively low cost and high accessibility makes laboratory mice an excellent preclinical model for glaucoma. The microbead occlusion model was introduced in 2010 as an inducible model of ocular hypertension in mice and is now one of the most extensively utilized models of rodent glaucoma. Subsequent modifications of the microbead model increased the magnitude and duration of IOP elevation, primarily through modification of injection materials. Despite its popularity, accessibility of the model is hindered by procedural consistency between users. Here we outline an updated and comprehensive protocol for execution of the microbead model that is focused on improving surgical and outcome measure consistency and on enabling single experimenter execution.

Key words Intraocular pressure, Glaucoma, Mouse model, Ocular hypertension, Rodent, Microbead

1 Introduction

The glaucomas are a family of optic neuropathies which together are the most common cause of irreversible blindness worldwide. Loss of visual function in glaucoma is due to dysfunction and degeneration of retinal ganglion cells (RGCs), and many features

The original version of the chapter has been revised. A correction to this chapter can be found at https://doi.org/10.1007/978-1-0716-4140-8_23

Supplementary Information The online version contains supplementary material available at https://doi.org/10.1007/978-1-0716-4140-8_20.

Tatjana Jakobs and Paloma B. Liton (eds.), *Glaucoma: Methods and Protocols*, Methods in Molecular Biology, vol. 2858, https://doi.org/10.1007/978-1-0716-4140-8_20,

of this pathologic process remain poorly understood, necessitating the need for animal models of the disease.

Ocular hypertension (OHT) is the primary modifiable risk factor for glaucoma and the primary characteristic of most preclinical glaucoma models. Many groups have described various methods for inducing OHT in various species, including mice, rats, tree shrews, rabbits, cows, and nonhuman primates. Here we focus on the microbead model in mice, for several reasons. First, mice offer extensive genotype and phenotype diversity at relatively low cost and high accessibility. Second, the microbead occlusion model of OHT, first introduced in 2010 [1], is now widely used in mice. The basic premise of the model is that normal aqueous humor drainage can be artificially impeded by physical blockade at the iridocorneal angle [1].

The initial protocol for microbead-induced OHT relied upon hydrodynamic forces of aqueous humor flow to passively deposit injected microbeads in the outflow pathway [1, 6], which typically resulted in a 20% elevation in IOP that lasted for 4 weeks [1]. Subsequently, the protocol was adjusted to increase the duration and magnitude of IOP elevation [2–5]. The most widely utilized modification is the use of magnetic microbeads, in which magnetic microbeads are injected intracamerally and then manually "steered" by an externally applied magnetic field to deposit the microbeads in the iridocorneal angle [3, 7]. This active process reduces errant deposition of microbeads elsewhere in the anterior chamber [3], important for optical imaging of posterior ocular tissues, and produces a stable IOP elevation of ~85% over 6 weeks [7]. Selection of the passive or active method of microbead deposition should primarily consider the desired magnitude and duration of IOP elevation.

Although it is a popular model, the laboratory use of the microbead model is hindered by variable outcomes, which in our experience is primarily due to interuser variability in two procedural elements—intracameral microbead injection and IOP measurement, as discussed below.

1. *Intracameral microbead injection:* Both passive and active versions of the microbead model require delivery of microbeads into the anterior chamber via intracameral injection. Historically, this has required two well-trained experimenters working together to achieve successful and consistent intracameral injections: one to position the injector and one to administer the injection [6]. This process makes the procedure laborious and increases the potential for variability between end-users. These drawbacks are more severe in the magnetic microbead model due to its more complex and time-consuming protocol.
2. *IOP measurement.* Accurate, noninvasive, longitudinal measurement of IOP, typically performed by tonometry in rodents, is important in OHT models [8–10]. Accurate and consistent

measurement of IOP in mice is challenging, including in the microbead model of OHT [8], and depends on precise alignment of the tonometer with the center of the cornea and proper calibration and operation of the tonometer [8]. The TonoLab tonometer, which is specifically calibrated for rodents, has improved the accuracy of noninvasive IOP measurement in mice [11, 12]. However, even with this device, successful and consistent alignment of the tonometer with the center of the cornea, while possible, is technically challenging in awake mice [6]. Sedation immobilizes the mouse and thus greatly facilitates proper alignment of the tonometer but can artificially lower IOP in a time-dependent manner [13, 14]. The window of time in which IOP is reliable under anesthetized conditions is variable and must be empirically determined for each laboratory. Thus, the methodology for IOP measurement is complex and requires considerable skill and experience.

Here, we outline an updated protocol for the microbead model of OHT that utilizes a novel, integrated platform for surgical procedures and hands-free IOP measurements. This protocol enables a single experimenter to carry out all procedures, while improving consistency in microbead delivery and IOP measurements. We include details for use of both magnetic and nonmagnetic microbeads, as well as procedures for accurate IOP measurements under anesthesia. These updated protocols require custom manufacturing of equipment; thus, access to machining and three-dimensional printing facilities is necessary. We note that the use of a manual injection apparatus does not require access to such manufacturing capabilities and that protocols for execution of the nonmagnetic and magnetic microbead models using a manual injection apparatus are described by Calkins et al. (2018) [6] and Ito et al. (2016) [7]. However, our experience is that custom manufacturing is well worthwhile to obtain better long-term results with the microbead model of OHT.

This protocol is intended to provide a comprehensive starting guide for execution of the microbead model of OHT. If difficulties are experienced in establishing the model, hands-on training with an experienced lab is highly recommended. Variables such as micropipette preparation and injection angle can have a profound effect on success of the model and are readily identified by observation and training.

2 Materials and Assembly

Appropriate sterilization protocols should be used throughout this protocol, including utilization of single-use or sterilized instruments and aseptic preparation of solutions. The procedure below requires approval by an Institutional Animal Care and Use Committee, and its practice should adhere to applicable animal welfare codes and regulations.

2.1 General

1. Micropipette puller (*see* **Note 1**).
2. Microelectrode beveler (BV-10, Sutter Instruments).
3. (Optional) Coarse diamond abrasive plate (104C, Sutter Instruments).
4. Rebound tonometer and disposable probes (TONOLAB, iCare). We modified our tonometer, so that it can be actuated by a separate foot switch, thereby avoiding hand motion when acquiring IOP measurements.
5. Focal light source for surgery (dual gooseneck LED recommended).
6. Nonserrated, straight, or curved forceps (approximately 2 mm) for eye positioning. The use of curved vs. flat forceps is a matter of individual preference and comfort.
7. Magnetic Microbead Protocol only: 0.25″ cubic N52 neodymium magnet connected to a thin stainless-steel Allen key.

2.2 Anesthesia and Animal Support

1. A gas anesthesia system for use in mice, including an induction chamber and nose cone (*see* **Note 2**).
2. Animal temperature controller—low voltage (TCAT-2LV, Physiotemp; *see* **Note 3**)
3. Heat plate (HP-4M, Physiotemp; *see* **Note 3**)
4. Heat plate (HP-4M, Physiotemp; *see* **Note 3**)

2.3 Integrated Surgical and IOP Platform

1. CAD drawings for platform assembly (*see* Supplemental Material).
2. Threaded connecting rod (6516 K121, McMaster-Carr).
3. Threaded connecting rod (6516 K4, McMaster-Carr).
4. Round aluminum rod, ½" OD x 12″ long (83,048, K&S).
5. M3 x 50 mm screws and compatible nuts.
6. Manual rotation stage (Thorlabs, RP01).
7. Manual rotation stage (Thorlabs, RP03).
8. Linear stage (Newport, TSX-1D).
9. Optical breadboard plate (Newport, SA2-08x08).
10. Knob (McMaster-Carr, 6479 K35).
11. Foot-long aluminum 90-degree angle for part 2 (McMaster-Carr, 8982 K145).
12. Aluminum slab for part 3 (McMaster-Carr, 1651 T7, 6"x6").
13. Aluminum disk for part 4 (McMaster-Carr, 1610 T12, Ø 0.5″).

14. Stainless-steel plate. All the components of the integrated surgical and IOP platform will be ultimately placed on this plate, which will serve as the base for the magnetic stands. Thus, plate dimensions should be chosen accordingly. Use a type of stainless steel with magnetic properties.
15. Velcro straps.
16. Breadboard mounting feet (Newport, SA2-FT-70).

2.4 Injection Apparatus

1. Stereo microscope (*see* **Note 4**).
2. Syringe pump (Harvard Apparatus, PHD ULTRA 70–3006).
3. Foot switch for syringe pump (Harvard Apparatus, 702,215).
4. Injection assembly (World Precision Instruments, MMP-KIT).
5. Gastight 25 μL syringe (Hamilton, 1702LT).
6. Manual micromanipulator (World Precision Instruments, M3301) with magnetic base.

2.5 Consumable Materials

1. Charcoal canisters (isoflurane waste container).
2. 4-inch thin-wall glass capillaries with filament (1.5 OD/1.12 ID)
3. 0.6 ml microcentrifuge tubes, autoclaved
4. 1.5 ml microcentrifuge tubes, autoclaved
5. Sterile vacuum filter units (250 ml, pore size = 0.22 μm) for sterilization of solutions.
6. 5 cc disposable syringe

2.6 Reagents

1. 70% ethanol (for sterilization).
2. 95% O_2/5% CO_2-EM compressed gas (in cylinder).
3. Isoflurane.
4. Mineral oil, light (NF/FCC).
5. Polystyrene microspheres (*see* **Note 5**):
   5a. Nonmagnetic: 15 μm (1 x 10^6 beads/mL stock solution; ThermoFisher Cat#F8844). Store at 4 °C.
   5b. Magnetic: 1:1 mixture of 2 μm (1.2 x 10^{10} beads/mL) and 6 μm (4 x 10^8 beads/mL) magnetic polystyrene microbeads with PEG-COOH surface groups (micromer-M, Micromod, Rostock, Germany). Store at room temperature.
6. Phosphate-buffered saline (PBS) without sodium azide.
7. 1% tropicamide ophthalmic solution (dilation drops).
8. 0.5% proparacaine hydrochloride ophthalmic solution (anesthetic drops). Store at 4 °C.
9. 0.5% moxifloxacin hydrochloride ophthalmic solution (antibiotic drops).

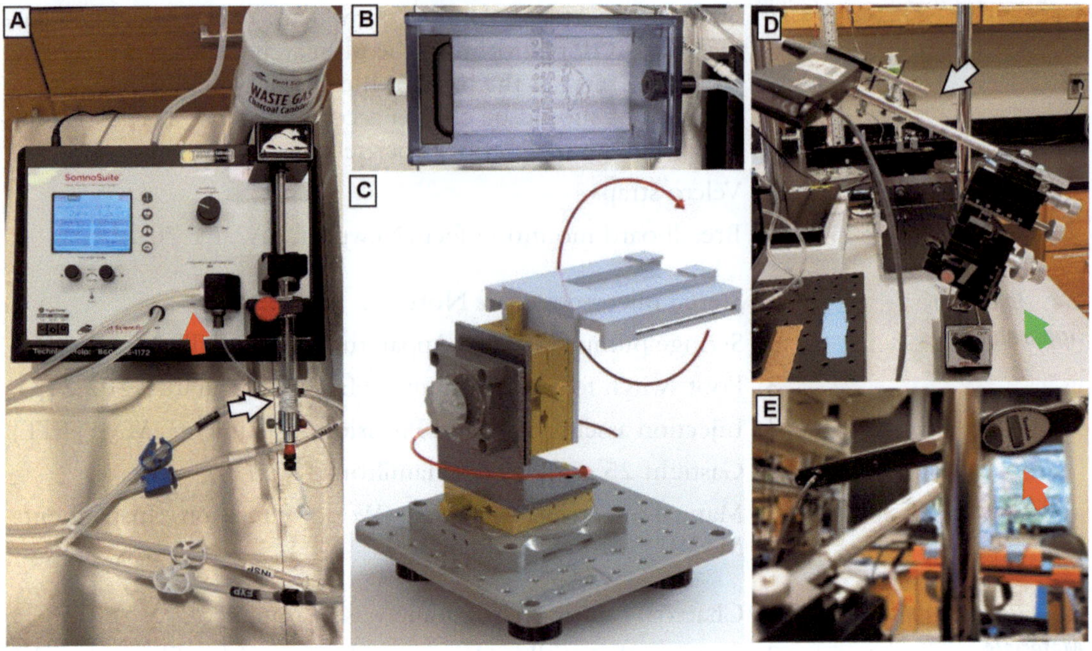

Fig. 1 Anesthesia and platform assemblies. (**a**) Photographs of SomnoSuite anesthesia system. The glass syringe (white arrow) is mounted on a syringe pump that delivers anesthetic liquid to the vaporizer. Red arrow indicates gas anesthetic outlet from the vaporizer to both the induction chamber and the nose cone. Color-coded clips are used to redirect the gas. Waste is purged into a charcoal filter canister (top-right corner of the photograph). (**b**) Induction chamber. (**c**) Custom-made surgical platform. Refer to the assembly files for complete instructions. This platform allows for linear movement in three dimensions and rotation, with axes shown in the rendered image as red arrows. The heat plate can be slid into the groove on the white top surface. (**d**, **e**) IOP measurement setup which includes TonoLab tonometer (red arrow), a micromanipulator (green arrow), and a custom-made mounting apparatus (white arrow)

2.7 Anesthesia Apparatus Assembly

1. Follow manufacturer's instructions for assembly of the anesthesia apparatus. Assembly occurs only once at initial setup of the equipment (Fig. 1a, b).

2.8 Injection and Tonometry Apparatus Assembly

The preparation of this equipment requires access to 3D printers (part 1) and machining facilities (parts 2-4). CAD files for parts 1-4 are provided in the supplementary materials. A commercial device was incorporated in the original prototype of our injection platform but is no longer available on the market. Therefore, we have re-designed the platform to include only parts that can be easily procured.

1. Assemble the machined parts according to the "assembly CAD file" provided in the supplementary materials (Fig. 1c).
2. Fabricate the tonometer holder using the instructions in the assembly CAD file. Attach the tonometer to a micromanipulator using the tonometer holder (Fig. 1d, e).

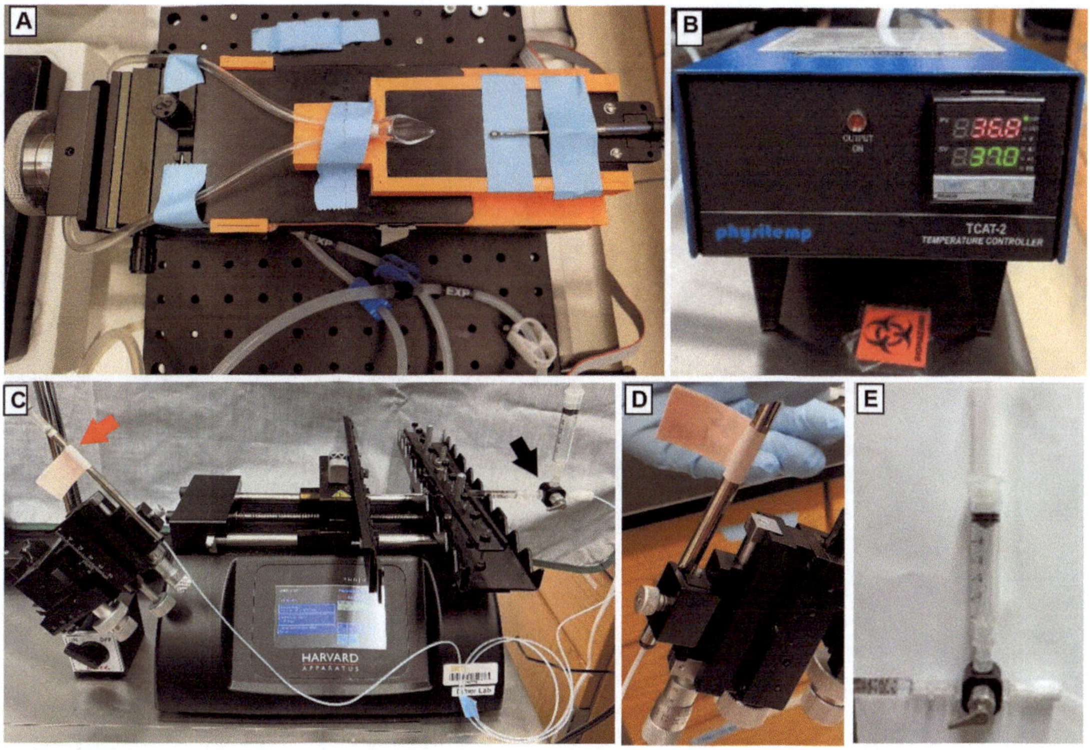

Fig. 2 Injection assembly. (**a**) Photograph showing a heat plate (black) installed on the three-dimensional printed platform of the surgical setup (orange). Nose cone (on the left) is taped to the platform. (**b**) Animal temperature controller. (**c**) Injection assembly and syringe pump. Black arrow indicates the three-way valve connected to a 5 ml syringe filled with mineral oil on the top and a Hamilton microsyringe to the left. The remaining outlet from this valve is connected by tubing to the commercial injection assembly (red arrow). (**d**) Closer view of the commercial injection apparatus in panel C (red arrow). (**e**) Closer view of the three-way valve in panel C (black arrow)

3. Secure the heat plate by sliding it into part 1 of the assembly and tape the nose cone for the anesthesia assembly to the heat plate (Fig. 2a).
4. Wire the heat plate to the controller according to the manufacturer's instructions (Fig. 2b).
5. Secure the needle side of the injection assembly on a micromanipulator (Fig. 2c,d).
6. Connect the opposite side of the injection assembly to the Hamilton syringe using a three-way valve (Fig. 2c, e). Mount the Hamilton syringe on the syringe pump (Fig. 2c).
7. Place the stereomicroscope (if using) in a position that allows easy observation of the rotational platform.

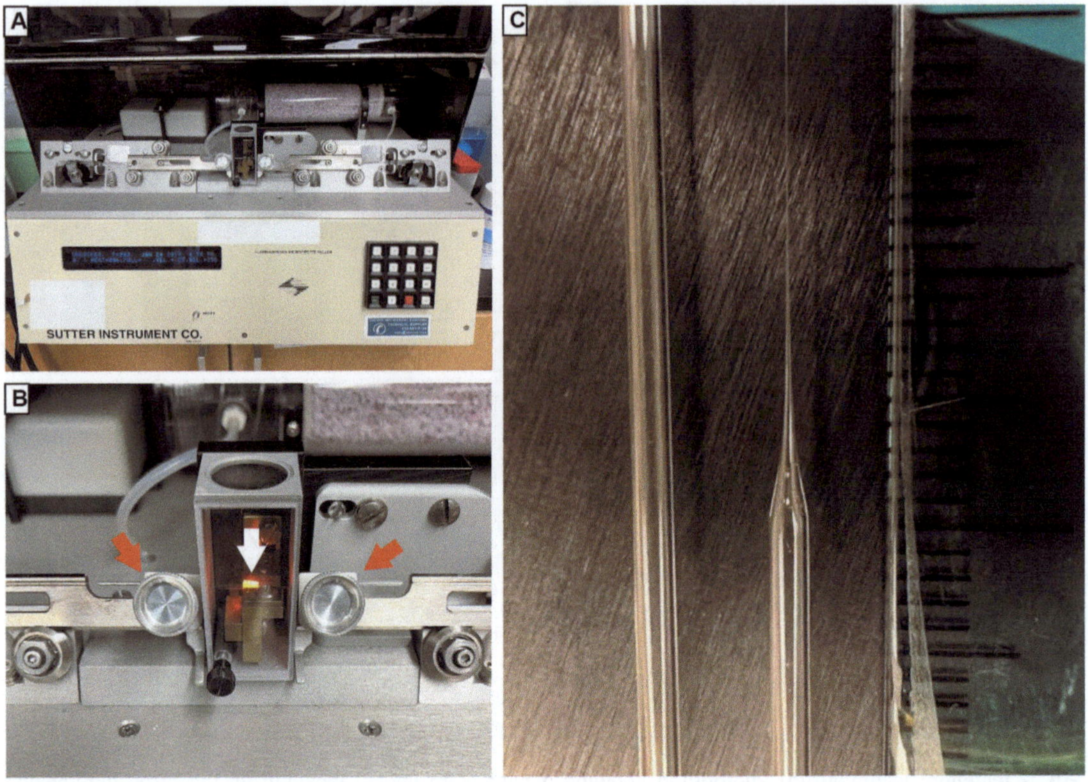

Fig. 3 Production of glass micropipettes. (**a**) Photograph of microelectrode puller. (**b**) Photograph of a glass capillary secured in the puller. White arrow indicates location of the heating element. Red arrows show the micropipette clamped on both sides to the pulling arms. (**c**) Photograph of the pulled (right) and original (left) micropipettes. Ruler subdivisions are in millimeters

2.9 Micropipette Preparation

1. Use a glass micropipette puller to create micropipettes for microbead and saline injection (Fig. 3a). Determine appropriate settings for your instruments (*see* **Note 6**).
2. Insert a glass capillary into the holder and secure with screws. Press the "pull" button to heat the filament (Fig. 3b).
3. When the glass electrode separates into two micropipettes, loosen screws and remove (Fig. 3c).
4. Tribeveling of the micropipette tip increases the repeatability and efficiency of injections.

   4a. Mount the coarse diamond abrasive plate on the microelectrode beveler's rotational platform, according to the manufacturer's instructions. Add a few drops of deionized water on the abrasive surface as lubricant.

   4b. Use a pair of fine scissors with thin blades to score and break the tip of the micropipette (Fig. 4a). The exact distance of the break point to the tip depends on the profile and taper length of the pulled micropipette, but a final lumen diameter of ~100 μm is desired.

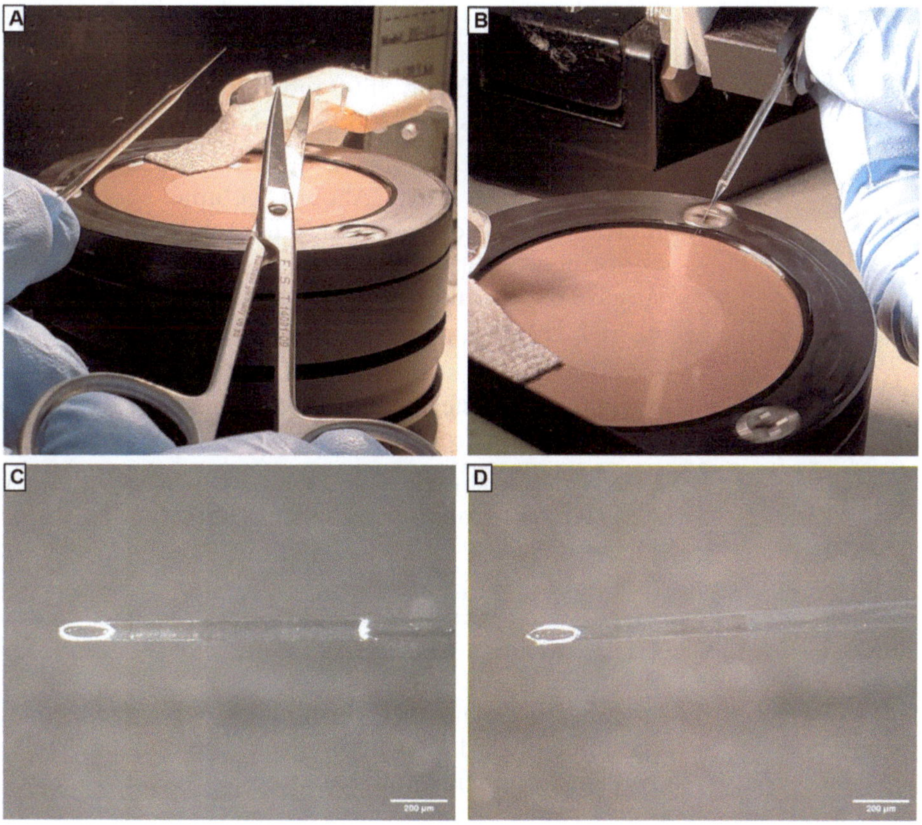

Fig. 4 Micropipette trimming. (**a**) Photograph of a trimmed micropipette and the fine scissors used to break it. (**b**) The beveling setup, including the diamond abrasive plate, the beveler rotational system, and the trimmed micropipette approaching the surface at 25° angle. (**c**) A micropipette after beveling on the main side (part "b" of the tribeveling approach). The appearance of elliptical cross-section signals the completion of this step. (**d**) Micropipette after tribeveling. The cross-sectional profile should be free of jagged surfaces and have a fine pointed tip

4c. Bring the micropipette tip in contact with the plate at 25 degrees. Allow for a smooth surface to develop (*see* **Note 7,** Fig. 4b). Once the lumen shows an elliptical cross section visible under the microscope, the micropipette is ready for the next step (Fig. 4c).

4d. Axially rotate the micropipette by approximately 70 degrees to expose the side of the beveled surface to the abrasive plate. Once half of the rounded tip is ground down, return to the original position, and then rotate 70 degrees in the opposite direction. Grind down the glass until the rounded tip turns into a sharp pointed tip (*see* **Note 8,** Fig. 4d).

2.10 Reagent Preparation—Microbeads

1. For polystyrene microbeads, proceed to **step 3**.
2. For ferromagnetic microbeads, sterilize by autoclaving for 20 min at 121 °C and 3500 mbar pressure followed by rinsing five times using sterile HBSS (*see* **Note 9**) [15].
3. Using aseptic technique, aliquot microbeads into a 0.6 ml microcentrifuge tube. Aliquot volume should be slightly more than the volume needed for total number of injections performed. Solution remaining in the aliquot at the end of the surgical day should be discarded.
4. Sterilize PBS using vacuum sterilization filter units. Sterile solution can be stored at 4 °C for 1 month. Using aseptic technique, transfer 300 μL of sterilized PBS to a 0.6 ml microcentrifuge tube.
5. Place 1 ml of 70% ethanol in a 1.5 ml microcentrifuge tube for sterilization of micropipettes after insertion in the injection apparatus.

3 Methods

3.1 IOP Measurements

Baseline measurements of IOP should be obtained for all animals being studied (including naïve controls). To obtain reliable, hands-free IOP measurements under anesthesia:

1. Weigh the animal and input the corresponding value into the SomnoSuite anesthesia device. The device will automatically set the flow rates based on the animal weight (*see* **Note 10**).
2. Position the tonometer horizontally to avoid any component of gravitational force affecting the measurements (the device will give an error otherwise). Ensure the working range of the micromanipulator allows the tonometer to be suitably placed, that is, there is sufficient reach and adjustment over the animal's head when the animal is placed in the nose cone (Fig. 5a).
3. Place the animal in the induction chamber, and set 2% isoflurane to be delivered at 500 ml/min to the chamber. Monitor the animal closely and, once it is immobile, check for a loss of righting reflex by rotating it to the supine position (*see* **Note 11**).
4. Run "flush" to clear excess anesthetic from the tubing. Redirect the flow to the nose cone and run the preprogrammed settings for the delivery of 1% isoflurane (*see* **Note 12**). Take the animal out of the induction chamber, and place over the heat pad with the head affixed to the nose cone. Secure the head with the velcro straps (*see* **Note 13**).

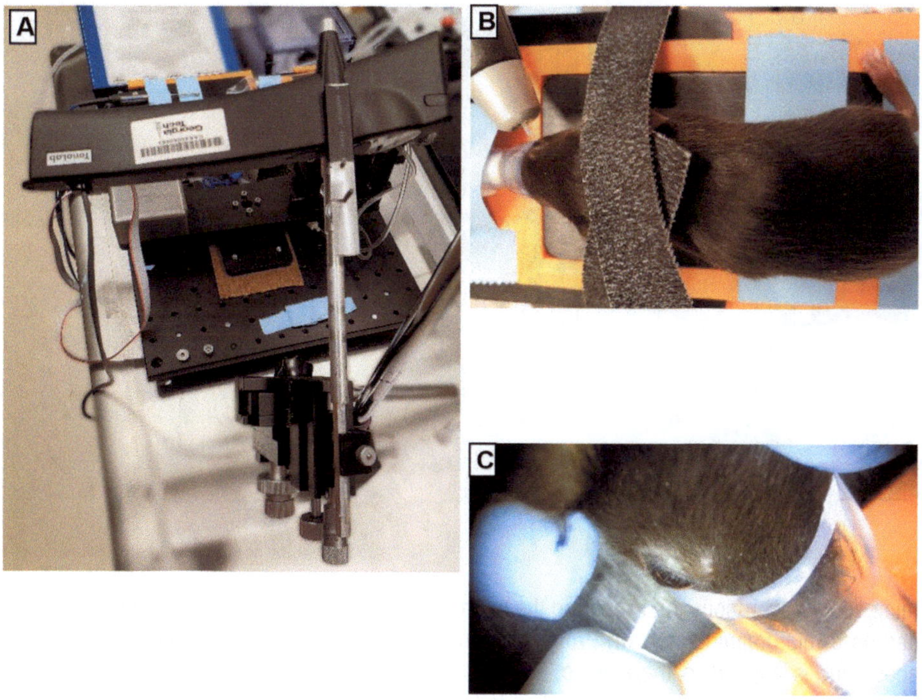

Fig. 5 IOP measurement. (**a**) Horizontal orientation of the tonometer in the tonometer holder. (**b, c**) Alignment of the tonometer probe perpendicular to the center of the cornea. Velcro straps attached to the surgical platform (hands-free, **b**) or a gentle, manual hold (**c**) may be used to immobilize the head in the desired position

5. Position the tonometer tip perpendicular to the center of the cornea. Check from both the top and the side to ensure proper positioning, since the readings are sensitive to tip misplacement/misalignment (*see* **Note 14**, Fig. 5b, c).
6. Read IOP (*see* **Notes 14** and **16**).
7. Quickly rotate the stage and repeat for the contralateral eye, if desired.
8. Turn off the anesthesia, unstrap the animal, and place over a heated pad to recover.

3.2 Intracameral Injections

The integrated surgical and IOP platform enables a single experimenter to conduct intracameral microbead injections by utilizing foot controls.

(a) Injection Procedure for Nonmagnetic Microbeads

1. Insert and tighten the prepared micropipette into the injection assembly mounted on the micromanipulator (*see* **Note 17**, Fig. 6a).
2. Fill the micropipette with mineral oil by depressing the plunger of the 5 cc syringe attached to the side port of the three-way valve (Fig. 2c). Ensure no bubbles are

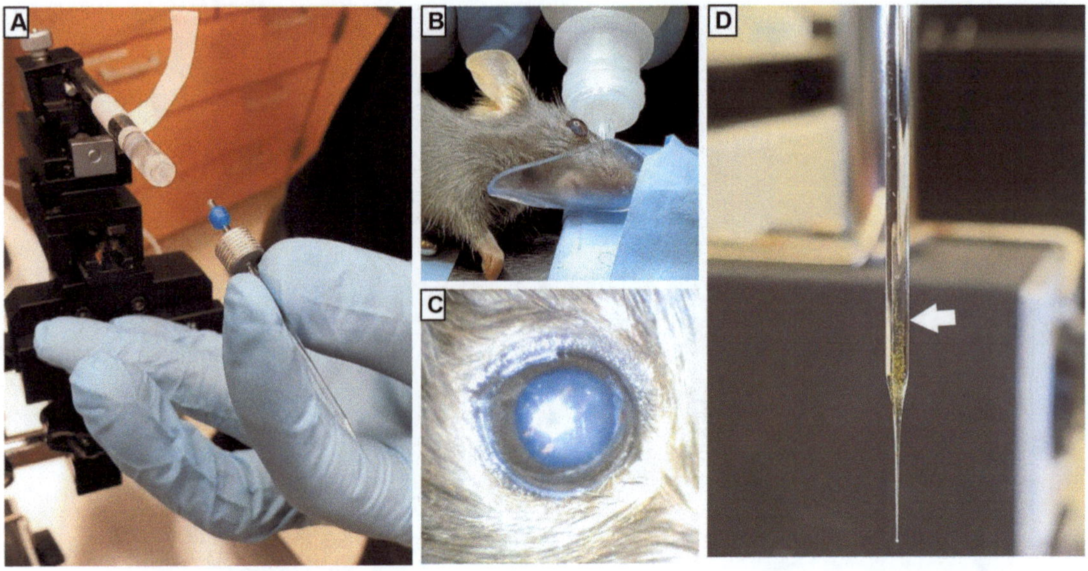

Fig. 6 Preinjection preparations. (**a**) Preparing the micropipette to be loaded into the injection apparatus, which is mounted on a micromanipulator. (**b**) Proper placement of the mouse on the surgical platform. A drop of topical anesthetic is applied to the eye. (**c**) The desired pupil dilation is achieved after application of 1% tropicamide. (**d**) The desired volume of microbeads (yellow) loaded in the micropipette after rinsing the inner lumen with sterile PBS. White arrow indicates the meniscus formed at the interface between the mineral oil and microbead solution

present throughout the line and that oil beads form at the tip of the micropipette. Use a Kimwipe to remove excess mineral oil from the tip.

3. Apply one drop of 1% tropicamide ophthalmic solution to each eye (*see* **Notes 18** and **19**).
4. Place the animal in the induction chamber and deliver 2.5% isoflurane via the anesthesia system until righting reflex is lost (*see* **Note 20**).
5. Divert isoflurane flow to the nose cone. Transfer the animal to the heat pad and affix the nose cone. Orient the animal on its side with the cornea to be injected facing up (Fig. 6b). Secure the animal with Velcro straps.
6. Set syringe pump to zero (zero out) and sterilize the tip of the micropipette by submerging it in the microcentrifuge tube filled with 70% ETOH.
7. For bilateral microbead injections, wet the internal surface of the micropipette by submerging the tip of the micropipette in the microcentrifuge tube of sterile saline. Set the automatic syringe pump to load 2 μL of sterile saline into the micropipette (*see* **Notes 21** and **22**). Eject and discard 1.5 μL of the sterile saline from the micropipette.
8. Check dilation (Fig. 6c) and reapply 1% tropicamide ophthalmic solution, if necessary (*see* **Note 23**).

9. Set the automatic syringe pump to the desired injection volume at a flow rate of 18 μL/min. Load the solution for injection (sterile saline or microbeads), using the desired injection volume plus a volume of 0.5ul (*see* **Note 24**). Keep the tip of the micropipette submerged in the solution until the proper volume of solution is loaded. Check the location of the meniscus where the injectable solution interfaces with the mineral oil to ensure the proper volume is loaded (Fig. 6d).
10. Apply local anesthesia (0.5% proparacaine hydrochloride ophthalmic solution, one drop) directly to the eye and wait for 1 min.
11. Proptose the eye with curved or flat-edge forceps (*see* **Note 24**; Fig. 7a).

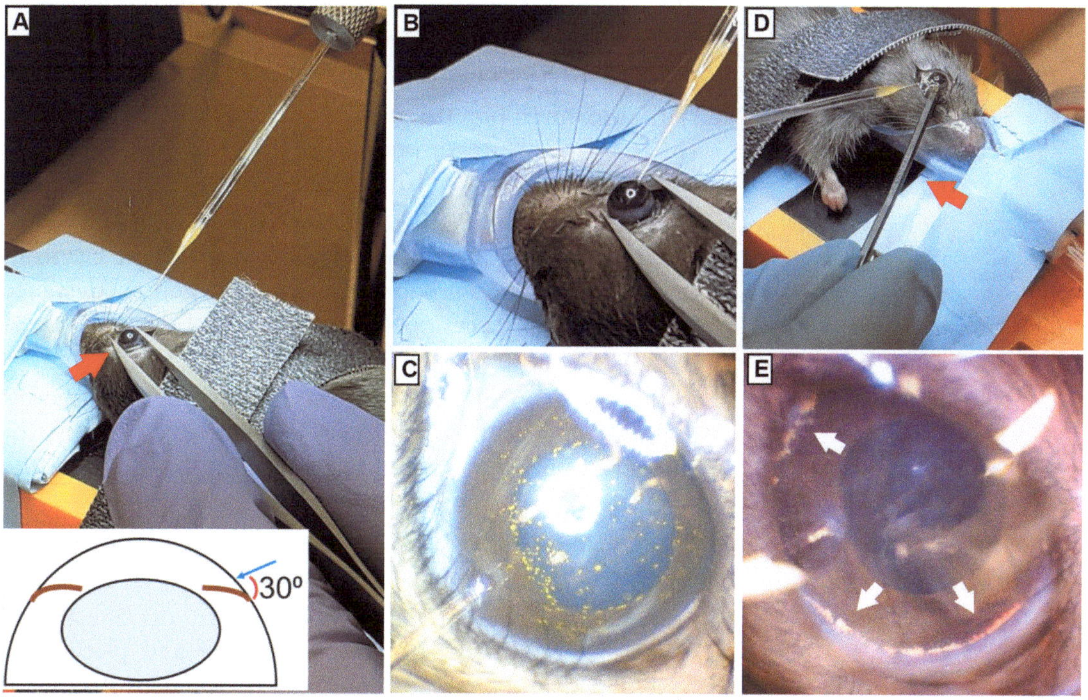

Fig. 7 Microbead injection. (**a**) Photograph of eye being proptosed with forceps. Arrow indicates the "brace" position generated by the back arm of the forceps. Inset: Schematic illustrating the orientation of the micropipette with respect to the limbus. (**b**) Photograph of the first 5–7 s of microbead injection. The eye is braced by forceps until the desired volume of microbead solution is delivered. Note that the micropipette is inserted in the cornea at an ~30° angle from the limbus. (**c**) Photograph of the second 10–15 s of microbead injection. Forceps are removed and the micropipette remains until microbeads disperse. (**d**) Magnetic apparatus (arrow) pointing at the limbus for delivery of magnetic microbeads. The experimenter encircles the limbus with the magnet in a fashion described in the main text, for a circumferentially uniform delivery. (**e**) Accumulation of magnetic microbeads at the angle (arrows) upon the completion of delivery. Micropipette is kept inside the anterior chamber until the microbeads are stabilized in place. Procedures in panels (**a**–**c**) incorporate nonmagnetic microbeads while panels (**d**–**e**) are magnetic

12. With the eye stabilized by the forceps, align the tip of the micropipette with the far edge of the dilated iris (Fig. 7a, b). A 30^0 angle of approach with respect to the limbus is typically successful for smooth penetration of the cornea and clearance of the iris (Fig. 7b). The five-axes design of this platform (linear XYZ movement and two rotational axes, Fig. 1c) allows for free movement of the surgical bed in three-dimensional space to achieve proper alignment of the eye with the micropipette tip while the latter remains stationary.
13. While stabilizing the eye with the forceps (*see* **Note 25**), advance the micropipette in a continuous motion until the cornea is punctured (*see* **Note 26**).
14. With the eye still proptosed, use the foot pedal control of the automatic syringe pump to inject the desired volume. The eye should remain proptosed and gently supported by the forceps until the desired injection volume is delivered into the anterior chamber (*see* **Notes 27** and **28**).
15. With the micropipette still in the cornea, wait another 15–20 s to ensure dispersion of the microbeads in the anterior chamber (*see* **Note 29**, Fig. 7c).
16. Slowly withdraw the micropipette from the cornea. Stabilize the eye using forceps as a brace to prevent the eye from traveling with the micropipette, applying gentle resistance in the opposite direction to that employed during corneal puncture.
17. Apply one drop of 0.5% proparacaine hydrochloride ophthalmic solution and one drop of 0.5% moxifloxacin hydrochloride ophthalmic solution (antibiotic) directly to the cornea.
18. If performing bilateral injections, use the rotational platform to flip the animal and repeat **steps 8–17**.
19. Upon completion of all injections, turn off anesthesia. Remove the animal from the nose cone and place on a heated pad and then in a clean cage for recovery. With isoflurane anesthesia, the animal will awake within minutes.
20. Monitor the animal for signs of distress, as per the approved IACUC protocol.

(b) Injection procedure for magnetic microbeads: The procedure for magnetic microbead injection is identical to that of non-magnetic microbeads, with the following exceptions:

Step # 9: Set the syringe pump to deliver an injection volume of 0.4 μL at 2.4 μL /min.

Step #14: Divide the eye into imaginary quadrants. Hold the magnetic steering apparatus (a permanent magnet attached to a thin stainless-steel Allen key) over the cornea in the targeted quadrant (*see* **Note 30**, Fig. 7d). Press the foot pedal to inject 0.4 μL of the microbeads. "Collect" the injected microbeads on the cornea using the magnetic steering apparatus. Slowly drag the microbeads to the irideocorneal angle, and distribute them uniformly to cover the entire circumference of the quadrant (Fig. 7e). Repeat for each quadrant (total injection volume equals 1.6 μL).

3.3 Monitoring and Model Maintenance

1. The cornea may temporary become cloudy 24–48 h after surgery. Beyond 48 h, there should be no visible difference in the cornea between saline- and microbead-injected eyes. However, microbeads will remain visible in the anterior chamber of microbead-injected animals (Fig. 8).

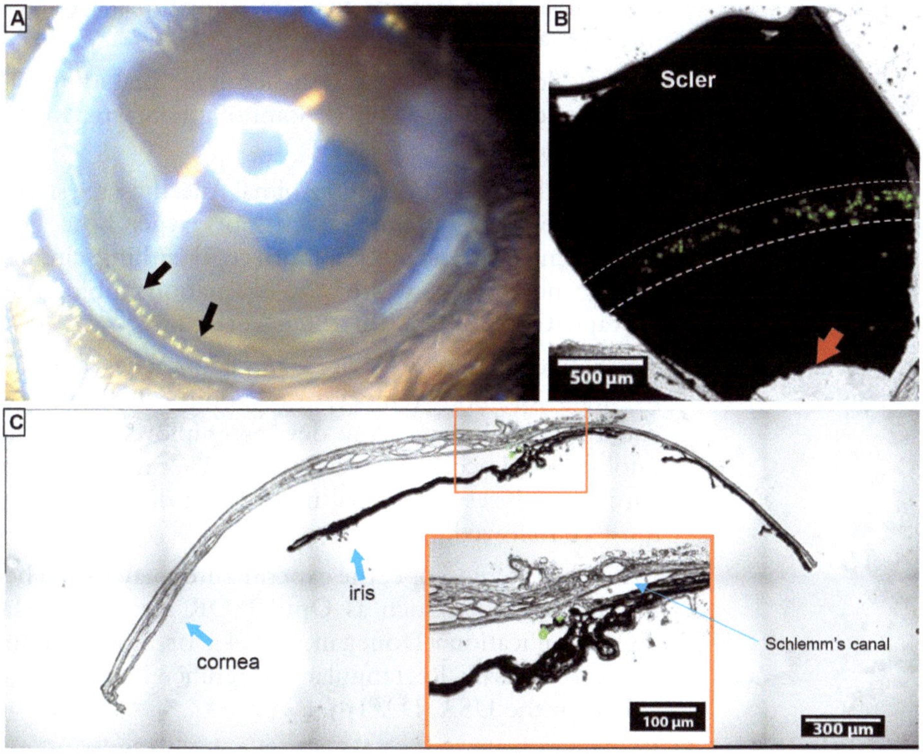

Fig. 8 Postop evaluation of microbead delivery. (**a**) Yellow nonmagnetic microbeads are deposited at the angle (arrows). Image is taken using a surgical microscope 24 h after surgery. (**b**) Fluorescent image of the nonmagnetic microbeads located at the limbus. Eye was enucleated 24 h after surgery, fixed in 10% formalin, and four incisions were made resulting in an anterior segment flat mount. Fluorescent image is merged with a light micrograph for one quadrant; green pseudocolor shows the fluorescent microbeads. Red arrow indicates the pupillary margin and dashed lines show the putative limbal region. (**c**) Cross-sectional (sagittal) view of the angle 24 h after nonmagnetic microbead (green fluorescence) injection. Insert outlined by red box shows a magnified view of the angle

2. To assess the efficacy of microbead injections and to monitor model progression, IOP measurements should be taken for at least three consecutive days following intracameral injection followed by 1–2 times per week for the remainder of the experiment (*see* **Notes 31** and **32**). IOP measurements should be taken as outlined in Subheading 3.1.
3. The duration of IOP elevation can be extended by reinjection prior to the loss of ocular hypertension following the same procedures above (*see* **Note 33**).

4 Notes

1. A horizontal (i.e., P-97, Sutter Instruments) or vertical (i.e., PC-100, Narishige) electrode puller may be utilized.
2. Any gas anesthesia system with mouse nose cone adaptors is acceptable. Two systems that are compatible with microbead injection are the following:
   - Low-flow anesthesia system for mice including induction chamber and nose cones (SomnoSuite Starter Kit for Mice, Kent Scientific).
   - V-1 Tabletop Laboratory Animal Anesthesia System with an accessory kit containing a ten-foot oxygen hose, flowmeter, oxygen flush assembly, vaporizer, breathing circuit, chamber, nosecones, waste gas evacuation tubing, and two VaporGuard filters (901,806; VetEquip).
3. A variety of materials, devices, and approaches are available to maintain core body temperature, monitor depth of anesthesia, and track vital signs. Any devices employed must allow for unobstructed access to eyes. All IACUC guidelines and standard procedures for animal monitoring during gas anesthesia must be followed.
4. In lieu of a stereoscope, the experimenter may wear a headband mount magnifier, such as OptiVISOR Headband Magnifier, 2X Magnification (Donegan, DA-4), or 3.5x Magnification, Optical Glass, Rectangular Magnifier-Headband Mount (Made in the USA, DA-10).
5. Frequently agitate the microbead solution by tapping to prevent aggregation and sticking, particularly just before use. Alternatively, the microbead sample can be vortexed prior to injection.
6. Protocols for pulling micropipettes should be optimized for the specific instrument utilized, as variation between pullers (i.e., position and type of filament) can influence settings. Refer to the manufacturer's directions for settings. As a

guide, example settings from a horizontal pipette puller and a vertical pipette puller are provided below:

(a) P-97 Model from Sutter Instruments (Shorter Taper).

P = 500 units.

Heat = 490 units.

Pull = 30 units.

Velocity = 120 units.

Time = 200 units

(b) P-97 Model from Sutter Instruments (Longer Taper).

P = 200 units.

Heat = 806 units.

Pull = 0 units.

Velocity = 25 units.

Delay = 250 units

(c) PC-100 Model from Narishige.

P = 500 units.

Heat = 650 units.

Pull = 30 units.

Velocity = 120 units.

Time = 200 units

7. For the BV-10 beveling system, Sutter Instruments recommends bubble formation over the abrasive plate as the best method for assessing progression of the beveling surface. However, we have found that monitoring the noise caused by griding the glass is an easier and more reliable technique. When the micropipette contacts the abrasive plate, noise is initially heard but slowly fades as the beveled surface smoothens.
8. It is recommended to increase the angle between the micropipette and the abrasive plate to 45° when sharpening the sides to engage only the very tip of the micropipette and keep the rest of the profile intact. Grind the sides just enough so that a pointed tip is achieved. Overgrinding can result in jagged surfaces which can prevent a clean puncture through the cornea.
9. When using magnetic microbeads, hold a strong magnet close to the microbead tube to avoid loss of beads during the rinse steps.
10. If the anesthesia equipment does not autoregulate isoflurane flow, the optimal flow rate must be determined empirically based on depth of anesthesia and latency to anesthesia. If the animal shows sign of agonal breathing, increasing the flow rate may help alleviate the symptom.

11. The loss of righting reflex is an indicator of the start of unconsciousness or light anesthesia. With progression of anesthesia, the episcleral venous pressure drops, which leads to a decrease in the IOP. Therefore, the animal should be transferred to the nose cone immediately after the loss of righting reflex, and the measurements should be taken as quickly as possible. In our experience, the average measurement time (from the end of induction to the end of measurements) for both eyes is 2–3 min.
12. If isoflurane/O_2 mixing is performed manually, the optimal mix and duration for anesthesia induction may need to be optimized. The guidelines provided in this protocol for both induction and maintenance of anesthesia can be utilized to determine optimal mixing for manually regulated anesthesia.
13. The mouse's head should be immobilized, but Velcro straps should not be overtightened. Excess force applied by the Velcro straps can artificially affect the IOP. The experimenter can alternatively choose to hold the animal's head with one hand. While this handgrip method increases the control over the orientation of the center of the cornea with respect to the tonometer probe tip, caution must be taken not to apply excessive force which may result in an artificial spike in the IOP.
14. Proper maintenance of the TonoLab tonometer is critical for accurate IOP measurement. The instrument must be routinely cleaned, and probes replaced, as specified in the operating manual.
15. The TonoLab tonometer (iCare) is programmed to provide a final IOP measurement after six rebound readings. A long beep signals calculation of the "final" IOP measurement, which is an average of four rebound repetitions with the highest and lowest readings omitted. If the user prefers to record each IOP measurement and manually calculate the average IOP, it is important to note that only the IOP measurement from the first rebound (e.g., reading "1.15" on the display) is a pure measurement. IOP measurements displayed for rebounds 2–5 are a running average based on the current reading and individual readings from the previous rebound(s). For example, the IOP measurement for rebound #3 (e.g., reading "3. 16" on the display) is an average of the individual measurements for rebounds 1, 2, and 3. To record only individual measurements, the IOP measurement displayed for reading 1. 15 should be recorded after the first rebound and the device cleared (00 on the display) for repeated measurement. For additional information and support, refer to the Tonolab User Manual (https://tonovet.com/products/icare-lab/lab-brochure/).

16. IOP in mice fluctuates diurnally [16, 17]. To reduce variability and ensure accurate, longitudinal assessment of IOP, it is critical that all IOP measurements be conducted at a specific time of the day within a limited time window, usually taken as 2 h. Also, users should be alert to the possibility of IOP spikes after injection (*see* **Note 32**).
17. Micropipettes are prone to breakage and become dull with repeated use. Use one micropipette per animal to reduce the risk of ocular injury and prevent contamination between animals.
18. To deliver eye drops to an awake mouse, scruff the mouse with your nondominant hand, as you would for delivery of an intraperitoneal injection. Hold the animal upright and deliver the eye drop with your dominant hand, tilting the animal slightly to the left or right.
19. If performing injections in multiple animals on a single day, procedure times can be shortened by dilating several mice simultaneously. Covering the housing cage to darken the environment will also hasten dilation after application of the dilation drops.
20. Based on the depth of anesthesia required, a higher percentage (2.5%) of isoflurane anesthetic is utilized for intracameral injection than for IOP measurements (2.0%).
21. When performing bilateral saline injections, it is not necessary to prewet the micropipette. Load 0.5ul more than the desired injection volume of sterile saline and proceed with intracameral injection of the sterile saline.
22. When performing unilateral microbead and saline injections in a single animal, the saline should be injected first to avoid contamination of saline injections with microbeads. It is also not necessary to prewet the micropipette, as the saline injection will serve this purpose.
23. Intracameral injection with insufficient dilation can lead to iris injury and intraocular bleeding. Sufficient dilation is achieved when approximately 75% or more of the anterior chamber is free of iris.
24. Volumes anywhere from 1–4 μL of microbeads have been utilized for this model [1, 2, 4, 5]. The most common injection volume is 1.5 μL.
25. During proptosis and stabilization, forceps should never squeeze the eye from both directions, which can cause ocular injury and impact aqueous fluid dynamics. Proptosis is achieved by applying slight, downward pressure to the eyelids on either side of the eye. Stabilization of the eye against

rotation during cannulation is achieved by slight inward pressure on the back arm of the forceps, directly opposite the micropipette.

26. Advancement of the micropipette should be slow and steady. Stopping or intermittent motions, particularly at the point of puncture, can cause breakage of the micropipette or corneal abrasion. Tribeveling of micropipettes substantially improves ease of corneal puncture.
27. Ensure that the entire volume of microbeads is delivered prior to retraction of the micropipette. The microbead solution is a suspension, which often requires additional time to fully exit the micropipette after it is dispensed by the syringe pump.
28. If a clog of the micropipette is observed or suspected, the eye can be very subtly shifted (not squeezed) with the forceps to promote flow of the solution. If this is unsuccessful, the micropipette should be withdrawn from the eye and the surgery terminated. Reinjection can be attempted when anterior chamber volume returns to normal, typically 24–36 h later.
29. Nonmagnetic microbeads should disperse throughout the anterior chamber and begin collecting in the iridocorneal angle. If microbeads remain near the injection site for longer than 30 s, ensure that forceps are not applying pressure to the eye, which can impede aqueous humor dynamics.
30. The magnetic steering apparatus provides a focused magnetic field for directed delivery of microbeads to the outflow pathway, which reduces off-target delivery. The strength of the magnetic force can be altered by changing the distance between the magnet and the tip of the Allen key. Ideally, the magnetic force should be enough to prevent the microbeads from falling onto the lens or the iris but not so strong as to cause microbead clump formation.
31. To ensure proper sealing of the cornea and prevent corneal injury, wait 24 h between intracameral injections and IOP measurements.
32. Intracameral injection of either microbeads or saline results in substantial changes in fluid volume of the anterior chamber. This is true for successful injections and for those resulting in significant efflux of aqueous humor, that is, corneal puncture without solution delivery. These changes in anterior chamber volume can result in either a substantial increase or decrease in IOP in the first 24–36 h after injections. Additionally, a rat model of ocular hypertension has previously been shown to experience significantly higher elevation in dark phase IOP as compared to the light phase. This phenomenon has been associated with the decrease in outflow facility in this hypertensive

model which exacerbates the effect of increased aqueous humor formation rate during dark phase on IOP elevation [18].

33. Subsequent injections should puncture the cornea in a different area than the original injection. Corneal wound healing from a prior injection as well as subsequent IOP elevations will increase corneal stiffness, thereby making corneal puncture more difficult.

References

1. Sappington RM et al (2010) The microbead occlusion model: a paradigm for induced ocular hypertension in rats and mice. Invest Ophthalmol Vis Sci 51(1):207–216
2. Cone FE et al (2010) Differential susceptibility to experimental glaucoma among 3 mouse strains using bead and viscoelastic injection. Exp Eye Res 91(3):415–424
3. Samsel PA et al (2011) A novel method for the induction of experimental glaucoma using magnetic microspheres. Invest Ophthalmol Vis Sci 52(3):1671–1675
4. Frankfort BJ et al (2013) Elevated intraocular pressure causes inner retinal dysfunction before cell loss in a mouse model of experimental glaucoma. Invest Ophthalmol Vis Sci 54(1): 762–770
5. Chen H et al (2011) Optic neuropathy due to microbead-induced elevated intraocular pressure in the mouse. Invest Ophthalmol Vis Sci 52(1):36–44
6. Calkins DJ, Lambert W, Formichella CR, WM ML, Sappington RM (2018) Microbead occlusion model in mice (Chapter 9). Methods in molecular biology: methods in glaucoma research. Springer Publishing, Inc. Methods Mol Biol 1695:23–39. https://doi.org/10.1007/978-1-4939-7407-8_3
7. Ito YA, Belforte N, Cueva Vargas JL, Di Polo A (2016) A magnetic microbead occlusion model to induce ocular hypertension-dependent glaucoma in mice. J Vis Exp 109:e53731. https://doi.org/10.3791/53731. PMID: 27077732; PMCID: PMC4841308
8. Hu Y, Danias J (2018) Noninvasive intraocular pressure measurement in animals models of glaucoma. Methods Mol Biol 1695:49–61. https://doi.org/10.1007/978-1-4939-7407-8_5. PMID: 29190017; PMCID: PMC5815315
9. Morris CA, Crowston JG, Lindsey JD, Danias J, Weinreb RN (2006) Comparison of invasive and non-invasive tonometry in the mouse. Exp Eye Res 82(6):1094–1099. https://doi.org/10.1016/j.exer.2005.12.001. Epub 2006 Feb 7. PMID: 16466714
10. Filippopoulos T, Matsubara A, Danias J, Huang W, Dobberfuhl A, Ren L, Mittag T, Miller JW, Grosskreutz CL (2006) Predictability and limitations of non-invasive murine tonometry: comparison of two devices. Exp Eye Res 83(1):194–201. https://doi.org/10.1016/j.exer.2005.12.005. Epub 2006 Mar 24. PMID: 16564045
11. Pease ME, Cone FE, Gelman S, Son JL, Quigley HA (2011) Calibration of the TonoLab tonometer in mice with spontaneous or experimental glaucoma. Invest Ophthalmol Vis Sci 52(2):858–864. https://doi.org/10.1167/iovs.10-5556
12. Saeki T, Aihara M, Ohashi M, Araie M (2008) The efficacy of TonoLab in detecting physiological and pharmacological changes of mouse intraocular pressure--comparison with Tono-Pen and microneedle manometery. Curr Eye Res 33(3):247–252. https://doi.org/10.1080/02713680801919716. PMID: 18350435
13. Qiu Y, Yang H, Lei B (2014) Effects of three commonly used anesthetics on intraocular pressure in mouse. Curr Eye Res 39(4): 365–369. https://doi.org/10.3109/02713683.2013.845224. Epub 2013 Nov 11. PMID: 24215504
14. Tsuchiya S, Higashide T, Hatake S, Sugiyama K (2021) Effect of inhalation anesthesia with isoflurane on circadian rhythm of murine intraocular pressure. Exp Eye Res 203:108420. https://doi.org/10.1016/j.exer.2020.108420. Epub 2020 Dec 24. PMID: 33359512
15. Gerberich BG, Hannon BG, Brown DM, Read AT, Ritch MD, Schrader Echeverri E, Nichols L, Potnis C, Sridhar S, Toothman MG, Schwaner SA, Winger EJ, Huang H, Gershon GS, Feola AJ, Pardue MT, Prausnitz MR, Ethier CR (2022) Evaluation of spatially targeted scleral stiffening on neuroprotection in a

rat model of glaucoma. Transl Vis Sci Technol 11(5):7. https://doi.org/10.1167/tvst.11.5.7. PMID: 35536721; PMCID: PMC9100482

16. Aihara M, Lindsey JD, Weinreb RN (2003) Twenty-four-hour pattern of mouse intraocular pressure. Exp Eye Res 77(6):681–686. https://doi.org/10.1016/j.exer.2003.08.011

17. Savinova OV, Sugiyama F, Martin JE, Tomarev SI, Paigen BJ, Smith RS, John SW (2001) Intraocular pressure in genetically distinct mice: an update and strain survey. BMC Genet 2:12. https://doi.org/10.1186/1471-2156-2-12

18. Jia L, Cepurna WO, Johnson EC, Morrison JC (2000) Patterns of intraocular pressure elevation after aqueous humor outflow obstruction in rats. Invest Ophthalmol Vis Sci 41(6):1380–1385

Chapter 21

Continuous Wireless Telemetric Measurement of Intraocular Pressure (IOP), Ocular Perfusion Pressure (OPP), and Cerebrospinal Fluid Pressure (CSFP) in Nonhuman Primates (NHPs)

J. Crawford Downs

Abstract

Intraocular pressure (IOP) and cerebrospinal fluid pressure (CSFP) telemetry in large animal models can be used to determine the exact IOP, CSFP, translaminar pressure, and translaminar pressure gradient exposure that each normal and treated eye is subjected to relative to its fellow eye. In this way, it is possible to determine the independent contributions of each of these parameters (mean and/or transient fluctuations) to the risk of both the onset and rate of progression of glaucoma. Importantly, we have shown that IOP and CSFP fluctuate continuously by up to 100% over the course of the day, so snapshot cage-side IOP measurements are unable to adequately capture the pressure in the eye; CSFP is not measurable noninvasively at all. Implementation of IOP and CSFP telemetry will allow us to precisely determine the pressure insult in each eye of each animal and thereby unravel the true mechanisms underlying pressure-induced damage to the retinal ganglion cells in glaucoma.

Key words Lamina cribrosa, Mechanical stress, Long-term IOP monitoring, Intraocular pressure fluctuations

1 Introduction

Glaucoma is a leading cause of irreversible blindness worldwide, and the management of glaucoma represents one of most important public health problems facing eye care delivery in the United States [1–3]. Although elevated intraocular pressure (IOP) is one of the most important glaucoma risk factors, many glaucoma patients do not exhibit high IOP during their clinic visits [4, 5]. That said, lowering mean IOP further in these "normotensive" glaucoma patients is still effective in slowing glaucoma progression [4]. In addition, a significant number of patients continue to lose vision despite achieving "normal" IOP levels with IOP-lowering therapy [6, 7]. Large clinical studies have also

Tatjana Jakobs and Paloma B. Liton (eds.), *Glaucoma: Methods and Protocols*, Methods in Molecular Biology, vol. 2858,
https://doi.org/10.1007/978-1-0716-4140-8_21,

identified many ocular hypertensive patients who never develop glaucoma even after years of elevated IOP [6, 7]. One possible explanation for the murkiness in the IOP-glaucoma relationship is that we know very little about true IOP in patients due to limitations inherent to current snapshot measurement techniques and that IOP fluctuations play an important role in disease pathophysiology. IOP fluctuates over time [8–15], and when one considers both the frequency and magnitude of IOP fluctuations, it becomes clear that a single IOP measurement taken during normal clinic hours is insufficient to characterize true IOP and hence the real pathology and risk of disease progression in glaucoma patients. Long-term IOP fluctuations have been reported to be a strong predictor for glaucoma progression, especially in normotensive patients with low mean IOP levels [16, 17]. A recent clinical study has shown that fluctuations in circumlimbal corneal stretch measured with the TriggerFish contact lens sensor, presumably associated with transient IOP fluctuations, is associated with visual field progression in glaucoma patients [15]. Finally, the UK Glaucoma Treatment Study investigators recently reported that ocular pulse amplitude (OPA) was an independent predictor of rapid glaucoma progression in patients, in addition to mean IOP [18].

The mechanisms of glaucomatous damage to the retinal ganglion cells (RGC) are not fully understood. The RGCs and their axons transmit visual information from the retina to the brain, and the RGC axons pass out of the eye through the scleral canal at the optic nerve head (ONH). The ONH is spanned by a fenestrated connective tissue structure known as the lamina cribrosa (LC) that provides structural support for the laminar RGC axons as the they leave the eye [19]. The preponderance of evidence suggests that RGC axons are damaged in the laminar region of the ONH in glaucoma [20–24]. Among the known risk factors, one of the most consistent is elevated intraocular pressure (IOP), although the safe IOP threshold in each eye varies widely as mentioned previously.

There have been conflicting reports as to whether ocular perfusion pressure (OPP) contributes to glaucoma risk [25–35]. It is important to note that most previous studies have either used snapshot IOP measurements or contact lens sensors, which can only measure circumferential corneal stretch related to IOP fluctuations and cannot be calibrated to IOP itself. These IOP measurement methods either fail to quantify IOP fluctuations (tonometry) or cannot be calibrated to true IOP (contact lens sensor). Only contact lens "IOP" sensors have been able to capture the frequency of transient IOP fluctuations over periods longer than a few seconds, but they can only be used for discrete 24 hour periods and cannot quantify the IOP magnitude [15, 36]. Blood pressure is also generally measured with sphygmomanometry at the brachial artery that captures BP at a single time point using an indirect measurement that is error prone [37]. As a result, studies of the role of OPP dynamics in glaucoma have been impractical to date.

Retrobulbar cerebrospinal fluid pressure (CSFP) surrounding the optic nerve partially counteracts IOP at the LC through the translaminar pressure (TLP = IOP − CSFP) [38–54]. While IOP acts on the entire globe and affects ONH biomechanics through both laminar and scleral canal stress and strain, CSFP only acts on the retrolaminar optic nerve. Recent retrospective clinical studies and animal experiments have reported that higher CSFP (measured with a single lumbar puncture) is protective against glaucoma, and low CSFP increases glaucoma risk [39, 40]. Prospective clinical studies have found that CSFP decreases with age and is lower in patients with both primary open-angle glaucoma and normal tension glaucoma compared with either healthy controls or patients with ocular hypertension [51, 55]. However, TLP estimates in these reports are extrapolated due to their CSFP and IOP measurements occurring at different time points, sometimes months apart [41]. In addition, since the LC bears the bulk of the pressure load in the ONH due to its high stiffness relative to the surrounding neural tissues, thickness of the LC plays a critical role in the distribution of stress and strain in the ONH through the translaminar pressure gradient (TLPG = TLP/LC thickness), adding a morphological component to TLP. Given the interplay between IOP and CSFP acting on the ONH, it is plausible that the translaminar pressure (TLP = IOP − CSFP) is more relevant to glaucoma than either of these pressures alone, although IOP and CSFP may affect the ONH differently according to some numerical simulations [50, 56] and experimental studies [57].

Given the potential roles of mean IOP, OPP, and CSFP and their fluctuations and dysregulation in glaucoma patients, it is critical to study disease characteristics in glaucoma models that closely recapitulate the true character of these critical pressures. The nonhuman primate (NHP) is the only animal in which experimental IOP elevation can be used to develop an optic neuropathy that is clinically and histologically indistinguishable from human glaucoma [59–62]. NHPs develop experimental glaucoma in 3–-12 months after moderate chronic IOP elevation from normal (11–14 mmHg) to 22–35 mmHg. This accelerated time course allows for rapid testing of new technologies and treatments prior to undergoing human device development and long-duration human clinical trials. The NHP glaucoma model is also unilateral, leaving an untreated control eye for longitudinal comparison. In this model, unilateral, noninvasive lasering of the trabecular meshwork (TM) induces unilateral chronic IOP elevation. The model has been widely used and is powerful because the NHP eye shares many of the contributing risk factors for ONH susceptibility in human glaucoma, such as ONH connective tissue architecture, blood flow, a wide age range, and connective tissue stiffness. Clinical Heidelberg Spectralis 2 spectral-domain optical coherence tomography (SD-OCT) imaging is easily accomplished in the NHP with settings similar to those in patients.

1.1 Indwelling Bilateral IOP, ICP/CSFP, and OPP Telemetry

Very little is known about IOP, OPP, CSFP, and TLP dynamics, as characterization of the true, 24 hour pressures in individual eyes have been impossible due to the lack of accurate continuous measurement of both IOP and CSFP in patients or large animal models of glaucoma, such as NHPs. Changes in IOP, CSFP, and TLP occur very frequently and at multiple time scales, yet it is unknown if these fluctuations impact glaucoma development and/or progression [52, 53, 63–65]. To address this critical barrier, we have developed and validated a fully implantable, wireless telemetry system that can measure IOP, intracranial pressure (ICP, a surrogate measure of CSFP) continuously in NHPs to characterize IOP, OPP, CSFP, TLP, and TLPG dynamics over long periods [63–65]. This system will be used to study the independent contributions of these pressures to glaucoma development and progression using continuous wireless telemetry in Rhesus macaque monkeys, a powerful large animal model of glaucoma with a fenestrated collagenous LC similar to humans. The NHP model of glaucoma allows for baseline characterization prior to induction of unilateral IOP elevation, and IOP/CSFP telemetry allows quantification of cumulative differential IOP/TLP exposure in the glaucoma eyes relative to their fellow control eyes. We can then determine if baseline IOP fluctuation, CSFP, and TLPG contribute to glaucoma susceptibility and progression, with all analyses taking the true differential IOP exposure in fellow eyes within animals into account.

Our previous studies using IOP, OPP, and CSFP telemetry in NHPs have shown that transient IOP fluctuations in NHPs occur ~10,000 times per waking hour and comprise 6–16% of the total IOP-related mechanical energy the eye must absorb, depending on the animal. In addition, NHPs exhibit a strong diurnal IOP cycle that is of similar magnitude to humans despite sleeping upright, showing that they are a suitable model for translational studies. Using NHPs equipped with telemetry systems, we have shown that (1) transient IOP fluctuations occur ~10,000 times per waking hour and comprise 6–16% of the total IOP-related mechanical energy the eye must absorb, depending on the NHP [63]; also, transient IOP fluctuations exhibit a strong diurnal cycle [63, 66]; (2) NHPs exhibit a strong diurnal TLP cycle (driven primarily by ICP/CSFP) that is of similar magnitude to humans despite sleeping upright, showing that NHPs are a suitable model for TLP studies [64]; (3) while IOP is the only modifiable and readily measurable pressure-based risk factor for glaucoma, the rank order of TLP and TLPG differed greatly from the rank order of IOP, demonstrating that a comprehensive view of relevant risk factors is warranted [65]. Finally, there is tremendous variability among NHPs in IOP, CSFP, TLP, and TLPG and their transient and diurnal fluctuations, which allows for rigorous testing of hypotheses regarding the independent contributions of these factors to glaucoma in the NHP model.

1.2 Important Considerations for Telemetric Measures of Physiologic Variables

There are several telemetry systems for animal and patient monitoring available commercially. Critical variables one needs to consider are the following:

- Sampling frequency (how often the parameter is measured), which is dependent on the character of the signal itself, for example, does it fluctuate on short time scales and do those fluctuations need to be captured?
- Movement in tissues/organs in which pressures need to be measured, and how that is to be accomplished without disrupting the tissues/organ or the transducer and its wiring
- Duty cycle (the period of time measurements are acquired and if there are breaks between sampling periods)
- Number of channels/variables monitored and whether video or sound is also necessary
- Radio frequency interference resulting from sources in the room, caging, the animal's body, or other implants nearby
- Data transmission distance and wireless protocol, which affect the amount of energy required to reliably stream data to a receiving antenna
- Antenna location, especially when monitoring species like NHPs that can interact with exposed hardware and wiring
- Size of the implant's electronics and battery package, which is determined by a combination of the animal's body size, length of study, sampling frequency, duty cycle, number of data channels, and transmission range
- Transducer calibration to a reference standard to correct for drift error and assess linearity, including the frequency of those calibrations, and how drift/linearity correction will be applied to the raw telemetry data
- Location of transducer relative to tissue/organ of interest, for example, should an IOP transducer be in the eye itself or adjacent to the eye and connected to the eye with a tube
- Detection and filtering of signal noise and dropout, as well as smoothing if there is any jitter in the data stream
- Data summarization—mean, time intervals, time-window averaging, detection, and characterization of transients (magnitude, duration, area/impulse)

2 Materials

2.1 TSE-Systems Stellar Implant Systems

Our current Stellar XXL Implant system is commercially available from TSE-Systems (Chesterfield, MO, USA) and consists of a titanium battery and electronic case with integral suture loops, an antenna, and helically wound, silicone-encased wire leads to each transducer that allow for stretch. Transducers in our system allow for monitoring up to three pressures simultaneously in each animal: bilateral IOP plus either carotid artery blood pressure (BP) or intraparenchymal intracranial pressure (ICP) that is a surrogate measure for retrobulbar CSFP (Fig. 1). Animal motion and body temperature sensors are also integrated into each implant. The implants include a single-use C-cell Li-Ion battery, which will power a three-pressure implant for ~28 months on a 33% duty cycle (data acquisition at 250 Hz for 40 s of every 2 min period, 24 h/day). The implants do not store data on board the device and transmit continuously during data acquisition via a wireless link to a ceiling-mounted antenna/access point that is wired via UAB to a data acquisition computer. In our hands, these implants generally yield <5% dropout/noise when two antennas are ceiling mounted above a standard 6′ × 6′ NHP cage wherein the NHP has the full cage space to roam.

2.2 Data Acquisition

Telemetry implants are controlled through the TSE-Systems Stellar Commander software utility that wirelessly connects the hardware access point to the implant through the transceiver in the animal's

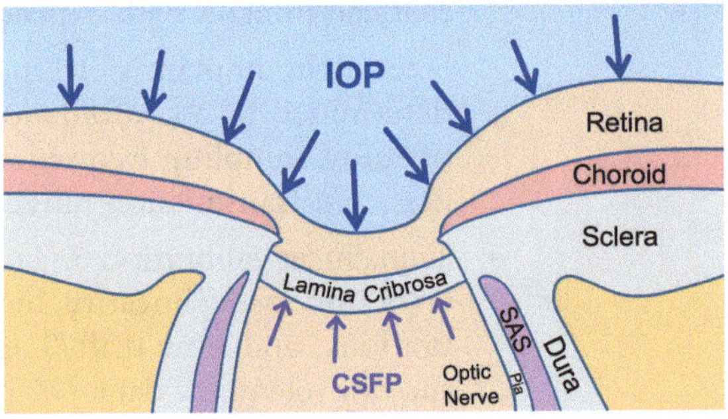

Fig. 1 Mechanical stress and strain are a constant presence within the ONH at all levels of IOP, CSFP, and TLP. IOP and cerebrospinal fluid pressure (CSFP) act mechanically on the tissues of the eye, producing deformations, strain, and stress within the tissues. These deformations depend on the geometry and material properties of each individual eye. In a biomechanical paradigm, IOP- and CSFP-related stress and strain also induce connective tissue damage directly (laminar beam yield), or indirectly (ischemia), which damage axons and drives glaucomatous cupping and cell-mediated tissue remodeling processes that alter both the tissues' geometry and mechanical response to load. SAS, subarachnoid space. (Reproduced from Downs, [58] with permission)

battery/electronic package. Each implant transmits on a different frequency, which allows up to 16 implants to operate simultaneously in the same room without interference. Each hardware access point can accommodate up to eight telemetry implants via hardwired connections to antennas (model PA9-12, TE Connectivity, Berwyn, PA, USA) attached to a ceiling-mounted rail placed above the row of cages; at least one antenna is required for each NHP, and multiple antennas can be wired together in parallel to provide adequate coverage for large enclosures. Telemetry data are acquired and recorded using the NOTOCORD-hem data acquisition system (Instem, Philadelphia, PA, USA), and the access points include a barometric pressure sensor, so all pressure transducers include automatic atmospheric pressure compensation. This system acquires uncalibrated telemetry signals on a Windows 10 PC or laptop through a USB connection to the TSE Stellar hardware access point, along with time-synchronized HD video via Hikvision tilt-pan-zoom video cameras. Scheduling of telemetry data acquisition date, time, and duty cycle are accomplished in NOTOCORD-hem, which also provides data/video playback and analysis capabilities.

2.3 Materials for Surgical Implantation (All Sterile)

Gas sterilizer, ethylene oxide (EtO)

Sterile isotonic balanced salt solution (BSS), 500 mL IV bottle, with the following drugs added:

- 2 mL of Decadron (4 mg/mL)
  - 0.1 mL of Clindamycin (150 mg/mL)
  - 0.15 mL of Gentamicin (40 mg/mL)

70% ethanol

Luer-lock syringes (3 mL, 10 mL)

Syringe needles (27G, 18G)

Syringe cannula, stainless steel, 27G

IV infusion set tubing for bonneting

Tygon tubing, 1/8″ inner diameter with 1/32″ wall thickness for bonneting

Sterile surgical drapes

Tegaderm patches, frame style, 4″ × 4-3/4″

Sterile gauze pads

Sterile cotton tip applicators

Razek Craniotomy hand drill, gas sterilized

3/16″-diameter high-speed steel twist drill bit, gas sterilized

F-size high speed steel twist drill bit, gas sterilized

3/32″-diameter high speed steel twist drill bit, gas sterilized

5/16″ high speed steel bottoming tap with handle, gas sterilized
Scalpel (#10 and #15 blade)
Storz orbital retractor/elevator (double ended, 16 mm/25 mm)
Metzenbaum tonsil scissors
Crile/Rankin hemostatic forceps, 15.9 cm
Tenzel double-ended periosteal elevator
Storz Senn-Kanavel retractor
Surgical scissors
Jacobson micro mosquito forceps, curved
ALM retractor
Stryker 1.5 × 5 mm cross pin self-tapping maxillofacial bone screws
Sterile Philips-head screwdriver
Silk suture material (size 00)
Nylon monofilament suture (00)
Vicryl absorbable suture (8-0 and 4-0)
Braided polyester nonabsorbable suture (00)
Stainless steel wire (27G)
Vetbond skin adhesive
Bone wax
Ophthalmic antibiotic ointment with Neomycin, Polymyxin B Sulfate, Bacitracin Zinc
Bandages
Horseshoe-shaped gel pads, 1″ thick

3 Methods

3.1 Preparation

The implant systems (Fig. 2) are gas sterilized with EtO, and the IOP transducer reservoir and aqueous transduction tubes are dry, so they must be filled in a sterile manner just prior to surgical implantation. The IOP transducer filling procedure is performed on a sterile field in an aseptic procedure as follows:

1. Fill a 3 mL syringe equipped with a 27G blunt cannula with 70% ethanol and insert it into the fill tube.
2. Slowly fill the transducer reservoir with fluid, while holding the tube end vertically so that all bubbles exit the system.
3. Switch the 27G blunt cannula over to a 10 mL syringe filled with sterile BSS while holding the cannula and syringe Luer lock ends underwater in a small dish of sterile BSS to avoid introducing bubbles into the system.

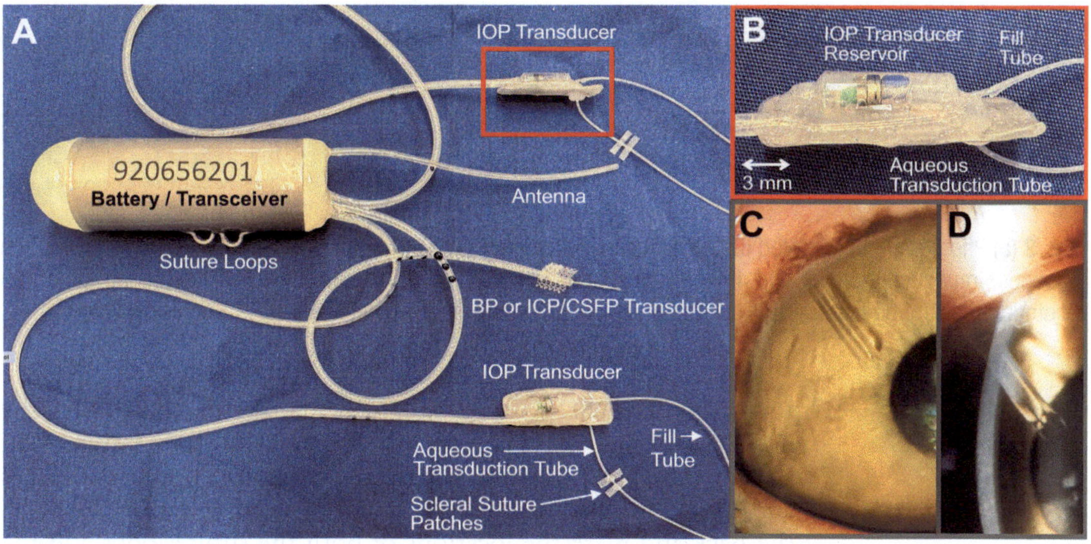

Fig. 2 (**a**) Photograph of the TSE-Stellar Total Implant System, showing the implant battery/electronics package, bilateral extraocular IOP transducers, and the BP/ICP/CSFP transducer. (**b**) Closeup photo of an IOP transducer showing the aqueous-filled IOP transducer reservoir and fill/aqueous transduction tubes. (**c** and **d**) Slit lamp photographs of the aqueous transduction tube implanted in the anterior chamber of a representative NHP eye. (Reproduced with permission from Jasien et al. [67])

4. Flush the transducer reservoir and tubing with at least 4 mL of BSS, running IOP telemetry to make sure you do not exceed 125 mmHg filling pressure.
5. Tie off fill tube end only adjacent to the end of the cannula with 00 sterile silk suture.
6. Cover the eye tube/scleral anchor patches with plastic tubing from an IV infusion set, with the distal end cut at a 45-degree angle to facilitate pulling through the orbital tissues; tie the outer tube tight to the inner aqueous transduction tube with 00 silk suture between scleral suture patches to hold the outer tubing on, and then tie that to the transducer baseplate with another silk suture, keeping the aqueous transduction and fill tube loops secured under the tie (Fig. 2).
7. After the IOP transducers are filled, secure all three transducers in custom stainless-steel bonnets equipped with sterile 00 silk suture loops that allow for pulling the transducers through subcutaneous tunnels without damage (Fig. 3).
8. Cover the BP/CSFP transducer with a length of 1/8″-inner-diameter Tygon tubing, fitted onto a custom stainless-steel bonnet plug (Fig. 3); slit the tube partway to facilitate transducer and lead mesh insertion, and then tie securely with 00 silk suture placed over the mesh (Fig. 3c).
9. Cover the bonneted implant and leads with a sterile towel.

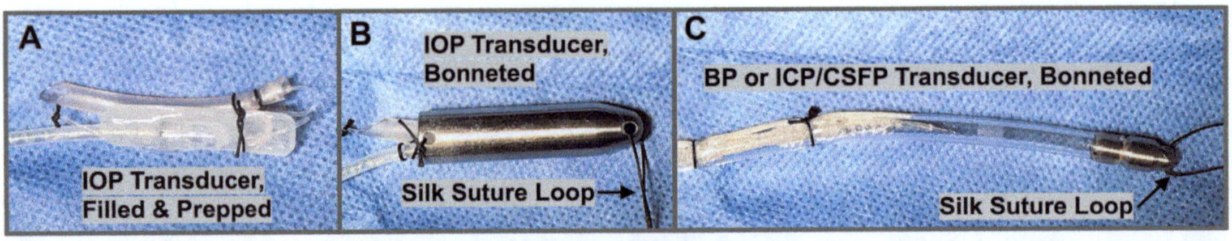

Fig. 3 (**a**) Photograph of the filled IOP transducer and tubes bundled in preparation for bonneting, showing the aqueous transduction tube and integrated scleral suture patches covered with a protecting tube. (**b**) Photograph of the bonneted IOP transducer. (**c**) Photograph of the bonneted BP/ICP/CSFP transducer

3.2 Surgical Implantation

Prep/shave animal and create aseptic field from the mid-back to the nose, dorsal side up. Then prep and drape the shaved area using U-drape, with back exposed; wrap the drape just under the brows and across the nose to cover the eyelids. Place the implant body on the back and mark the locations of both the suture loops and the pocket incision (~4 cm anterior to edge of the implant) with a surgical marker. With a large scalpel, open an ~8 cm pocket incision through the skin perpendicular to the dorsal midline and then use large scissors to blunt dissect a large subcutaneous pocket just above plane of the musculature. The pocket should be wide and deep enough to accommodate the implant and allow access on either side to tie the securing sutures. Create subcutaneous pocket ~8 cm deep and ~6 cm wide on the side of the neck for redundant lead.

Make a ~4 cm incision all the way to bone above each eye on the brow bone, extending from 1 cm medial to the jaw muscle pocket out to 0.5 cm from the canthus. Use a periosteal elevator to separate the periosteum from the underlying bone for the whole length of the incision, both above the incision past the edge of the muscle pocket and below the incision to the orbital entry. The opening into the orbit should be wide enough to accommodate an elevator spatula bent to the shape of the orbital roof, pushed into the orbit above the eye below the muscle pocket to shield eye from the orbitotomy drill. On top, peel the periosteum back along top of brow into the medial 1 cm of muscle pocket; relieve periosteum with scalpel parallel to the dorsal midline for 1.5 cm at top edge of muscle pocket. Use an elevator placed in pocket in the orbit to protect eye, hold back the muscle and skin with a Senn-Kanavel retractor, and then use a standard 3/16″-diameter twist drill bit in a Razek craniotomy hand drill to create an orbitotomy in the anterior medial corner of the muscle pocket; clean out the bone debris with a cotton-tipped applicator, and then remove protecting elevator in the orbit. Pack the incision with one-half of a 2″ × 2″ sterile gauze pad soaked in sterile BSS. Repeat on the other eye.

Shift focus back to the subcutaneous implant pocket on the back, and hold open pocket with an elevator, placing a 30-cm-long section of 00 nylon monofilament suture (Ethilon, Ethicon, Johnson & Johnson MedTech, New Brunswick, NJ, USA) under each of the suture loop locations, making sure to bite into deep muscle; secure the ends of each suture loop with a hemostat marked with one, two, or three bands of tape on the arm so you can keep track of the anterior-to-posterior order of the loops, two on each side and one in the center of the implant body. Place the implant body above the pocket and use curved mosquito hemostats to pass the sutures through the implant suture loops, and then resecure suture loop ends in the marked hemostats. Once all implant sutures are placed through the loops in the implant body, insert the implant in the tissue pocket, and then handtie each suture, proceeding posterior to anterior until all sutures are tied and ends are trimmed. Keep the implant leads covered in a sterile towel draped posteriorly over the back of the pocket to protect them from contamination and eliminate the possibility that a lead is mistakenly damaged while trimming the sutures.

Option 1: OPP—Initial Placement of BP Transducer A 2-cm-wide subcutaneous tunnel is blunt-dissected with large scissors down the right side of the neck to the farthest anterior point possible, with care taken that the tunnel is roughly midway between the lower jaw and the clavicle. The bonneted BP transducer is then inserted as far as possible to the anterior-most aspect of the tunnel and left there.

Option 2: ICP/CSFP Transducer Use a scalpel to cut ~3-cm-long incisions parallel to the dorsal midline above the locations of the craniotomies for the ICP transducer on the right side and the indwelling titanium calibration port on the left side. Scrape to bare bone with the scalpel and insert a retractor to keep the incision open and cranium exposed. Use a hand drill to create an F-sized craniotomy for the titanium port. Use a 5/16″ bottoming tap to thread the bone in the craniotomy, being careful to keep the tap perpendicular to the cranium. Clear the bone debris with a cotton-tipped applicator, nick the dura with an 18G needle, and install the titanium port by threading it into the cranium via the thread, tightening it to the cranial surface with a sterile wrench. Install the central lead screw into the brain parenchyma, along with a sterile silicone washer coated with antibiotic ointment using a sterile Philips-head screwdriver.

Use a large scissor to blunt dissect a subcutaneous lead tunnel from the transducer craniotomy incision toward the midline to the anterior edge of the implant body pocket; leave the scissors in place, and then pass a large hemostat under the scissors through the subcutaneous track to the implant pocket, and then withdraw the scissors. Grasp the suture loop on the ICP transducer bonnet with the hemostat and pull the bonneted transducer through the track to the craniotomy incision. Remove the bonnet, and then bend the transducer lead 90 degrees away from the plane of the open mesh such that the mesh patch will lay flat on the cranium when the transducer is inserted into the parenchyma. While holding the transducer back to avoid damage, use a hand drill to drill a 3/32″--diameter craniotomy for the transducer, clear the bone debris with a cotton-tipped applicator, nick the dura with an 18G needle, and insert the ICP transducer into the brain parenchyma. Seal the craniotomy with bone wax with a dull-edged spatula, and then secure the mesh patch to the skull using Stryker 1.5 × 5 mm cross pin self-tapping bone screws.

Initial Placement of IOP Transducers Create subcutaneous tunnels for the IOP transducer leads by blunt dissecting with scissors, working from the brow incisions back to the implant pocket on the back, being careful to avoid the ICP calibration port, ICP transducer lead, implant, and other leads. Leave the scissors in place, run the large hemostats under the scissors through the track, and then withdraw the scissors after the hemostats are in place. Grasp the suture loop on the IOP transducer bonnet with the hemostat, and pull the bonneted transducer through the track to the brow incision. Repeat for the other eye, and then pack both incisions with half of a 2″ × 2″ cotton gauze soaked with BSS. Pull slack out of the leads at the implant pocket, and place redundant leads in the pocket on the side of the neck that was created previously. Create a subcutaneous tunnel for the implant antenna along the midline of the skull, thread the antenna into the track, and then use a mattress suture to secure the antenna to the underside of the skin at the anterior edge of the implant pocket incision. Close the implant pocket incision, and the cranial port and ICP transducer incisions with two layers of subcutaneous sutures, and cover with Vetbond skin adhesive.

Cover the brow incisions with Tegaderm to maintain sterility, and then remove other drapes. Turn the animal on its back, placing horseshoe-shaped gel pads around the implant to shield it from table pressure. Prep and drape the surgical sites for aseptic technique.

Option 1: OPP—Final Placement of Carotid BP Transducer - Orient the chin such that the neck is extended, and the right side is slightly more exposed. Palpate the carotid artery to determine its location, and then use a scalpel to make a ~8-cm-long incision parallel to the midline above the artery. Blunt dissect to the artery, carefully avoiding the jugular vein and nerves, to isolate a 2.5 cm section of the carotid artery. Place prewetted, 15-cm-long sections of 00 silk suture under each end of the isolated artery, with the tail ends draped out of the incision. Prepare a 1″ 18G needle to pierce the artery by bending the hypodermic cutting edge and tip perpendicular to the needle shank with a large hemostat and inserting the swab end of a wooden-shanked cotton swab tightly into the needle hub. Locate the end of the preplaced bonneted transducer by palpation through the wall of the incision, and then blunt dissect to the transducer to bring it into the incision; remove the bonnet. With an assistant pulling up the silk sutures on both ends of the isolated artery, use the bent needle to pierce the anterior surface of the artery midway between the sutures, and then slide the transducer into the artery lumen toward the heart, momentarily relieving tension on the proximal suture to allow the transducer lead to pass by it and then retension on the suture. Once the transducer is past the proximal suture, verify that a strong cardiac pulse is seen in the BP telemetry signal. While continuing to hold tension in the sutures around the carotid artery to block blood flow, use gauze and cotton-tipped applicators to carefully remove all blood and fluid from the insertion site, and then apply several drops of Vetbond cyanoacrylate adhesive to the insertion site below the open mesh to seal the hole in the carotid. Slowly release suture tension to verify that there is no bleeding, and then remove the sutures. Place single mattress sutures with 00 silk around the lead insertion site, 2 cm toward the jaw from the insertion, and on the lead loop below the jaw, taking care to avoid nerves, vessels/veins, and the cheek pouch. Close the neck incision with two layers of 4-0 Vicryl suture.

Final Placement of IOP Transducers Position the animal's head to optimize the approach for the eye surgeon using gel positioners and towels. Prep the face and eyes for sterility, and then drape with a sterile adhesive eye surgery drape. Roll in the ophthalmic surgical microscope and open the drapes with Westcott scissors. The eye surgeon then opens the conjunctiva and Tenon's capsule in the superotemporal quadrant with Westcott scissors and blunt dissects to bare sclera to form a track back to the orbitotomy. A closed mosquito hemostat is then passed through the track into the orbitotomy, and the tips are cleared of tissue with a scalpel to allow the hemostat to grasp the 45-degree end of the bonnet tube containing the aqueous transduction tube of the IOP transducer. The bonnet tube is then pulled into the track to expose the near end of the bonnet tube at the eye, where the silk sutures are cut, freeing the bonnet, which is then removed, leaving the aqueous transduction tube and scleral suture patches exposed in the incision near the limbus. The suture patches are then secured to the sclera with 9-0 nylon monofilament suture. The tube is trimmed to length and inserted into the anterior chamber through a track created with a 25G needle, with care to place the tube in the center of the angle between the iris and the corneal endothelium. Tube length should be set such that ~2.5 mm is visible in the anterior chamber, and the tube does not impede imaging through the pupil or touch the corneal endothelium. The incision in the conjunctiva and Tenon's capsule is then closed with two layers of running 8-0 Vicryl absorbable suture. Repeat this procedure for the other eye.

After the ocular incisions are closed, the brow incisions are exposed by carefully cutting through the drape and Tegaderm with scissors, and a Stryker 1.5 × 5 mm cross pin self-tapping maxillofacial bone screw is placed through the stainless-steel mesh at the front of the IOP transducer baseplate into the brow ridge. The fill tube is plugged with a 2-mm-long piece of 27G stainless steel wire and tied tightly closed with 00-size braided polyester nonabsorbable suture (Ethibond Excel, Ethicon, Johnson & Johnson MedTech, New Brunswick, NJ, USA). Once the baseplate is secured to the bone, the brow incision is closed with two layers of 4-0 Vicryl absorbable suture (Ethicon, Johnson & Johnson MedTech, New Brunswick, NJ, USA), cleaned, and covered with Vetbond cyanoacrylate skin adhesive. The animal is then recovered and placed back in their cage with warming lamp support. Postoperative exams are done at days 3, 7, 14, 21, and 28 in which the eyes are examined with a slit lamp to detect any abnormality in anterior chamber tube position and assess for ocular infection and inflammation, along with a physical exam of all incision sites to ensure proper healing and treat any abnormalities or infection. During the entire heal-in period, the implant battery/electronics pack is bandaged, and all NHPs are jacketed in custom NHP jackets. In each postoperative exam, jackets and bandages are removed; the incision sites are examined, cleaned, and dressed with antibiotic ointment; sterile bandages are reapplied over the battery/electronic package; and a clean jacket is put on.

3.3 IOP, OPP, and ICP/CSFP Transducer Calibration

After 6–8 weeks of heal-in time, IOP and either OPP or ICP transducers are calibrated in a combined exam performed under general anesthesia. IOP and OPP calibrations are accomplished by raising or lowering a manometer bottle to precisely control IOP, so the IOP transducers can be calibrated at sequential static IOPs of 5–30 mmHg against the reference digital pressure gage [63, 68, 69] and the OPP to central retinal artery (CRA) intermittent or full collapse [69, 70]. The IOP and OPP calibration procedures take approximately 5 min each. Our published data show that there are no ill effects from this procedure [69], which induces short duration IOPs about one-tenth as large as those associated with rubbing one's eyes [71]. ICP/CSFP calibration is accomplished by comparing the indwelling Stellar ICP transducer reading against a clinical gold standard Codman ICP Express microsensor (Integra Life Sciences, Princeton, NJ, USA). IOP calibration is done every 2 weeks, and ICP/CSFP calibrations occur monthly.

IOP Calibration

Each animal is placed under anesthesia, and both eyes cannulated with a 27G scalp vein needle are placed through the cornea into the anterior chamber at the limbus. The needle tube is connected to a bottle of sterile isotonic saline solution via a sterile infusion set, and the connecting tube fitted with a NIST-calibrated inline pressure gage (model XP2i; Crystal Engineering, San Luis Obispo, CA) via a three-way stopcock as previously described [68]. This procedure has been shown to be safe for the animals and does not cause prolonged hypotony [72] or negative affects even when performed biweekly for 2 years [62, 73]. The bottle is lowered until the inline pressure gage reads 5 mmHg, allowed to stabilize, and then the telemetric IOP readings from the implanted transducers are recorded for comparison. The manometer-controlled IOP is raised in increments of 5 mmHg up to 30 mmHg and the telemetric IOP readings compared to that from the calibrated inline pressure gage at each step. The telemetric IOP data is recorded, and the readings from the calibrated inline transducer and the implanted transducer are compared to quantify IOP transducer signal drift and linearity.

OPP Calibration

Ocular perfusion pressure (OPP) is defined as the arterial blood pressure within the eye minus IOP, which is calculated directly from the continuous IOP and carotid artery BP telemetry data as follows [69, 70]. To calibrate OPP using the calibrated IOP telemetry data and the uncalibrated BP telemetry data, we measure central retinal artery (CRA) diastolic and systolic BP using ophthalmodynamometry (Fig. 3) as a function of continuous telemetric measurement of both IOP and carotid systolic and diastolic BP. By raising the IOP via manometry and observing the IOP levels at which momentary and full CRA collapse first occur in the live infrared video captured by NOTOCORD-hem in real time from the Heidelberg Spectralis OCT alongside the telemetry signals (Fig. 3), we calculate the CRA diastolic (Fig. 3b) and systolic BPs (Fig. 3c). We then calculated continuous OPP directly from the telemetric aortic BP and IOP data streams between OPP calibration exams in Eq. 1 as

$$\text{OPP} = \frac{(\text{CRA systolic BP} - \text{CRA diastolic BP})}{(\text{aortic systolic BP} - \text{aortic diastolic BP})} \times (\text{aBP} - \text{aortic systolic BP}) + \text{CRA systolic BP} - \text{IOP}, \quad (1)$$

where *aBP* and *IOP* denote the continuous carotid BP and IOP telemetry data, respectively. The arterial systolic and diastolic BP values in Eq. 1 are captured along with the CRA systolic and diastolic BPs at the time of OPP calibration. This allows OPP to be calculated directly from the IOP and arterial BP telemetry signals 250 times per second [69]. Note that Eq. 1 scales the arterial pulse pressure amplitude measured with telemetry in a remote large artery (aorta, carotid, or femoral) to the smaller pulse pressure in the CRA, accounts for the higher overall BP in the remote large artery relative to the smaller CRA, and corrects for any drift or error in the telemetry arterial BP transducer reading itself [70].

ICP/CSFP Calibration

Every 4 weeks, the cranial port site is shaved to calibrate CSFP, scrubbed with three successive washes of betadine and Quatricide, and covered with a sterile drape. The skin over the port is opened with a scalpel, the central lead screw is removed, and a sterile, calibrated Codman ICP Express Microsensor (DePuy Synthes, Raynham, MA) is inserted into the brain parenchyma of the full depth of the lead screw shaft and then retracted ~1 mm. A sterile silicone washer coated with antibiotic ointment placed around the Codman microsensor lead is used to seal the microsensor lead to the interior sidewall of the port bolt to prevent CSF fluid egress, maintain ICP during tilt, and prevent contaminants from entering the cranium. The animal is then tilted from the baseline prone position (0°) to +45° (head up) incline position and −45° (head down) decline position and then back to the prone position in 15° increments, with care taken to allow for pressure stabilization at each step while ICP/CSFP is continuously recorded from both the indwelling Stellar telemetry sensor and the adjacent Codman Microsensor at 250Hz with NOTOCORD-hem data acquisition software (Fig. 4) [64]. After data collection, the sensor is removed, and the port is resealed with a new sterile lead screw and silicone washer coated in triple antibiotic ointment, and then the skin is sutured closed over the port and allowed to heal. We have not experienced any infections or complications from over 60 CSFP calibrations done in 4 NHPs over 12 months that were used in our recent publications [64, 65, 74]. Total combined exam time is approximately 2 h and 30 min, after which the dexmedetomidine anesthesia is reversed with Antisedan and the animal is returned to its cage for immediate recovery. Each position is held until the pressures of both sensors are stable, and the values are compared to assess Stellar pressure transducer drift against the Codman Microsensor gold standard. There is remarkable agreement between ICP measured with the Codman microsensor and indwelling Stellar telemetry transducer during these procedures (Fig. 5). Although the transducers are linear, the initial prone position is used as the calibration reference for consistency.

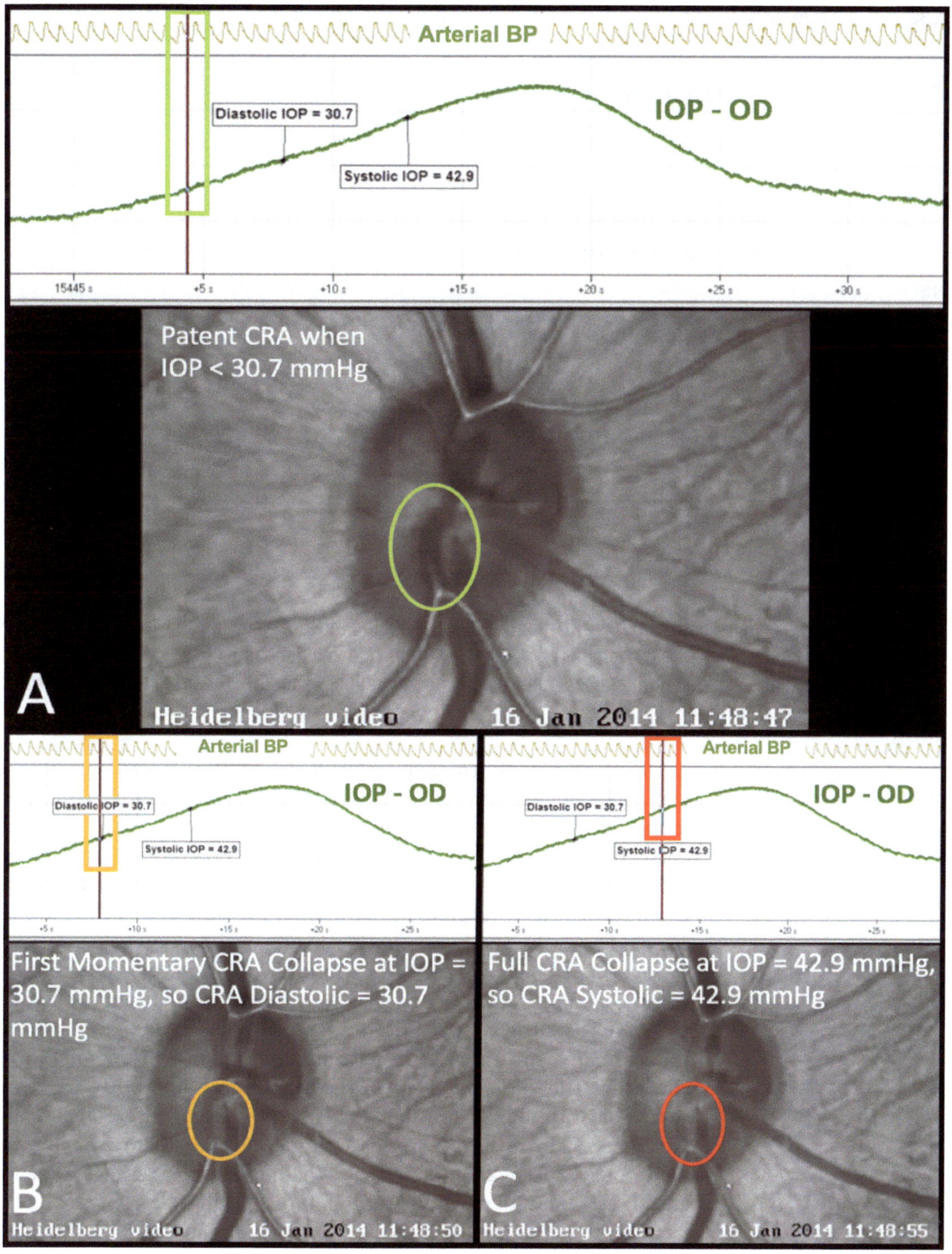

Fig. 4 (**a**) IOP is manually elevated while IOP and carotid artery BP are monitored via telemetry and the ONH is visualized in real time using the infrared image from the Heidelberg Engineering Spectralis OCT device (Spectralis, Heidelberg Engineering, Heidelberg, Germany). The ONH video from the Spectralis is slaved into the NOTOCORD-hem data acquisition system along with the telemetry data stream; CRA patency is monitored. (**b**) The CRA first collapses momentarily at 30.7 mmHg when IOP equals CRA BP, so CRA diastolic BP is 30.7 mmHg. (**c**) The CRA fully collapses at 42.9 mm Hg when IOP equals CRA BP, so CRA systolic BP is 42.9 mmHg. (Reproduced from Markert et al. with permission [69])

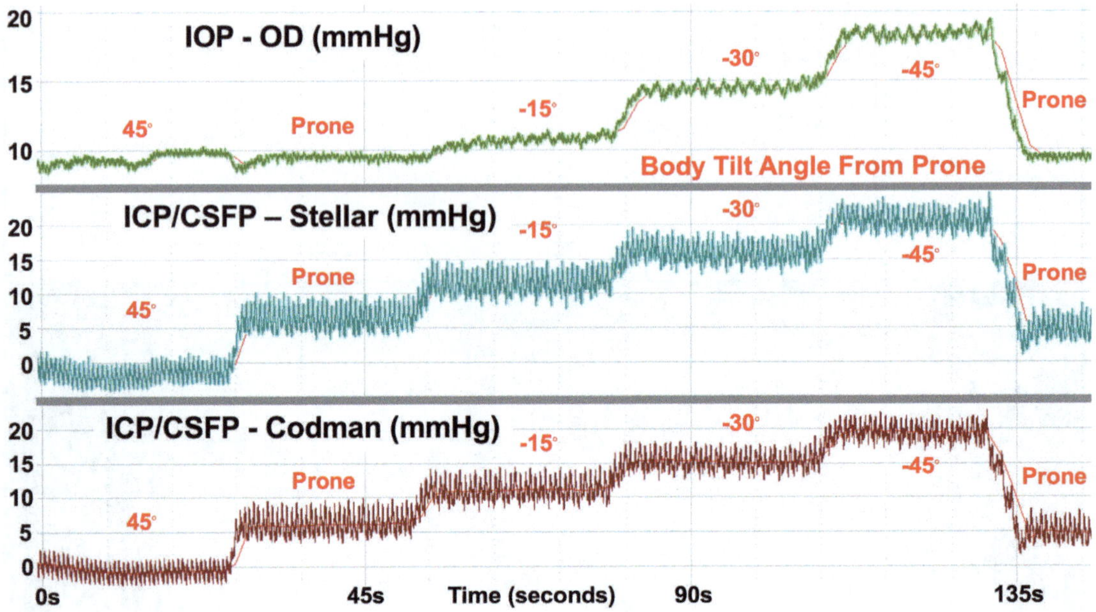

Fig. 5 Labeled screenshot from NOTOCORD-hem data acquisition software showing the IOP and ICP/CSFP signals from the indwelling Stellar telemetry transducers (top and middle) and the Codman ICP Express microsensor (bottom), acquired during a body tilt transducer calibration procedure. (Adapted from Jasien et al. [74], with permission)

ICP and IOP transducer drift is similar at approximately 2 mmHg per month; IOP and ICP data are calibrated to either manometric or clinical gold standards. All pressure data are drift-corrected continuously between calibration procedures via custom software postprocessing routines that assume linear drift between calibrations. Also, changes in barometric pressure are tracked in the animal rooms by the telemetry hardware, and barometric compensation occurs in real time. After calibration, it is then possible to begin telemetry data collection. The continuous IOP radiotelemetry signal is subject to signal transmission loss when the animal moves away from the ceiling-mounted antenna or orients its body such that the signal must pass through significant body mass to reach the antenna. As a result, the data are digitally filtered using an automated algorithm to eliminate signal loss and ensure maximum data quality. Only 24-h periods in which at least 75% of the data in all 24 1-h increments remain after filtering are used for analyses. This approach generally results in a <5% data rejection rate overall.

3.4 Data Summarization: Quantification of Mean and Transient Pressures

First, raw IOP and ICP/CSFP data is calibrated as described above, filtered for noise and signal dropout, and then subjected to a dual-band finite impulse response (FIR) filter to identify transient IOP fluctuation peaks and troughs for quantification in the larger dataset. The full methodology is described in our previous publications [63, 69]. The low-band FIR filter is tuned to identify slower transient IOP fluctuations such as ocular pulse amplitude and CSFP cardiac pulse, while the high-band FIR filter is tuned to identify higher-frequency IOP/CSFP fluctuations from sources such as blink and saccade. The FIR filter was only used to identify the transient IOP fluctuation trough positions in the IOP data stream, with the peaks identified by searching for the largest pressure value between adjacent troughs, to avoid false identification of double peaks such as those shown at time = 2.6 s in Fig. 6. Transient pressure fluctuations are quantified by identifying each pressure peak surrounded by two troughs (Fig. 6); the two troughs were averaged into a single baseline value. The peak-to-baseline difference is catalogued and counted as the magnitude of an individual transient pressure fluctuation. Transient IOP/CSFP magnitude frequency is plotted in a histogram by magnitude bin within each eye. The limits of the smallest magnitude bin were determined by our minimum transient pressure magnitude detection resolution (0.6 mmHg). Larger bin cutoff values were selected arbitrarily, although they were chosen to roughly correspond to ocular pulse amplitude (OPA) at 0.6–2 mmHg and then blinks, saccades, and other sources at 2–5 mmHg, 5–10 mmHg, 10–15 mmHg, and >15 mmHg [63].

Quantification of IOP and CSFP Impulse

Total IOP/CSFP Impulse, defined as the area under the continuous pressure versus time curve, is an engineering-based metric that serves as a surrogate measure of the total amount of pressure-related energy the eye must withstand over time. IOP/CSFP Transient Impulse is quantified as the portion of Total IOP/CSFP Impulse associated with transient pressure fluctuations alone (Fig. 6, orange-shaded area for IOP as an example), calculated using the IOP troughs and peaks identified in earlier analysis steps. IOP Transient Impulse is a surrogate measure of the energy the ocular coat must absorb due to transient IOP fluctuations, and the IOP Baseline Impulse (Fig. 6, green-shaded area) is a measure of the amount of IOP energy the eye must withstand due to momentary baseline IOP. The relative contribution of IOP Transient Impulse, calculated as a percentage of Total IOP Impulse, is averaged hourly over all days for all NHPs. This metric assesses the amount of transient IOP fluctuation-related energy relative to the total IOP-related energy each eye must absorb over time. Similar metrics are calculated for CSFP that capture the amount of transient CSFP-related energy the retrolaminar tissues must absorb over time.

Calculation of TLP and TLPG

Translaminar pressure (TLP) is calculated continuously as IOP-CSFP, which are both calibrated as described above [64]. The translaminar pressure gradient (TLPG) is calculated

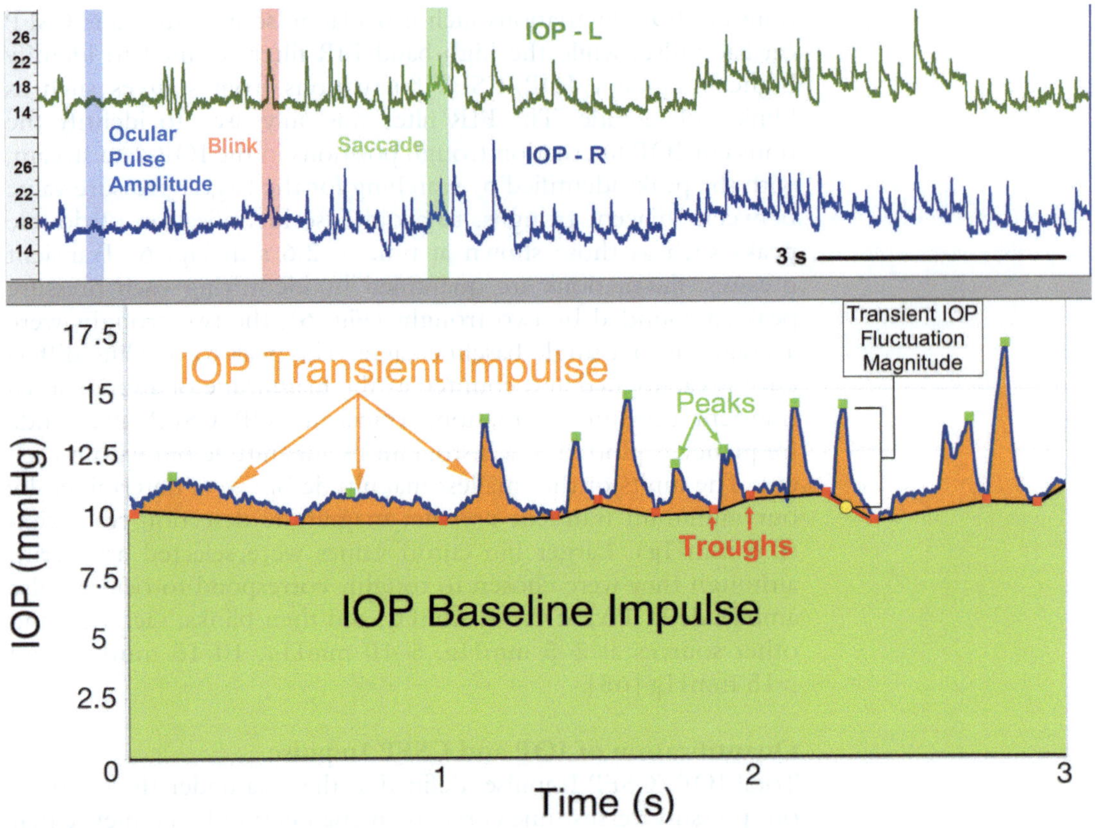

Fig. 6 Identification and quantification of frequency, magnitude, and impulse (energy) of transient IOP fluctuations. (*Top*) Screenshot of ~11 s of continuous telemetry data showing IOP in the left (L) and right (R) eyes of an NHP, with transient IOP fluctuations associated with blinks, saccades, and ocular pulse amplitude shown with red, green, and blue shading, respectively. (*Bottom*) Area under the IOP versus time curve, which represents total IOP impulse, a surrogate measure for the cumulative IOP-related mechanical energy the eye must withstand and absorb over time. The green-shaded area represents the IOP Baseline Impulse, which is a measure of the IOP energy the eye must withstand due to momentary baseline IOP, and the orange-shaded area represents the IOP transient impulse, which is a measure of the IOP energy the eye must withstand due to transient IOP fluctuations alone. (Adapted from Markert et al. [69] and Turner et al. [63] with permission)

continuously as TLP/LC thickness for each eye as described in our recent publication [65] and measured and updated biweekly with any changes in LC thickness that occur longitudinally due to glaucoma progression.

Quantification of IOP, CSFP, and TLPG means and Transients for Inclusion in Statistical Models We collect continuous IOP and ICP/CSFP telemetry data sampled at 33% duty cycle (40 s of every 2-min period) during both the normative and glaucoma periods for each NHP. Transient IOP, CSFP, and TLPG fluctuations are characterized using three methods as shown in Fig. 7: (1) time-window averaging to characterize mean values by 10-min,

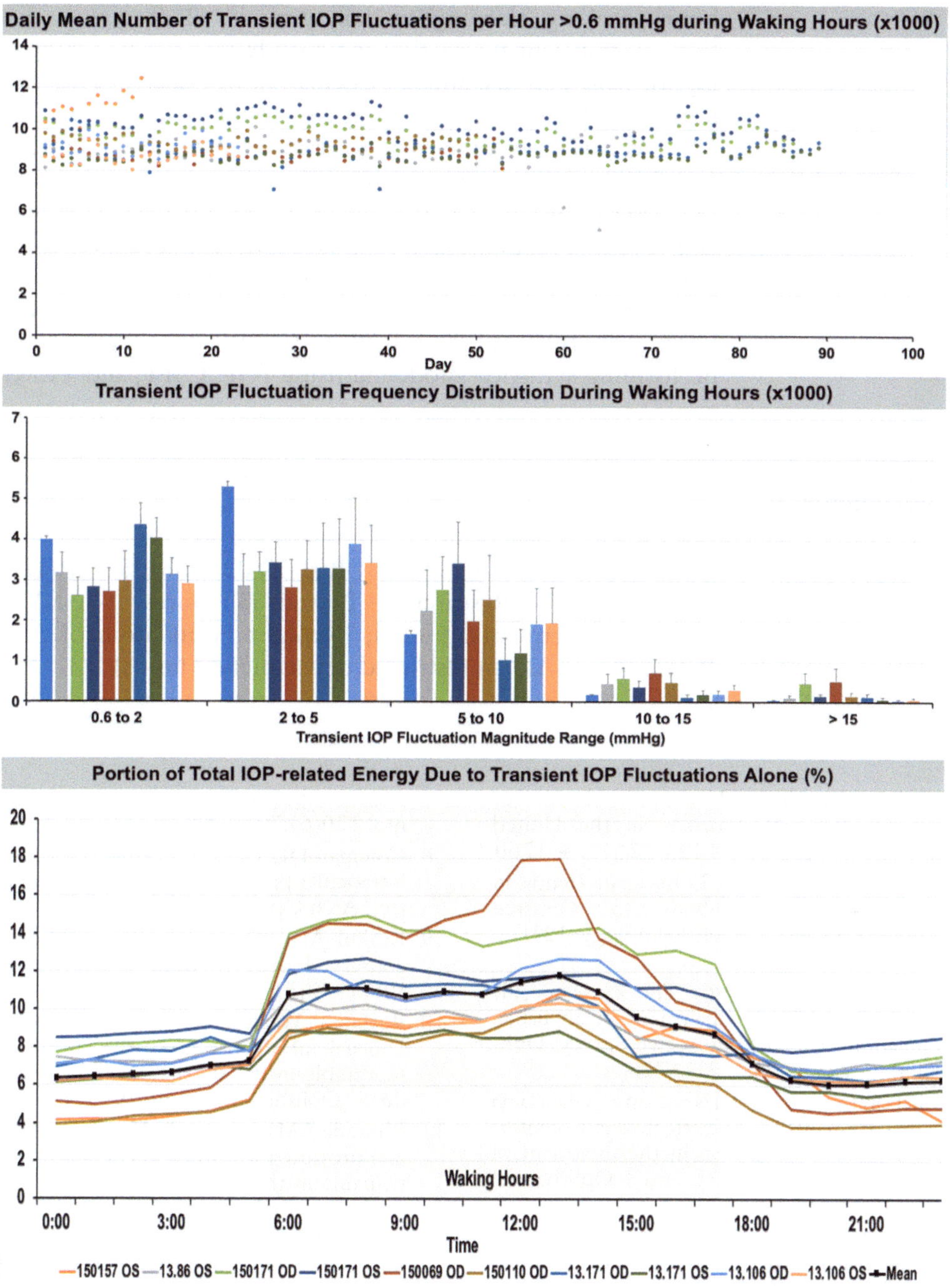

Fig. 7 Example summary IOP telemetry data for several NHP eyes averaged over multiple days, showing the average number of transient IOP fluctuations per waking hour (*top*), frequency distribution of transient IOP fluctuations binned by magnitude per waking hour (*middle*), and the mean percent transient IOP impulse plotted by hour (*bottom*), which represents the percentage of total IOP-related energy the eye must absorb over time that is due to transient IOP fluctuations alone. (Adapted from Jasien et al. [67] with permission)

hourly, waking/sleeping, or daily periods; (2) frequency distributions of transient fluctuation magnitude by hourly, waking/sleeping, or daily periods; and (3) calculation of transient IOP and TLP impulse, which is the percentage of the area under the IOP and CSFP versus time curves that are associated with transient IOP and CSFP fluctuations alone; this parameter is a measure of the mechanical energy that the eye must absorb from transient IOP and CSFP fluctuations alone. These methods are described in detail in our recent publications [63–65, 69]. Note that we are not using TLP directly in our statistical models, since it is highly autocorrelated with IOP (TLP = IOP − CSFP), and therefore we are performing statistical modeling using IOP, CSFP, and TLPG.

Acknowledgments

Grant Information: NIH R01-EY026035-05 (JCD) and P30-EY003039; Research to Prevent Blindness, NY, NY (unrestricted departmental funds); EyeSight Foundation of Alabama, Birmingham, AL (unrestricted departmental funds)

References

1. Rein DB et al (2006) The economic burden of major adult visual disorders in the United States. Arch Ophthalmol 124(12):1754–1760
2. Malihi M et al (2014) Long-term trends in glaucoma-related blindness in Olmsted County, Minnesota. Ophthalmology 121(1): 134–141
3. Rahmani B et al (1996) The cause-specific prevalence of visual impairment in an urban population. The Baltimore Eye Survey. Ophthalmology 103(11):1721–1726
4. Collaborative Normal-Tension Glaucoma Study Group (1998) The effectiveness of intraocular pressure reduction in the treatment of normal-tension glaucoma. Am J Ophthalmol 126(4):498–505
5. Anderson DR, S. Normal Tension Glaucoma (2003) Collaborative normal tension glaucoma study. Curr Opin Ophthalmol 14(2):86–90
6. Kass MA et al (2010) Delaying treatment of ocular hypertension: the ocular hypertension treatment study. Arch Ophthalmol 128(3): 276–287
7. Kass MA et al (2002) The Ocular Hypertension Treatment Study – a randomized trial determines that topical ocular hypotensive medication delays or prevents the onset of primary open-angle glaucoma. Arch Ophthalmol 120(6):701–713
8. Coleman DJ, Trokel S (1969) Direct-recorded intraocular pressure variations in a human subject. Arch Ophthalmol 82(5):637–640
9. Realini AD et al (2006) Does IOP follow a conserved daily rhythm? Invest Ophthalmol Vis Sci 47(5):4464
10. Realini T, Weinreb RN, Wisniewski SR (2010) Diurnal intraocular pressure patterns are not repeatable in the short term in healthy individuals. Ophthalmology 117(9):1700–1704
11. Bhorade AM et al (2009) Variability of intraocular pressure measurements in observation participants in the ocular hypertension treatment study. Ophthalmology 116(4):717–724
12. Realini T, Weinreb RN, Wisniewski S (2011) Short-term repeatability of diurnal intraocular pressure patterns in glaucomatous individuals. Ophthalmology 118(1):47–51
13. Allison K, Patel D, Alabi O (2020) Epidemiology of glaucoma: the past, present, and predictions for the future. Cureus 12(11):e11686
14. Turner DC et al (2017) The magnitude and time course of IOP change in response to body position change in nonhuman primates

measured using continuous IOP telemetry. Invest Ophthalmol Vis Sci 58(14):6232–6240

15. De Moraes CG et al (2016) Visual field change and 24-hour IOP-related profile with a contact lens sensor in treated glaucoma patients. Ophthalmology 123(4):744–753
16. Kim JH, Caprioli J (2018) Intraocular pressure fluctuation: is it important? J Ophthalmic Vis Res 13(2):170–174
17. Asrani S et al (2000) Large diurnal fluctuations in intraocular pressure are an independent risk factor in patients with glaucoma. J Glaucoma 9(2):134–142
18. Rabiolo AMG, Crabb DP, Garway-Heath DF, on behalf of the United Kingdom Glaucoma Treatment Study Investigators (2024) Relationship between intraocular pressure fluctuation and visual field progression rates in the United Kingdom Glaucoma Treatment Study. Ophthalmology
19. Downs JC, Girkin CA (2017) Lamina cribrosa in glaucoma. Curr Opin Ophthalmol 28(2): 113–119
20. Zeimer R (1995) Biomechanical properties of the optic nerve head. In: Glaucoma, pp 107–121
21. Quigley HA, Addicks EM (1981) Regional differences in the structure of the lamina cribrosa and their relation to glaucomatous optic nerve damage. Arch Ophthalmol 99(1): 137–143
22. Howell GR et al (2007) Axons of retinal ganglion cells are insulted in the optic nerve early in DBA/2J glaucoma. J Cell Biol 179(7): 1523–1537
23. Nickells RW et al (2012) Under pressure: cellular and molecular responses during glaucoma, a common neurodegeneration with axonopathy. Annu Rev Neurosci 35:153–179
24. Downs JC (2015) Optic nerve head biomechanics in aging and disease. Exp Eye Res 133:19–29
25. Quaranta L et al (2016) Twenty-four-hour intraocular pressure and ocular perfusion pressure characteristics in newly diagnosed patients with normal tension glaucoma. Eye (Lond) 30(11):1481–1489
26. Choi J et al (2006) Effect of nocturnal blood pressure reduction on circadian fluctuation of mean ocular perfusion pressure: a risk factor for normal tension glaucoma. Invest Ophthalmol Vis Sci 47(3):831–836
27. Choi J et al (2007) Circadian fluctuation of mean ocular perfusion pressure is a consistent risk factor for normal-tension glaucoma. Invest Ophthalmol Vis Sci 48(1):104–111
28. Choi J et al (2013) Relationship between 24-hour mean ocular perfusion pressure fluctuation and rate of paracentral visual field progression in normal-tension glaucoma. Invest Ophthalmol Vis Sci 54(9):6150–6157
29. Graham SL, Drance SM (1999) Nocturnal hypotension: role in glaucoma progression. Surv Ophthalmol 43(Suppl 1):S10–S16
30. Kim YK et al (2010) Circadian blood pressure and intraocular pressure patterns in normal tension glaucoma patients with undisturbed sleep. Korean J Ophthalmol 24(1):23–28
31. Lee NY et al (2017) Fluctuation in systolic blood pressure is a major systemic risk factor for development of primary open-angle glaucoma. Sci Rep 7:43734
32. Leske MC (2009) Ocular perfusion pressure and glaucoma: clinical trial and epidemiologic findings. Curr Opin Ophthalmol 20(2):73–78
33. Leske MC et al (2002) Incident open-angle glaucoma and blood pressure. Arch Ophthalmol 120(7):954–959
34. Memarzadeh F et al (2010) Blood pressure, perfusion pressure, and open-angle glaucoma: the Los Angeles Latino Eye Study. Invest Ophthalmol Vis Sci 51(6):2872–2877
35. Xu L, Wang YX, Jonas JB (2009) Ocular perfusion pressure and glaucoma: the Beijing Eye Study. Eye (Lond) 23(3):734–736
36. Mottet B et al (2013) 24-hour intraocular pressure rhythm in young healthy subjects evaluated with continuous monitoring using a contact lens sensor. JAMA Ophthalmol 131(12):1507–1516
37. Chung E et al (2013) Non-invasive continuous blood pressure monitoring: a review of current applications. Front Med 7(1):91–101
38. Jonas JB, Berenshtein E, Holbach L (2003) Anatomic relationship between lamina cribrosa, intraocular space, and cerebrospinal fluid space. Invest Ophthalmol Vis Sci 44(12): 5189–5195
39. Berdahl JP et al (2008) Intracranial pressure in primary open angle glaucoma, normal tension glaucoma, and ocular hypertension: a case-control study. Invest Ophthalmol Vis Sci 49(12):5412–5418
40. Berdahl JP, Allingham RR, Johnson DH (2008) Cerebrospinal fluid pressure is decreased in primary open-angle glaucoma. Ophthalmology 115(5):763–768
41. Berdahl JP, Allingham RR (2010) Intracranial pressure and glaucoma. Curr Opin Ophthalmol 21(2):106–111
42. Berdahl JP, Ethier CR, Allingham RR (2009) Cerebrospinal fluid pressure and glaucomatous

optic disc cupping. Graefes Arch Clin Exp Ophthalmol 247(9):1289–1290. author reply 1291-4

43. Berdahl JP, Yu DY, Morgan WH (2012) The translaminar pressure gradient in sustained zero gravity, idiopathic intracranial hypertension, and glaucoma. Med Hypotheses 79(6): 719–724
44. Morgan WH, Yu DY, Balaratnasingam C (2008) The role of cerebrospinal fluid pressure in glaucoma pathophysiology: the dark side of the optic disc. J Glaucoma 17(5):408–413
45. Morgan WH et al (2002) Optic disc movement with variations in intraocular and cerebrospinal fluid pressure. Invest Ophthalmol Vis Sci 43(10):3236–3242
46. Morgan WH et al (1998) The correlation between cerebrospinal fluid pressure and retrolaminar tissue pressure. Invest Ophthalmol Vis Sci 39(8):1419–1428
47. Morgan WH et al (1995) The influence of cerebrospinal fluid pressure on the lamina cribrosa tissue pressure gradient. Invest Ophthalmol Vis Sci 36(6):1163–1172
48. Yang D et al (2014) Optic neuropathy induced by experimentally reduced cerebrospinal fluid pressure in monkeys. Invest Ophthalmol Vis Sci 55(5):3067–3073
49. Morgan WH et al (2008) Glaucoma and cerebrospinal fluid pressure. Ophthalmology 115(12):2317–2318. author reply 2318
50. Hua Y, Voorhees AP, Sigal IA (2018) Cerebrospinal Fluid Pressure: Revisiting Factors Influencing Optic Nerve Head Biomechanics. Invest Ophthalmol Vis Sci 59(1):154–165
51. Ren R et al (2010) Cerebrospinal fluid pressure in glaucoma: a prospective study. Ophthalmology 117(2):259–266
52. Liu KC et al (2020) Current concepts of cerebrospinal fluid dynamics and the translaminar cribrosa pressure gradient: a paradigm of optic disk disease. Surv Ophthalmol 65(1):48–66
53. Wostyn P et al (2015) Glaucoma and the role of cerebrospinal fluid dynamics. Invest Ophthalmol Vis Sci 56(11):6630–6631
54. Killer HE, Flammer J, Miller NR (2008) Glaucoma and cerebrospinal fluid pressure. Ophthalmology 115(12):2316–2317. author reply 2317
55. Fleischman D et al (2012) Cerebrospinal fluid pressure decreases with older age. PLoS One 7(12):e52664
56. Karimi A et al (2022) Relative contributions of intraocular and cerebrospinal fluid pressures to the biomechanics of the lamina cribrosa and laminar neural tissues. Invest Ophthalmol Vis Sci 63(11):14
57. Feola AJ et al (2017) Deformation of the lamina cribrosa and optic nerve due to changes in cerebrospinal fluid pressure. Invest Ophthalmol Vis Sci 58(4):2070–2078
58. Downs JC (2020) Neural coupling of intracranial pressure and aqueous humour outflow facility: a potential new therapeutic target for intraocular pressure management. J Physiol 598(8):1429–1430
59. Quigley HA, Addicks EM (1980) Chronic experimental glaucoma in primates. II. Effect of extended intraocular pressure elevation on optic nerve head and axonal transport. Invest Ophthalmol Vis Sci 19(2):137–152
60. Quigley HA, Addicks EM (1980) Chronic experimental glaucoma in primates. I. Production of elevated intraocular pressure by anterior chamber injection of autologous ghost red blood cells. Invest Ophthalmol Vis Sci 19(2):126–136
61. Quigley HA et al (1980) The mechanism of optic nerve damage in experimental acute intraocular pressure elevation. Invest Ophthalmol Vis Sci 19(5):505–517
62. Burgoyne CF (2015) The non-human primate experimental glaucoma model. Exp Eye Res 141:57–73
63. Turner DC et al (2019) Transient intraocular pressure fluctuations: source, magnitude, frequency, and associated mechanical energy. Invest Ophthalmol Vis Sci 60(7):2572–2582
64. Jasien JV et al (2020) Diurnal cycle of translaminar pressure in nonhuman primates quantified with continuous wireless telemetry. Invest Ophthalmol Vis Sci 61(2):37
65. Jasien JV et al (2020) Quantification of Translaminar Pressure Gradient (TLPG) with continuous wireless telemetry in Nonhuman Primates (NHPs). Transl Vis Sci Technol 9(12):18
66. Jasien JV et al (2019) Cyclic pattern of Intraocular Pressure (IOP) and transient IOP fluctuations in nonhuman primates measured with continuous wireless telemetry. Curr Eye Res 44(11):1244–1252
67. Jasien JV et al (2020) Comparison of extraocular and intraocular pressure transducers for measurement of transient intraocular pressure fluctuations using continuous wireless telemetry. Sci Rep 10(1):20893
68. Downs JC et al (2011) 24-hour IOP telemetry in the nonhuman primate: implant system performance and initial characterization of IOP at multiple timescales. Invest Ophthalmol Vis Sci 52(10):7365–7375
69. Markert JE et al (2018) IOP, IOP transient impulse, ocular perfusion pressure, and mean

arterial pressure relationships in nonhuman primates instrumented with telemetry. Invest Ophthalmol Vis Sci 59(11):4496–4505

70. Wilson KI et al (2020) Intra-subject variability and diurnal cycle of ocular perfusion pressure as characterized by continuous telemetry in nonhuman primates. Invest Ophthalmol Vis Sci 61(6):7
71. Turner DC, Girkin CA, Downs JC (2019) The magnitude of intraocular pressure elevation associated with eye rubbing. Ophthalmology 126(1):171–172
72. Jasien JV et al (2017) The Magnitude of hypotony and time course of intraocular pressure recovery following anterior chamber cannulation in nonhuman primates. Invest Ophthalmol Vis Sci 58(7):3225–3230
73. Fortune B et al (2013) Onset and progression of peripapillary retinal nerve fiber layer (RNFL) retardance changes occur earlier than RNFL thickness changes in experimental glaucoma. Invest Ophthalmol Vis Sci 54(8):5653–5661
74. Jasien JV et al (2020) Effect of Body position on Intraocular Pressure (IOP), Intracranial Pressure (ICP), and Translaminar Pressure (TLP) via continuous wireless telemetry in Nonhuman Primates (NHPs). Invest Ophthalmol Vis Sci 61(12):18

Chapter 22

In Vitro and In Vivo Methods for Studying Retinal Ganglion Cell Survival and Optic Nerve Regeneration

Yuqin Yin and Larry I. Benowitz

Abstract

Glaucoma is marked by a progressive degeneration of the optic nerve and delayed loss of retinal ganglion cells (RGCs), the projection neurons of the eye. Because RGCs are not replaced and because surviving RGCs cannot regenerate their axons, the visual loss in glaucoma is largely irreversible. Here we describe methods to evaluate treatments that may be beneficial for treating glaucoma using in vitro cell culture models (immunopanning to isolate neonatal RGCs, dissociated mature retinal neurons, retinal explants) and in vivo models that test potential treatments or investigate underlying molecular mechanisms in an intact system. Potentially, the use of these models can help investigators continue to improve treatments to preserve RGCs and restore visual function in patients with glaucoma.

Key words Retina, Retinal ganglion cells, Optic nerve, Glaucoma, Cell culture, Explants, Trophic factors, Axon regeneration, Cell signaling mechanisms, Quantitative methods

1 Introduction

Like most pathways in the mature central nervous system (CNS), the optic nerve cannot regenerate if injured [1]. Consequently, victims of traumatic, ischemic, or degenerative optic nerve damage suffer lifelong visual losses. Retinal ganglion cells (RGCs), the projection neurons of the eye, show little ability to extend axons distal to the site of nerve damage and begin to die after a few days [2]. Over the past few decades, many studies have identified factors that suppress or promote RGC survival and optic nerve regeneration. These studies have been motivated by the centrality of vision in our lives, the high prevalence of disorders that affect vision, and the likelihood that factors and pathways discovered using the optic nerve as a model system will afford insights into mechanisms to enhance regeneration in other parts of the CNS. Of particular relevance here is the significance of this research to glaucoma.

Tatjana Jakobs and Paloma B. Liton (eds.), *Glaucoma: Methods and Protocols*, Methods in Molecular Biology, vol. 2858, https://doi.org/10.1007/978-1-0716-4140-8_22,

Visual loss in glaucoma is most commonly associated with elevated intraocular pressure (IOP) which, in current thinking, leads to changes in astrocytes and inflammatory cells at the lamina cribrosa/optic nerve head that impair axonal function and ultimately lead to RGC death [3–5]. Whereas glaucoma therapy primarily aims at decreasing intraocular pressure, this approach fails to slow disease progression in many patients and does not protect RGCs that have begun to die nor does it restore axonal function. Consequently, glaucomatous loss of vision remains irreversible, and early detection and treatment are of great importance.

The methods described below enable the investigator to evaluate agents that are neuroprotective for RGCs and/or that promote axon regeneration in cases in which the cell bodies are still viable. Hopefully these methods will enable us to discover better ways to reverse optic nerve damage and restore the transmission of information from the eye to the brain.

1.1 In Vitro Methods

Many studies aimed at identifying factors that promote RGC survival and axon regeneration, or investigating the mechanisms that underlie the effects of such factors, begin with in vitro experiments. Three in vitro methods have been used to study RGC survival and axon outgrowth: purified neonatal RGC cultures, mixed adult retinal cell cultures, and retinal explants.

Purified RGC Cultures This method uses young postnatal RGCs (prior to P12) and enables one to investigate the direct effects of various factors on RGCs in the absence of other cell types. However, this method is not suitable for studying adult RGCs due to the low survival of mature RGCs after purification.

RGCs are purified from a whole retina cell suspension through "immunopanning," a two- step method that utilizes antibody-mediated plate adhesion. This procedure yields a highly pure population of RGCs (>99%), with a recovery rate ranging from 25% to 50% depending on the vigor used in the washing step and other factors. This technique was first used in rat RGC purification and has been modified for mouse RGCs as well.

Immunopanning RGCs was developed by Barres [6] and modified by others.

Mixed RGC Cultures Although purified adult RGCs do not survive well in culture, they do survive in mixed retinal cultures, enabling one to investigate factors and signaling pathways that promote RGC survival and/or axon regeneration [7, 8]. In order to distinguish from other retinal cells, RGCs are prelabeled by retrograde transport of a dye (usually Fluorogold) injected into the superior colliculus one week prior to preparing the culture. Mixed retinal cultures are mostly derived from rats [8–10]. Recently the mice with their RGCs genetically fluorescent-labeled [11, 12] have been used in the mixed culture. Especially when combined with an automated imaging and analysis system, this method makes the adult RGC culture easy to be carried out.

Retinal Explant Culture Retinal explant cultures can be viewed as a model that is intermediate between dissociated retinal cell cultures and the in vivo model. Retinal explants have been used to study processes such as retinal differentiation [13], neurodegeneration [14], and neurite outgrowth [15]. The major advantage of explant cultures is that cells are maintained within a seminormal environment, with preservation of cell-cell interactions, while maintaining a higher level of experimental control than in animal models [16]. Thus, retinal explant cultures provide a good platform for the identification and validation of novel neuroprotective or proregenerative factors. In general, however, they do not allow one to conclude that any observed effects are due to the direct action of agents on RGCs.

Neurite outgrowth from the explants is commonly visualized by phase microscopy or fluorescent immunostaining. A disadvantage of the former is that no objective distinction can be made between glial and neuronal processes, which can lead to inaccurate assessments of neurite outgrowth. This distinction can be made using antibodies to neuron-specific markers such as βIII-tubulin or neurofilament proteins, although there can still be a question as to the identity of the neurons from which the neurites originate. The use of transgenic animals that express a fluorescent protein in RGCs, such as Thy1- YFP mice [17], may allow for better identification of RGC axons provided that levels of Thy1 promoter activity, and thus of YFP expression, do not decline appreciably as a result of retinal dissection and the inevitable transection of RGC axons [18, 19]. Using Vglut2-tdTomato mice [11, 12] would be a good option for visualizing bright red fluorescence in the cell body and process from RGCs.

1.2 In Vivo Methods

Although in vitro cell cultures have been invaluable for mechanistic studies, for screening growth factors, evaluating effects of inhibitory substrates, and other purposes, in vivo studies provide the clearest evidence that a given treatment may be clinically relevant to promoting RGC survival and/or optic nerve regeneration. In addition, current methods allow for precise, quantitative evaluation of the effect size. In recent years, numerous labs have explored ways to promote RGC survival and to stimulate optic nerve regeneration using the in vivo model. The methods for an in vivo study include establishing a nerve injury model, delivering the treatment via intraocular injection, and applying appropriate methods to evaluate RGC survival and axon regeneration. Many earlier studies had used a peripheral nerve graft model which has been described in detail [20], but this model is seldom used since the discovery that, with suitable stimulation, RGCs can be induced to extend lengthy axons through the optic nerve itself [21, 22].

1.3 Evaluation of Optic Nerve Regeneration

Following optic nerve injury and treatment, animals usually survive from two weeks up to a few months for the study of short-term or long-term treatment effects on RGC survival and axon regeneration. There are several ways to evaluate axon regeneration: GAP-43 immunostaining in longitudinal sections through the optic nerve and manual counting of axons; anterograde tracing of regenerating axons with cholera toxin B fragment (CTB), in some cases combined with immunostaining; a tissue-clearing technique to visualize axons in unsectioned nerves; or genetically labeling RGCs with an axonally transported protein linked to a fluorescent dye. Each of these methods has its advantages and can be combined to use in the studies.

GAP-43 Immunostaining GAP-43 is a prototypical growth-associated protein with an apparent molecular mass ~43 kDa (true size ~24 kDa). It is dramatically upregulated in RGCs and their axons when the cells are in a growth state and downregulated in normal uninjured or nongrowing nerve fibers [23, 24]. Therefore, GAP-43 is a reliable indicator for RGC axons that are actively regenerating injured axons (Fig. 1).

CTB Anterograde Tracing Cholera Toxin B subunit (CTB) is a sensitive neuronal tracer with unique features. It stains axons and terminals in great detail, so that single axons can be followed over long distances and their arbors reconstructed in their entirety. As an

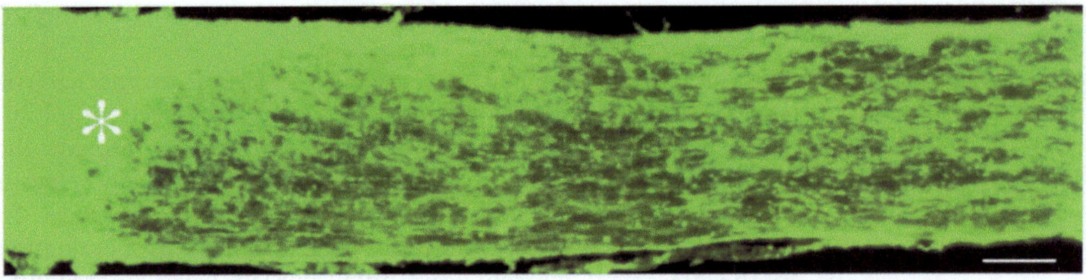

Fig. 1 GAP-43-positive axons in mouse optic nerve. Three weeks after optic nerve crush and intraocular injection of an AAV2-shPten virus plus oncomodulin and CPT-cAMP, many GAP-43-positive axons extent past the crush injury site (*asterisk*) into the optic nerve. Scale bar: 60 μm. (Y. Yin, L.B. Benowitz, unpublished)

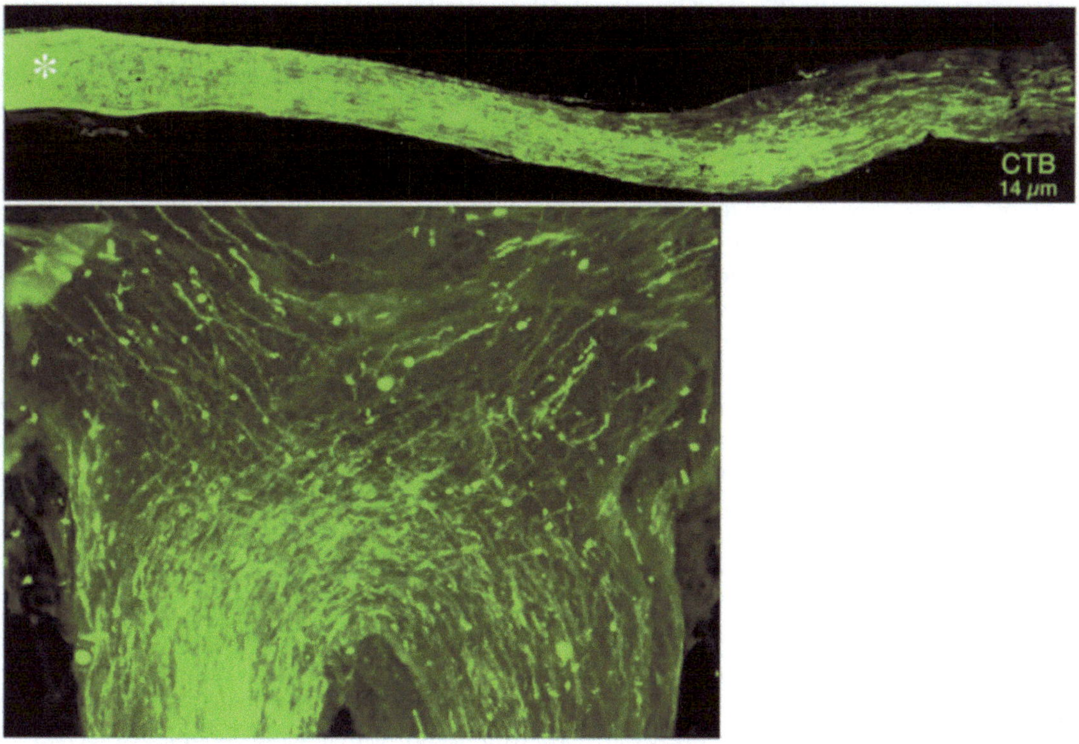

Fig. 2 CTB-positive axons regenerating through the optic nerve and into the optic chiasm. *Top:* Axons are visualized in a longitudinal section through the optic nerve (14 μm thick) 6 weeks after nerve crush followed by intraocular injection of an adeno-associated virus expressing an shRNA to knock down expression of the *pten* gene (AAV2-shPten), a shH10-oncomodulin virus, AAV2-c/a-Adenylate Cyclase, and the chemokine stromal cell-derived factor 1 (SDF1) [10]. *Bottom:* Regenerating axons entering the optic chiasm. Axons were labeled with unconjugated CTB and were visualized by anti-CTB immunostaining. Note clear morphology and high resolution (composite of five 14 μm sections: Y. Yin, H-Y. Gilbert, L.B. Benowitz, unpublished)

anterograde tracer, two types of CTB are often used to visualize regenerating axons: fluorescence-conjugated CTB or unconjugated CTB [25–27]. Usually, CTB is injected intravitreally 2–4 days before the animal is perfused to allow for transport from the cell body to the terminals. If injecting the fluorescent-conjugated CTB, the regenerating axons can be visualized under the fluorescent microscope right after the nerve sectioning. Therefore, the latter method is popular in many labs though the cost is relatively high if used in a large number of samples. In cases in which unconjugated CTB is used, the label can be visualized by immunostaining, as in the sample shown below in which numerous CTB-positive axons regenerate along the entire length of optic nerve and enter the optic chiasm (Fig. 2).

Tissue Clearing and Light Sheet Fluorescence Microscopy in Unsectioned Optic Nerves Longitudinal sectioning of the optic nerve can result in sections showing axon fragments that disappear out of the plane of section and a loss of three-dimensional information, especially when studying axon turning or branching in the nerve or the trajectory of axons that enter the brain. Several methods for optical clearing of tissue have been developed that overcome some of these problems. Many studies have described a method involving an organic solvent-based clearing protocol that allows for three-dimensional visualization the axon regeneration patterns after optic nerve injury in mice [28, 29]. This method consists of axon labeling with conjugated CTB in vivo, whole-tissue dehydration after tissue fixation, tissue clearing, and imaging with light-sheet fluorescent microscopy (LSFM) to visualize the pattern of optic nerve regeneration in adult tissues. This method is able to provide better understanding of three-dimensional axon growth pattern but requires special microscopy techniques. It may also underestimate the numbers of weakly labeled regenerating axons.

1.4 Quantification of Axon Growth

Axon growth can be quantified by counting the number of GAP-43-positive (or CTB-positive) axons extending 0.5 and 1 mm (or other prespecified distances) from the end of the nerve injury site in at least four longitudinal sections per case. Using a calibrated ocular to measure distance, the cross-sectional width of the nerve is measured at the point at which the counts are taken and is used to calculate the number of axons per millimeter of nerve width (axons/mm). The number of axons per millimeter is then averaged over the four sections. Σa_d, the total number of axons extending distance d in a nerve having a radius of r (determined empirically as half the greatest cross-sectional width), is estimated by summing over all sections having a thickness *t* (commonly 14 μm in our material) [22]:

$$\Sigma a_{\mathrm{d}} = \pi r^2 [\text{average axons per mm width}]/t$$

This calculation is widely used in the field. However, several points need to be noted. First, the average number of axons should be divided by the nerve width (axons/mm) for the calculation. Second, many published papers appear to have erroneously used the nerve width (diameter) for r instead of the radius (1/2 diameter) to calculate the area πr^2, which leads to a fourfold higher number of regenerating axons. This can be seen by comparing the images of regenerating axons vs. the numbers of axons reported in graphs from different labs. r should be ½ of the greatest width seen on sections in a given nerve. After calculating the total axon number in each case, the group means and SEMs are then obtained and the appropriate statistical tests applied to determine the significance of intergroup differences.

2 Materials

2.1 Materials for In Vitro Methods

1. For purification of postnatal RGCs via immunopanning.
2. Materials for retrograde labeling before immunopanning (optional).
3. Fast blue (1% in H_2O).
4. 10 μL Hamilton syringe.

2.2 Materials for Preparing Retinal Cell Suspensions

1. Earle's Balanced Salts Solution (EBSS containing Ca^{2+} and Mg^{2+}, pH 7.4).
2. Ovomucoid solution (egg white inhibitor, 13 mg/3 mL).
3. Papain (about 40–45 mg protein/mL, 30 U/mg).
4. Rabbit antirat macrophage antiserum (Cedarlane, CLAD51240).
5. Minimum Essential Medium Eagle (MEM) with 0.05% bovine serum albumin (BSA).
6. Nitex mesh.

2.3 Materials for Preparing Plastic Petri Dishes for Panning

1. Two 150 × 15 mm petri dishes (Falcon 1058).
2. Two 100 × 15 mm petri dishes (Falcon 1029).
3. Affinity-purified goat antimouse IgM, μ-chain-specific (1 mg/mL).
4. Affinity-purified goat antirabbit IgG H+L (1 mg/mL).
5. T11D7 supernatant (monoclonal supernatant containing IgM antibodies directed against Thy1.1 (the cell line is available from ATCC, no. TIB 103, name T11D7e2).
6. IgM Thy1.2 antibody for panning of mouse cells (Accurate Chemical Co., Cat No. MAS 731; or MCA01, Serotec).
7. Tris-HCl (50 mM, pH 9.5).
8. Dulbecco's phosphate-buffered saline (DPBS).

2.4 Materials for Panning

1. Nitex mesh.
2. MEM.
3. Trypsin in EBSS (0.125%).
4. Fetal Calf Serum (FCS).
5. Materials for evaluation of neurite outgrowth in purified RGC cultures.
6. Calcein (a fluorescent dye to stain live cell bodies and processes).
7. Hoechst 33342 (a fluorescent dye to stain nuclei).

8. Paraformaldehyde (4%).
9. Appropriate antibodies.
10. Cellomics Kinetiscan.

2.5 For Mixed Adult Rat RGC Cultures

1. Materials for mixed rat RGC cultures.
2. Fluorogold (FG, 2% in saline solution).
3. 10 μL Nanofil syringe.
4. Stereotaxic frame.
5. L-15 medium.
6. $NaHCO_3$.
7. 24-well plates.
8. HEPES (1 M).
9. Transferrin (stock: 2 mg/mL in H_2O).
10. Superoxide Dismutase (stock: 30,000 U/mL in H_2O).
11. Catalase (stock: 1 mg/mL in H_2O).
12. Gentamicin (stock: 10 mg/mL).
13. Insulin (stock: 5 mg/mL in H_2O).
14. Bovine serum albumin (BSA).
15. HKPPST: every 12 mL of 25X HKPPST consists of hydrocortisone (60 μL of stock at 500 nM), kynurenic acid (56.8 mg), putrescine dihydrochloride (968 μL of stock at 2.5 mM), progesterone (60 μL of stock at 500 nM), sodium selenite (90 μL of stock at 750 nM), and 6. 3, 3′, 5-triiodo-L-thyronine (T3) (60 μL of stock at 7.5 nM).
16. Papain suspension.
17. L-cysteine (stock: 3 mg/10 μL H_2O).
18. DNase (stock: 1 mg/mL in H_2O).
19. Paraformaldehyde (4%).
20. Poly-L-lysine solution.

2.6 Materials for Mixed Adult Mouse RGC Cultures

1. L-15 medium.
2. Neurobasal A.
3. B27.
4. 96-well plates.
5. Gentamicin (stock: 10 mg/mL).
6. Bovine serum albumin (BSA).
7. Papain suspension.
8. L-cysteine (stock: 3 mg/10 μL H_2O).

9. DNase (stock: 1 mg/mL in H_2O).
10. Paraformaldehyde (4%).
11. Poly-L-lysine solution.

2.7 Materials for In Vivo Methods

2.7.1 Optic Nerve Crush and Intraocular Injection

1. Ketamine (75 mg/kg for rats, 100 mg/kg for mice) and Xylazine (10 mg/kg for rats or mice).
2. Microsurgical tools.
3. Jewelers' forceps #5.
4. Sutures 10-0.
5. Needle 30G 1/2′ or fine tip glass catheters.
6. Polysporin ointment.
7. Isoflurane.

2.7.2 Materials for Animal Perfusion, Tissue Preparation, and GAP43 Immunostaining

1. Isoflurane.
2. Heparinized saline (10 unit/mL).
3. Paraformaldehyde (4%).
4. Sucrose (30%).
5. Superfrost Plus glass slides.
6. Polyclonal anti-GAP-43 antibody made in sheep.
7. Tris-buffered saline (TBS).
8. Methanol.
9. Donkey serum.
10. TBS_2T (TBS containing 2× NaCl and 0.1% Tween-20).
11. Solution A (5% donkey serum, 2% BSA in TBS_2T).
12. AlexaFluor 488 donkey antisheep IgG.

2.7.3 Materials for Whole-Mount Retina Staining and Quantification of RGC Survival After Optic Nerve Regeneration

1. Paraformaldehyde (4%).
2. Phosphate-buffered saline (PBS).
3. Goat serum.
4. Triton X-100.
5. Rabbit anti-βIII-tubulin antibody.
6. TUJ1 (a monoclonal antibody to -βIII-tubulin, Covance, MMS-435p).
7. Fluorescent secondary antibody goat antirabbit or goat antimouse IgG.
8. ImageJ software.

3 Methods

3.1 In Vitro Methods

3.1.1 Immunopurified Postnatal RGC Cultures

1. Retrograde Labeling of RGCs in Postnatal Rats (Optional)

To check the purity of isolated cells, retrograde labeling of RGCs is a reliable indicator. Postnatal animals are anesthetized, and under visual guidance, 4 μL of Fast Blue solution is injected through a 10 μL Hamilton syringe into the brachium of the superior colliculus bilaterally (*see* **Note 1**). Injections are performed through the skull, which is exposed on the dorsal surface by making a small longitudinal incision in the skin midline. It is not necessary to use a stereotactic device. In P6–P8 animals, the needle can be accurately positioned 2 mm lateral to the midsagittal sinus just anterior to its intersection with the transverse sinus at a depth of 4 mm. With these coordinates, the injection site lies at the intersection of the dorsal midbrain and diencephalon [30].

3.1.2 Preparing Retinal Cell Suspensions

1. One to ten rats (P8–P10) from a Sprague/Dawley or Long/Evans litter are used.
2. After removing the lens and vitreous humor, the dissected retinas are stored at room temperature in EBSS until the retinas are dissected from all animals.
3. After incubation with papain for 30 min, retinas are rinsed once and then triturated in an ovomucoid solution containing antirat-macrophage antiserum (1:100).
4. After allowing the cell suspension to incubate with the antiserum for 20 min, cells are centrifuged, resuspended in 10 mL MEM/BSA, and filtered through Nitex mesh, and MEM/BSA is added to a final volume to about 15 mL.

3.1.3 Preparing Plastic Petri Panning Dishes

1. One day before panning, prepare two 150 mm Petri dishes for antimacrophage panning. To each dish, add 20 mL Tris-HCl with 60 μL of the secondary antibody and affinity-purified goat antirabbit IgG, and store overnight at 4 °C.
2. One day before panning, prepare two 100 mm Thyl/T11D7 panning dishes for RGC adhesion. To each dish, add 10 mL Tris-HCl with 30 μL of Goat antimouse IgM; keep at 4 °C overnight (*see* **Note 2**).
3. On the day of panning, rinse 150 mm Petri dishes three times with DPBS, and then add 10 mL DPBS to each and set aside at RT until use.
4. Rinse 100 mm Petri dishes three times with DPBS, add 8–10 mL of T11D7 supernatant, and incubate at RT for at least 2 h. Before panning, rinse the dishes three times with DPBS.

3.2 Panning

1. Incubate the retinal cell suspension on the first antimacrophage dish for 45 min. Gently agitate the dish every 15–20 min or so to ensure access of all the cells to the bottom of the dish. Transfer the cell suspension to the second antimacrophage dish for 45 min (agitate gently every 15 min).
2. Collect the cell suspension, filter through Nitex mesh to remove small clumps that formed on the antimacrophage dishes; incubate half of the cell suspension on each of the two T11D7-dishes for 45–60 min (agitate gently every 15 min) at RT or for 30 min in a 37 °C incubator.
3. Gently wash off nonadherent cells on the T11D7 dishes with 5–8 washes of MEM. Check under a microscope to make sure all of the nonadherent cells are gone; if not, wash a few more times. Do not wash too vigorously or you will wash off the RGCs.
4. To release the purified RGCs, add Trypsin-EBSS solution; incubate 8 min in 37 °C incubator or 10 min at RT. Transfer the trypsin/cell suspension to a 15 mL tube containing 30% FCS in DMEM to stop the digestion. Spin cells 15 min at 200× *g* to rinse out the traces of FCS and resuspend cells in preequilibrated RGC growth media. An average yield for P6 animals is 50–60K cells per animal, about 40K cells per P8 rat (*see* **Note 3**).

3.2.1 Evaluation of Neurite Outgrowth in Purified RGC Cultures

Purified RGCs can be grown in Neurobasal A plus B27 media for 3 days (10,000 cells per 96-well). Cells can be stained with Calcein (Fig. 3) and Hoechst 33342 and imaged in 25 fields per well using a Cellomics Kinetiscan (or equivalent), and neurite outgrowth can be calculated using the Cellomics Image Analysis Algorithm (or equivalent). Cultured cells can also be fixed 10 min with 4% paraformaldehyde at room temperature and immunostained with appropriate antibodies as required.

3.3 Mixed Adult Rat RGC Culture

3.3.1 Retrograde Labeling in Adult Rats

1. Adult rats (>200 g) are anaesthetized and immobilized in a stereotaxic frame, and the skin is incised to expose the top of the skull.
2. Drill two holes bilaterally 1.2 mm lateral to the midline 6.5 mm posterior to Bregma.
3. Slowly inject FG solution (8 μL) at a depth of 4.0 mm into the superior colliculi.

Leave the needle in situ for a few minutes and then withdraw slowly.

4. One week after the surgery, the animal is sacrificed and the two FG-labeled retinas are removed to prepare cell cultures.

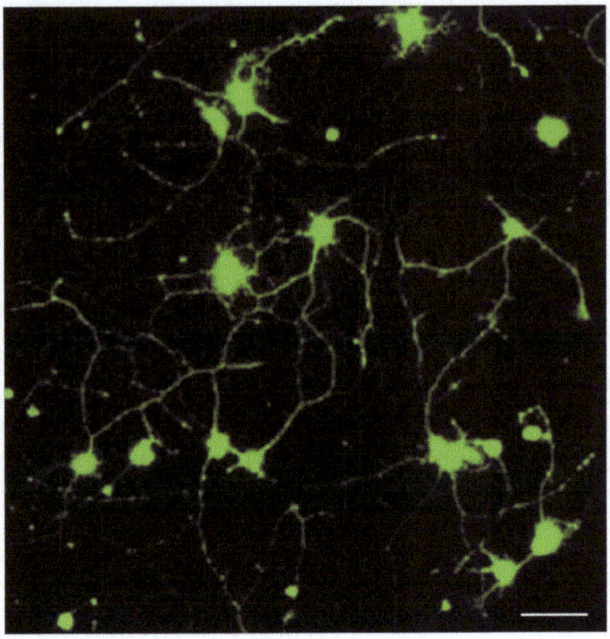

Fig. 3 Neurite outgrowth in purified postnatal day 6 mouse RGCs. With exposure to the growth factor oncomodulin combined with forskolin (to elevate cAMP) and mannose, many mouse RGCs isolated by immunopanning extend long processes in culture (Calcein staining). Scale bar: 40 μm [7]

3.3.2 Preparing the Culture Medium and Plates

1. Selection of medium: Instead of Neurobasal A plus B27, this culture uses a defined serum-free medium called Medium E. The reason of this selection is that Neurobasal A with B27 increases background growth levels, which could occlude the axon-promoting effects of factors being tested. L-15 medium is the base medium in this culture. Since it does not contain HCO_3^-, the pH will change when placed in a CO_2 incubator, and therefore, the medium must be supplemented with $NaHCO_3$ (22 mg per 10 mL); *see* **Note 4**.
2. Plates: Since RGCs represent only ~0.5% of the total cells in the retina, we typically use plates with larger wells (24- instead of 96-well plate) to enable us to obtain enough RGCs in each well for analysis. The plate is precoated with Poly- L-lysine for 30 min and then washed with dd H_2O once. The total volume of medium in each well of a 24-well plate is 400 μL and includes three parts: 100 μL of Medium E (4×), 250 μL of the experimental sample, and 50 μL of retinal cell suspension. L-15·$NaHCO_3$ is the basic medium for all three parts.

3. Medium E (4×):

L-15·$NaHCO_3$	3 mL
HKPPST	960 μL
HEPES	360 μL
Transferrin	120 μL
Superoxide dismutase	48 μL
Catalase	24 μL
Gentamicin	24 μL
Insulin	24 μL
BSA	240 mg

adjust pH to 7.4, bring volume up to 6 mL with L-15·$NaHCO_3$

4. Digestion solution:

L-15·$NaHCO_3$	6 mL
Papain	200 μL
1% BSA	28 μL
L-cysteine	10 μL
DNase	100 μL

adjust pH to 7.4, bring volume up to 10 mL with L-15·$NaHCO_3$

5. Washing solution

L15	25 mL
BSA	30 mg
DNase	200 μL

adjust pH to 7.4, bring volume up to 30 mL with L-15

6. Testing samples: Retinal cells from one rat are enough to test ten different samples (factors) in quadruplicate (10 × 4 = 40 wells). The samples are made with L-15·$NaHCO_3$.

3.3.3 Preparing Dissociated Retinal Cell Suspensions

Prelabeled rat retinas are dissected from the eyes and incubated in the digestion solution in a CO_2 incubator for 30 min. Gently wash retinas two times with 10 mL washing solution, and use the last 10 mL washing solution for the gentle trituration until all of the cells are dissociated. Centrifuge the cell suspension at 1000 rpm for

10 min; use L-15·$NaHCO_3$ to resuspend (2 mL medium for 2 retinas); *see* **Note 5**.

1. Plating Cells and Evaluating Axon Growth

Plate 50 μL cell suspension in each well together with 100 μL of 4× Medium E and 250 μL of test samples to make 400 μL in each well. After 3 days of growth in a CO_2 incubator, axon growth and cell survival can be quantified under fluorescent and phase microscopy. RGCs are first recognized by Fluorogold labeling, and then their axons are visualized under the phase contrast. Axon outgrowth is quantified as the percentage of FG-positive RGCs extending axons >30 μm (twice the average diameter of cultured RGCs). Based on prior experience, we do not count axons shorter than 30 μm in order to exclude spontaneous sprouting. Cells can be fixed with 4% paraformaldehyde 10 min at RT and stained with suitable antibodies as required by the experiment (Fig. 4).

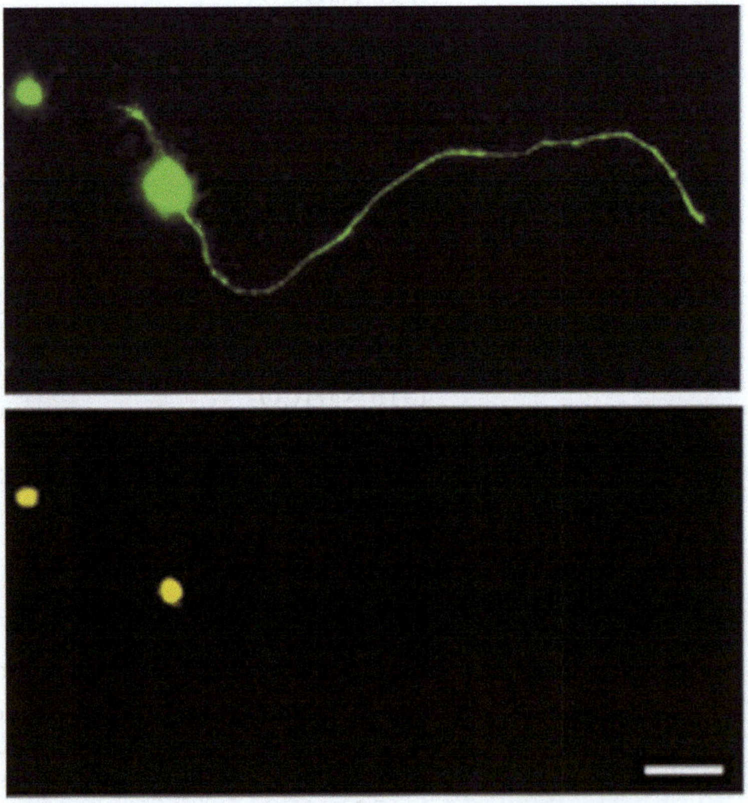

Fig. 4 Axon outgrowth in Fluorogold-labeled RGCs in a mixed retinal culture. Fluorogold was injected into the superior colliculus one week prior to sacrifice, retinal dissection, and dissociation. After a 3-day exposure in culture to oncomodulin, forskolin, and mannose, cells were fixed with 4% paraformaldehyde and stained with an antibody against GAP-43, a marker of axon outgrowth. Here, retrogradely labeled RGCs (bottom) are seen growing lengthy axons (upper image). Scale bar: 25 μm [8]

3.3.4 Mixed Adult Mouse RGC Culture

1. Genetically Labeled RGC Mouse Line

   In the retina, Vglut2 is specifically expressed in RGCs [11, 12]. A Vglut2-tdTomato mouse line (obtained by crossing a Vglut2-Cre line with a $STOP^{flx/flx}$-tdTomato line) exhibits RGCs expressing brightly fluorescent tdTomato, enabling RGCs to be readily recognized in dissociated mixed cultures.

2. Preparing the Culture Medium and Plates

   (a) Culture medium (4×):

Neurobasal A	5496 μL
B27(50X)	480 μL
Gentamicin	24 μL

   adjust pH to 7.4, bring volume up to 10 mL with Neurobasal A

   (b) Plates: with automated imaging system to record multiple areas of cell growth in each well, 96-well plates can be used to grow RGCs while providing enough information for the analysis. The plate is precoated with Poly-L-lysine for 30 min and then washed once with dd H_2O. The total volume of medium in each well of a 96-well plate is 200 μL and includes three parts: 50 μL of the culture medium (4×), 120 μL of the experimental sample, and 30 μL of retinal cell suspension.

   (c) Digestion solution:

Neurobasal A	6 mL
Papain	130 μL
1% BSA	28 μL
L-cysteine	20 μL
DNase	100 μL

   adjust pH to 7.4, bring volume up to 10 mL with Neurobasal A

   (d) Washing solution

L-15	30 mL
BSA	30 mg
DNase	200 μL

   adjust pH to 7.4, bring volume up to 30 mL with L-15

(e) Samples to be tested: Retinal cells from 3 mice are enough to test 19 different samples (factors) in quintuplicate ($19 \times 5 = 95$ wells). The samples are prepared in Neurobasal A.

3.3.5 Preparing the Dissociated Mouse Retinal Cell Suspension

Genetically labeled mouse retinas are dissected from the eyes and incubated in the digestion solution in a CO_2 incubator for 30 min. Gently wash retinas two times with 10 mL washing solution, and use the last 10 mL washing solution for the gentle trituration until all cells are dissociated. Centrifuge the cell suspension at 1000 rpm for 8 min; use Neurobasal A to resuspend (3 ml medium for six retinas).

3.3.6 Plating Cells and Evaluation of Axon Growth

Plate 30 μL of cell suspension in each well together with 50 μL of 4× culture medium and 120 μL of to-be-tested samples to make 200 μL in each well. Using the IncuCyte S3 Live Cell Automated Imaging and Analysis System, an automated bioassay is conducted for 3 days. Bright red fluorescent TdTomato-positive cells with their neurites are imaged, and neurite length and RGC survival are quantified with Neuronal Profiling software. Figure 5 is an example showing tdTomato-labeled RGCs after a 3-day culture.

3.4 In Vivo Methods

3.4.1 Optic Nerve Crush Model

The surgical approaches for rat and mouse optic nerve crushes are slightly different. The access to the rat optic nerve is through a skin incision on the top of the orbit and the Harderian gland around the optic nerve, whereas access to the mouse optic nerve is through the conjunctival sac which provides an easier surgical operation but a small, narrow exposure to the optic nerve.

3.4.2 Rat Optic Nerve Crush

1. Surgery is carried out under aseptic conditions.
2. Adult rats (>200 g body weight) are anesthetized using ketamine and xylazine injected intraperitoneally (IP).

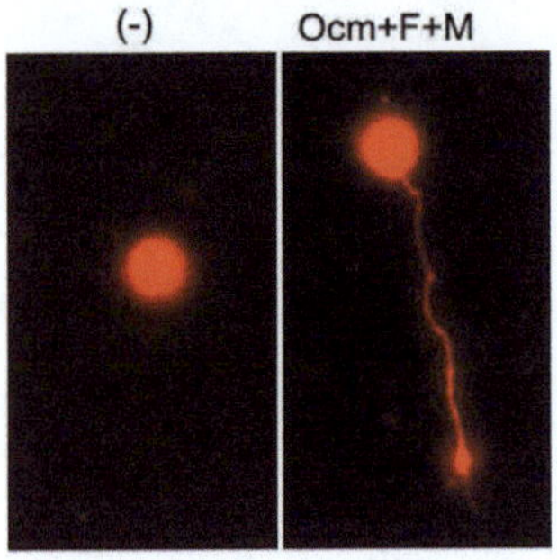

Fig. 5 Adult mouse RGC cultures. RGCs genetically labeled with tdTomato (red) treated with medium alone (-) or oncomodulin, forskolin, and mannose (Ocm + F + M) through an automated imaging and analysis system. (Y. Yin, L.B. Benowitz, unpublished)

3. The optic nerve is surgically exposed by retracting the overlying Harderian gland and resecting a minimal amount of muscle and connective tissue around the nerve, with extreme care taken not to damage the ophthalmic artery.
4. The epineurium surrounding the optic nerve is carefully slit, and the nerve is crushed 2 mm from the optic nerve head for 10 s using #5 jewelers' forceps.

3.4.3 Rat Optic Nerve Microcrush

To minimize overall tissue damage, a limited injury model called a microcrush has been developed [31]. Instead of using forceps, a microcrush lesion is made using a 10-0 suture to completely constrict the optic nerve by making a tight knot for 60 s and then releasing the suture. The microcrush causes much less of a cavity to form adjacent to the lesion site compared to conventional use of forceps while at the same time transecting all axons completely. In addition, the lesion site is sharply defined, which allows for accurate measurements of the distance of axon growth past the lesion site.

3.4.4 Intraocular Injection in Rat

After nerve crush or microcrush, depending on the experimental design, animals may receive an intraocular injection of growth factors, viruses, or other agents. A typical injection volume in rat is 5–10 μL per eye, with the same volume of aqueous withdrawn beforehand, or after making a small puncture on the cornea, to release excess pressure. The injection is delivered into the posterior chamber of the eye through a sterile 30 1/2G or thinner needle or a fine tip of glass catheter. The needle is left in situ for about 10 s for better distribution of the agent being injected and then withdrawn very slowly to avoid back-leakage. It is essential to avoid damaging the lens during the injections, since lens injury causes considerable inflammation that itself has massive effects in promoting RGC survival and axon regeneration [9, 22]. It is not necessary to dilate the pupil during the injection since the injection is made from the back of the eye. The surgical wound is sutured shut and swabbed with Polysporin ointment. The fundus is examined under a dissecting microscope for signs of ischemic damage or lens injury. Animals showing such damage are removed and sacrificed with an overdose of isoflurane.

Animals are allowed to recover from anesthesia and returned to their cages. In some experiments, agents are introduced prior to optic nerve injury. This occurs, for example, when attempting to affect changes that occur quickly after optic nerve injury or, in gene therapy studies, a lead time is required to allow a virally encoded gene to be expressed at sufficient levels.

3.4.5 Mouse Optic Nerve Crush and Intraocular Injection

1. Adult mice (8 weeks or older) are anesthetized with a combination of ketamine and xylazine given intraperitoneally.
2. Surgery is done under sterile conditions using a stereomicroscope.

3. A conjunctival incision is made over the dorsal aspect of the eye and then gently rotated the eye downward in the orbit.
4. The orbital muscles are slightly separated to expose the optic nerve at its exit from the eyeball, which is then crushed for 5 s with #5 jewelers' forceps near the back of the eye (within 0.5 mm) [25]. Care is taken not to damage the ophthalmic artery and retrobulbar sinus.
5. After the nerve crush, no suture is needed since the incision is very small and closes by itself after releasing all instruments from the eye.
6. Intraocular injections in mouse eyes are similar to those in rats except that the maximum volume is ~3 μL [25].

3.4.6 Animal Perfusion, Tissue Preparation, and Immunostaining for GAP-43 in Optic Nerve Sections

Animals are given an overdose of isoflurane and perfused intracardially with 50–100 mL of heparin-saline followed by 100–200 mL of 4% paraformaldehyde. The optic nerve is dissected out and placed in 4% paraformaldehyde again for postfixation (2 h at RT or 4 °C overnight). After immersion for several hours to overnight in 30% sucrose at 4 °C, the optic nerve is frozen in OCT (optimal cutting temperature), sectioned longitudinally on a Cryostat (14 μm thickness), mounted on Superfrost Plus glass slides, dried, and then ready to use for GAP-43 immunostaining. Unstained slides can be stored in −20 °C for many months. The detailed procedure is the following:

1. 5 min in TBS pH 7.4
2. 10 min in methanol (*see* **Note 6**)
3. 1 h in blocking solution (10% donkey serum in TBS)
4. Overnight in primary antibody (4 °C): sheep anti-GAP-43 in solution A (*see* **Note 7**).
5. Washing: on the second day, wash slides 1 h in TBS_2T, 4 °C; 1 h in solution A, RT; 1 h in TBS_2T, RT. Gently shake continuously (*see* **Note 8**).
6. 2 h in secondary antibody, RT: AlexaFluor 488 donkey anti-sheep IgG 1:500 in solution A.
7. 2 × 5 min wash in TBS_2T
8. 5 min wash in TBS

3.4.7 Evaluating RGC Survival

While using optic nerve to evaluate nerve regeneration, the retinas are used to determine RGC survival. After animal perfusion, the whole retinas are dissected out, and four partial cuts are made from the peripheral edge in order to open the retinal cup for flat-mounting (Fig. 5). Retinas are postfixed in 4% paraformaldehyde 2 h at RT and then rinsed with PBS and stored at 4 °C until immunostaining. Staining includes the following:

Three washes in PBS, 5 min for each of the following:

1. Blocking and permeabilization with 10% goat serum plus 0.2% Triton X-100, 1 h, RT, incubation with a rabbit anti-βIII-tubulin antibody (1:500) in PBS with 5% goat serum and 0.2% Trition X-100 overnight at 4 °C (*see* **Note 9**)
2. Three washes in PBS with 2% goat serum and 0.2% Triton X-100, 30 min. for each, RT, one wash in PBS, 10 min.
3. Fluorescent-conjugated antibody to rabbit IgG made in goat, 2 h at RT
4. Three washes in PBS

Within the ganglion cell layer, βIII-tubulin is expressed selectively in RGCs [9, 32, 33]. Immunopositive cells are counted using ImageJ software in 16 fields per retina in rats or 8 fields per retina in mice distributed in four quadrants of the eye at prespecified distances from the optic disc (red rectangles in Fig. 6). Cell survival is reported as the number of βIII-tubulin$^+$ cells per mm [2] averaged over all the fields sampled in each retina and then averaged across all cases within each experimental group.

Following optic nerve injury and regeneration, the expression level of βIII-tubulin can change, which can affect cell counting. The transcription factor Brn3a is a specific marker for RGCs in naïve or

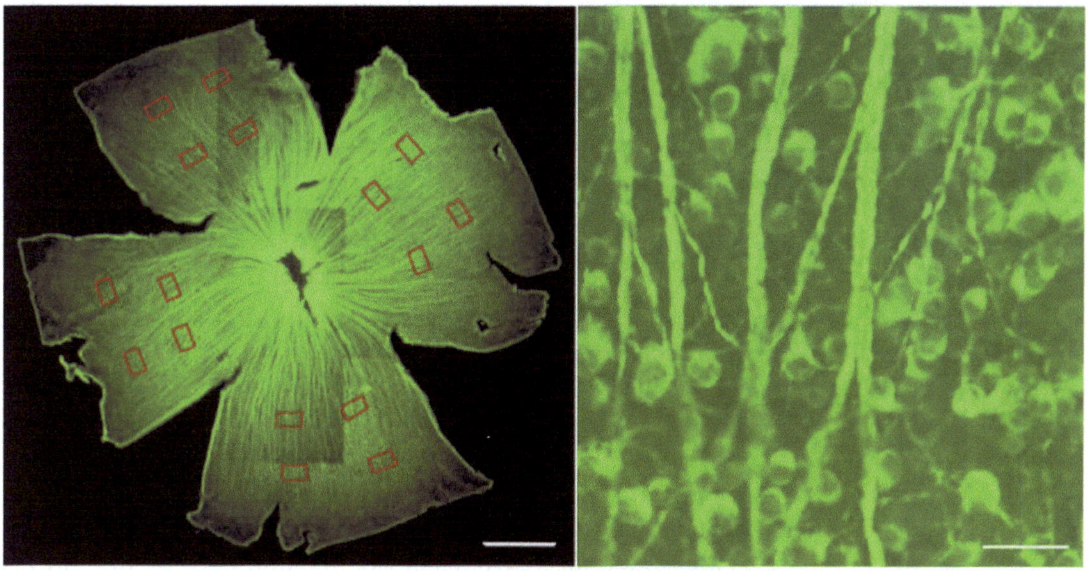

Fig. 6 Whole-mount rat retina immunostained for βIII-tubulin. The normal whole retina was dissected out from the eye and cut as following to open the cup. The red rectangles indicate the areas selected for RGC quantification (left). Immunostaining to βIII-tubulin shows strongly positive staining for RGC fiber bundles, cell bodies, and their fine processes (left and right). Scale bar: left, 500 μm; right, 40 μm. (Y. Yin, H-Y. Gilbert, L.B. Benowitz, unpublished)

optic nerve-injured retinas [34]. It stains RGC nuclei and cell numbers are easy to quantify with appropriate software. However, Brn3a does not exist in all of RGCs (about 80% RGCs express Brn3a), and levels of Brn3a decline sharply after optic nerve injury [35]. Therefore, detection of Brn3a (and/or 3b) may be combined with another marker to get a more accurate count for RGC survival. We have been using TUJ1 plus Brn3a co-staining and count cells that express either marker or

both as RGCs. This could become a routine way to accurately represent RGC survival after nerve injury and treatment. Other studies have used antibodies to a recently discovered RNA-binding protein that is expressed selectively in RGCs [36], though in our experience, its distribution becomes diffuse after nerve injury.

3.5 Conclusions

Preservation of injured retinal ganglion cells and regeneration of the optic nerve could benefit millions of patients with glaucoma as well as victims of traumatic or ischemic damage to the retina or optic nerve. The methods for testing potential therapeutics described here include in vitro and in vivo approaches. Whereas the former includes the use of purified RGC cultures (derived from neonatal animals), mixed retinal cultures, and retinal tissue explant cultures, the latter include the optic nerve injury models and methods to quantify the results of these studies. Application of these methods may someday lead to the development of treatments that can restore sight, arguably the most important of all our sensory faculties.

4 Notes

1. The injection should take place over a period of 1 min or so to allow for good spreading and uptake of the dye.
2. If purified RGCs are derived from mouse, the procedures are modified slightly.

   Usually P8–P10 CD1 mice or other Thy1.2-positive strains are used. Instead of IgM Thy1.1 antibody, an IgM Thy1.2 antibody is used for the panning dish (1:500).
3. During this procedure, cells should never be exposed to glutamate, aspartate, or glutamine since these are toxic to RGCs.
4. This is only necessary when the medium is to be used in the CO_2 incubator.

   Otherwise, as with the washing buffer used in the hood and exposing to air, no $NaHCO_3$ is added.
5. It is important to carry out the retinal dissection as quickly as possible, preferably within 5 min. During the trituration, it is better to add a small volume (e.g., 1 mL) of buffer at a time,

gently triturate, allow the cell clusters to settle down, transfer the dissociated cell suspension to another tube, and then add another small volume of buffer to triturate the remaining cell clusters until all cells are completely dissociated.

6. Methanol helps penetration and strengthens the staining intensity.
7. Our lab uses a custom-made polyclonal anti-GAP-43 antibody prepared in sheep [37].
8. The sheep anti-GAP-43 antibody requires extra-long washing to avoid background staining.
9. At times, TUJ1 (1:500), a monoclonal antibody to βIII-tubulin, gives a cleaner background.

References

1. Ramon y Cajal S (1991) Degeneration and regeneration of the nervous system, vol 5. Oxford University Press, Oxford
2. Bray GM, Vidal-Sanz M, Aguayo AJ (1987) Regeneration of axons from the central nervous system of adult rats. Prog Brain Res 71: 373–379
3. Lye-Barthel M, Sun D, Jakobs TC (2013) Morphology of astrocytes in a glaucomatous optic nerve. Invest Ophthalmol Vis Sci 54: 909–917. https://doi.org/10.1167/iovs.12-10109
4. Matsumoto H et al (2015) Membrane-bound and soluble Fas ligands have opposite functions in photoreceptor cell death following separation from the retinal pigment epithelium. Cell Death Dis 6:e1986. https://doi.org/10.1038/cddis.2015.334
5. Roh M et al (2012) Etanercept, a widely used inhibitor of tumor necrosis factor-alpha (TNF-alpha), prevents retinal ganglion cell loss in a rat model of glaucoma. PLoS One 7: e40065. https://doi.org/10.1371/journal.pone.0040065
6. Barres BA, Silverstein BE, Corey DP, Chun LL (1988) Immunological, morphological, and electrophysiological variation among retinal ganglion cells purified by panning. Neuron 1:791–803. https://doi.org/10.1016/0896-6273(88)90127-4
7. Yin Y et al (2009) Oncomodulin links inflammation to optic nerve regeneration. Proc Natl Acad Sci USA 106:19587–19592. https://doi.org/10.1073/pnas.0907085106. 0907085106 [pii]
8. Yin Y et al (2006) Oncomodulin is a macrophage-derived signal for axon regeneration in retinal ganglion cells. Nat Neurosci 9:843–852
9. Yin Y et al (2003) Macrophage-derived factors stimulate optic nerve regeneration. J Neurosci 23:2284–2293
10. Xie L et al (2022) Monocyte-derived SDF1 supports optic nerve regeneration and alters retinal ganglion cells' response to Pten deletion. Proc Natl Acad Sci USA 119: e2113751119. https://doi.org/10.1073/pnas.2113751119
11. Land PW, Kyonka E, Shamalla-Hannah L (2004) Vesicular glutamate transporters in the lateral geniculate nucleus: expression of VGLUT2 by retinal terminals. Brain Res 996: 251–254. https://doi.org/10.1016/j.brainres.2003.10.032
12. Engelund A, Fahrenkrug J, Harrison A, Hannibal J (2010) Vesicular glutamate transporter 2 (VGLUT2) is co-stored with PACAP in projections from the rat melanopsin-containing retinal ganglion cells. Cell Tissue Res 340: 243–255. https://doi.org/10.1007/s00441-010-0950-3
13. Wang SW, Mu X, Bowers WJ, Klein WH (2002) Retinal ganglion cell differentiation in cultured mouse retinal explants. Methods 28: 448–456. https://doi.org/10.1016/s1046-2023(02)00264-5
14. Manabe S et al (2002) Quantification of axotomized ganglion cell death by explant culture of the rat retina. Neurosci Lett 334:33–36. https://doi.org/10.1016/s0304-3940(02)01047-9
15. Lagreze WA et al (2005) The peptides ADNF-9 and NAP increase survival and neurite outgrowth of rat retinal ganglion cells in vitro.

Invest Ophthalmol Vis Sci 46:933–938. https://doi.org/10.1167/iovs.04-0766
16. Toops KA, Berlinicke C, Zack DJ, Nickells RW (2012) Hydrocortisone stimulates neurite outgrowth from mouse retinal explants by modulating macroglial activity. Invest Ophthalmol Vis Sci 53:2046–2061. https://doi.org/10.1167/iovs.11-8646
17. Feng G et al (2000) Imaging neuronal subsets in transgenic mice expressing multiple spectral variants of GFP. Neuron 28:41–51
18. Gasparini L et al (2011) Tau inclusions in retinal ganglion cells of human P301S tau transgenic mice: effects on axonal viability. Neurobiol Aging 32:419–433. https://doi.org/10.1016/j.neurobiolaging.2009.03.002
19. Bull ND et al (2011) Use of an adult rat retinal explant model for screening of potential retinal ganglion cell neuroprotective therapies. Invest Ophthalmol Vis Sci 52:3309–3320. https://doi.org/10.1167/iovs.10-6873
20. So KF, Aguayo AJ (1985) Lengthy regrowth of cut axons from ganglion cells after peripheral nerve transplantation into the retina of adult rats. Brain Res 328:349–354
21. Berry M, Carlile J, Hunter A (1996) Peripheral nerve explants grafted into the vitreous body of the eye promote the regeneration of retinal ganglion cell axons severed in the optic nerve. J Neurocytol 25:147–170
22. Leon S, Yin Y, Nguyen J, Irwin N, Benowitz LI (2000) Lens injury stimulates axon regeneration in the mature rat optic nerve. J Neurosci 20:4615–4626
23. Benowitz LI, Routtenberg A (1997) GAP-43: an intrinsic determinant of neuronal development and plasticity. Trends Neurosci 20:84–91
24. Skene JH (1989) Axonal growth-associated proteins. Annu Rev Neurosci 12:127–156
25. Kurimoto T et al (2010) Long-distance axon regeneration in the mature optic nerve: contributions of oncomodulin, cAMP, and pten gene deletion. J Neurosci 30:15654–15663. https://doi.org/10.1523/JNEUROSCI.4340-10.2010
26. de Lima S et al (2012) Full-length axon regeneration in the adult mouse optic nerve and partial recovery of simple visual behaviors. Proc Natl Acad Sci USA 109:9149–9154. https://doi.org/10.1073/pnas.1119449109.1119449109 [pii]
27. Moore DL et al (2009) KLF family members regulate intrinsic axon regeneration ability. Science 326:298–301. https://doi.org/10.1126/science.1175737. 326/5950/298 [pii]
28. Luo X, Yungher B, Park KK (2014) Application of tissue clearing and light sheet fluorescence microscopy to assess optic nerve regeneration in unsectioned tissues. Methods Mol Biol 1162:209–217. https://doi.org/10.1007/978-1-4939-0777-9_17
29. Myers A, Ford J, Decker S, Crawford F, Tzekov R (2021) Volumetric histological characterization of optic nerve degeneration using tissue clearing: literature review and practical study. J Histotechnol 44:206–216. https://doi.org/10.1080/01478885.2021.1938808
30. Potts RA, Dreher B, Bennett MR (1982) The loss of ganglion cells in the developing retina of the rat. Brain Res 255:481–486
31. Selles-Navarro I, Ellezam B, Fajardo R, Latour M, McKerracher L (2001) Retinal ganglion cell and nonneuronal cell responses to a microcrush lesion of adult rat optic nerve. Exp Neurol 167:282–289
32. Park K, Luo JM, Hisheh S, Harvey AR, Cui Q (2004) Cellular mechanisms associated with spontaneous and ciliary neurotrophic factor-cAMP-induced survival and axonal regeneration of adult retinal ganglion cells. J Neurosci 24:10806–10815. https://doi.org/10.1523/JNEUROSCI.3532-04.2004
33. Cui Q, Yip HK, Zhao RC, So KF, Harvey AR (2003) Intraocular elevation of cyclic AMP potentiates ciliary neurotrophic factor-induced regeneration of adult rat retinal ganglion cell axons. Mol Cell Neurosci 22:49–61
34. Nadal-Nicolas FM et al (2009) Brn3a as a marker of retinal ganglion cells: qualitative and quantitative time course studies in naive and optic nerve-injured retinas. Invest Ophthalmol Vis Sci 50:3860–3868. https://doi.org/10.1167/iovs.08-3267
35. Yukita M et al (2015) Molecular, anatomical and functional changes in the retinal ganglion cells after optic nerve crush in mice. Doc Ophthalmol 130:149–156. https://doi.org/10.1007/s10633-014-9478-2
36. Rodriguez AR, de Sevilla Muller LP, Brecha NC (2014) The RNA binding protein RBPMS is a selective marker of ganglion cells in the mammalian retina. J Comp Neurol 522:1411–1443. https://doi.org/10.1002/cne.23521
37. Benowitz LI, Apostolides PJ, Perrone-Bizzozero N, Finklestein SP, Zwiers H (1988) Anatomical distribution of the growth-associated protein GAP-43/B-50 in the adult rat brain. J Neurosci 8:339–352

Correction to: A Comprehensive Protocol for Microbead-Induced Ocular Hypertension in Mice

M. Reza Bahrani Fard, Nina Sara Fraticelli-Guzmán, Jessica Chan, A. Thomas Read, Andrew Feola, W. Daniel Stamer, Simon W. M. John, C. Ross Ethier, and Rebecca M. Sappington

Correction to:
Chapter 20 in: Tatjana Jakobs and Paloma B. Liton (eds.), ***Glaucoma: Methods and Protocols*****, Methods in Molecular Biology, vol. 2858,**
https://doi.org/10.1007/978-1-0716-4140-8_20

This book that was inadvertently published with one of the co-authors Nina Sara Protocol-Guzmán in Chapter 20 has been correctly updated as Nina Sara Fraticelli-Guzmán.

The updated version of this chapter can be found at
https://doi.org/10.1007/978-1-0716-4140-8_20

Tatjana Jakobs and Paloma B. Liton (eds.), *Glaucoma: Methods and Protocols*, Methods in Molecular Biology, vol. 2858,
https://doi.org/10.1007/978-1-0716-4140-8_23,

Index

A

B

C

D

E

F

G

H

I

Tatjana Jakobs and Paloma B. Liton (eds.), *Glaucoma: Methods and Protocols*, Methods in Molecular Biology, vol. 2858, https://doi.org/10.1007/978-1-0716-4140-8,